DICKENS'S FORENSIC REALISM

DICKENS'S FORENSIC REALISM

Truth, Bodies, Evidence

ANDREW MANGHAM

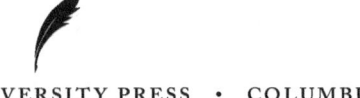

THE OHIO STATE UNIVERSITY PRESS • COLUMBUS

Copyright © 2016 by The Ohio State University.
All rights reserved.

Library of Congress Cataloging-in-Publication Data
Names: Mangham, Andrew, 1979– author.
Title: Dickens's forensic realism : truth, bodies, evidence / Andrew Mangham.
Description: Columbus : The Ohio State University Press, [2016] | Includes bibliographical references and index.
Identifiers: LCCN 2016036321 | ISBN 9780814213247 (printed case ; alk. paper) ISBN | 0814213243 (printed case ; alk. paper)
Subjects: LCSH: Dickens, Charles, 1812–1870—Criticism and interpretation. | Dead in literature. | Death in literature. | Human body in literature. | Medicine in literature. | Medical jurisprudence.
Classification: LCC PR4588 .M26 2016 | DDC 823/.8—dc23
LC record available at https://lccn.loc.gov/2016036321

Cover design by Laurence J. Nozik
Text design by Juliet Williams
Type set in Adobe Caslon

∞ The paper used in this publication meets the minimum requirements of the American National Standard for Information Sciences—Permanence of Paper for Printed Library Materials. ANSI Z39.48–1992.

9 8 7 6 5 4 3 2 1

FOR SAMI

Now I am disoriented and confused. I try in vain to find support; nothing seems solid, everything escapes me, deceives me. Our earthly hopes and desires are only vain fancies, our successes mere mirages that we try to grasp.

—*Théodore Géricault (1810)*

CONTENTS

	List of Illustrations	xi
	Acknowledgments	xiii
	Abbreviations	xv
	Introduction	1
Chapter 1	Contexts: Common Sense, Medicine, Law	21
Chapter 2	The Whole Truth: *Oliver Twist* and *Our Mutual Friend*	69
Chapter 3	Bodies: Early Journalism and *Bleak House*	120
Chapter 4	Collateral Evidence: *The Pickwick Papers* and *Great Expectations*	178
	Conclusion	226
	Bibliography	231
	Index	247

ILLUSTRATIONS

Figure 1.1	Frontispiece to *The Terrific Register*	39
Figure 1.2	George Cruikshank, "A Financial Survey of Cumberland" (1815)	57
Figure 3.1	"The Streets—Morning," *Sketches by Boz* (1836)	136
Figure 4.1	"Conviviality at Bob Sawyer's," *The Pickwick Papers* (1836–37)	187
Figure 4.2	"The Dying Clown," *The Pickwick Papers* (1836–37)	191
Figure 4.3	Illustration of the Prince de Condé's body as it was discovered, Taylor's *Principles and Practice of Medical Jurisprudence* (1865)	206

ACKNOWLEDGMENTS

For providing an environment in which it has been possible to write and think at my own pace, I would like to thank the Department of English Literature at the University of Reading. I am grateful to Alison Donnell for her unflagging encouragement and to the rest of my colleagues for their wonderful collegiality. I would like to thank Sally Shuttleworth, Anne-Marie Beller, Pamela K. Gilbert, Verity Hunt, Tatiana Kontou, and Rhianedd Smith for listening to me talk about the project, and I would like to thank Janice M. Allan and Holly Furneaux for putting aside time to read sections of this work and for offering a range of excellent suggestions.

There is no doubt that the range of inspiring PhD projects I have supervised at Reading has had an impact on the shape and texture of my thoughts: I owe particular debts to Verity Burke and Kate Robinson in this regard. I would like to thank my anonymous readers, who made invaluable comments while this book was still in manuscript form. Lindsay Martin at The Ohio State University Press has been tremendously supportive and positive throughout the publishing process. Julia Smith helped me prepare the manuscript for publication, and Jobi Zink at the Rosenbach Museum in Philadelphia assisted me in tracking down one of my images. Finally, I would like to thank my friends and family for their long-suffering patience. To Sami, thank you for offering support, love, and encouragement when I needed it most. This book is for you.

Part of my second chapter appeared as "Anatomical Sketches by Boz" in *The Dickensian* (107:1, 2011), and part of the third chapter was printed as "Pickwick's Interpolated Tales and the Examination of Suicide" in *19: Interdisciplinary Studies in the Long Nineteenth Century* 10 (2010). I would like to thank those journals and their editors for their kind permission to reprint the material here.

ABBREVIATIONS

Forster   John Forster, *The Life of Charles Dickens*, 2 vols. (1872–74; London: Chapman and Hall, 1876).
Journalism   *Dickens's Journalism*, vol. 1: *Sketches by Boz and Other Early Papers, 1833–39*, ed. Michael Slater (London: J. M. Dent, 1996).
               Dickens's Journalism, vol. 2: *"The Amusements of the People" and Other Papers: Reports, Essays and Reviews, 1834–51*, ed. Michael Slater (London: J. M. Dent, 1996).
               Dickens's Journalism, vol. 3: *"Gone Astray" and Other Papers from Household Words, 1851–59*, ed. Michael Slater (London: J. M. Dent, 1998).
               Dickens's Journalism, vol. 4: *"The Uncommercial Traveller" and Other Papers, 1859–70*, ed. Michael Slater and John Drew (London: J. M. Dent, 2000).
Letters   *The Letters of Charles Dickens*, vol. 1: 1820–39, ed. Madeline House and Graham Storey (Oxford: Clarendon Press, 1965).
               The Letters of Charles Dickens, vol. 2: 1840–41, ed. Madeline House, Graham Storey, and Kathleen Tillotson (Oxford: Clarendon Press, 1969).
               The Letters of Charles Dickens, vol. 3: 1842–43, ed. Madeline House, Graham Storey, and Kathleen Tillotson (Oxford: Clarendon Press, 1974).
               The Letters of Charles Dickens, vol. 4: 1844–46, ed. Kathleen Tillotson and Nina Burgis (Oxford: Clarendon Press, 1977).

The Letters of Charles Dickens, vol. 5: 1847–49, ed. Graham Storey, K. J. Fielding, and Anthony Laude (Oxford: Clarendon Press, 1981).

The Letters of Charles Dickens, vol. 6: 1850–1852, ed. Graham Storey, Kathleen Tillotson, and Nina Burgis (Oxford: Clarendon Press, 1988).

The Letters of Charles Dickens, vol. 7: 1853–55, ed. Graham Storey, Kathleen Tillotson, and Angus Easson (Oxford: Clarendon Press, 1993).

The Letters of Charles Dickens, vol. 8: 1856–58, ed. Graham Storey and Kathleen Tillotson (Oxford: Clarendon Press, 1995).

The Letters of Charles Dickens, vol. 9: 1859–61, ed. Graham Storey, Margaret Brown, and Kathleen Tillotson (Oxford: Clarendon Press, 1997).

The Letters of Charles Dickens, vol. 10: 1862–64, ed. Graham Storey, Margaret Brown, and Kathleen Tillotson (Oxford: Clarendon Press, 1998).

The Letters of Charles Dickens, vol. 11: 1865–67, ed. Graham Storey, Margaret Brown, and Kathleen Tillotson (Oxford: Clarendon Press, 1999).

The Letters of Charles Dickens, vol. 12: 1868–70, ed. Graham Storey, Margaret Brown, and Kathleen Tillotson (Oxford: Clarendon Press, 2002).

Stonehouse   J. H. Stonehouse (ed.), *Catalogue of the Library of Charles Dickens from Gadshill* (London: Piccadilly Fountain Press, 1935).

INTRODUCTION

Bodies are very unstable things in Dickens. In addition to the various characters with parts that are missing or defunct, like Wackford Squeers, Silas Wegg, Mr Smallweed, Mrs Skewton, Captain Cuttle, and Mrs Clennam, we find bodies that are taken apart (like the mangled remains of Mr Carker and Rigauld) and (re)assembled (like Mrs Jarley's waxworks or Mr Venus's French Gentleman). We encounter living bodies without souls, like the prisoners in "A Visit to Newgate" (1836) and *American Notes* (1842), and souls like Little Nell and Oliver Twist whose bodies seem barely capable of holding them in. More gruesomely, Dickensian bodies have a tendency to turn into slime and ash, such as when Miss Havisham is burned in *Great Expectations* (1860–61), or when the inhabitants of a city churchyard threaten to sully the appropriated dress of Lady Dedlock. Mr Krook, the drunken Lord Chancellor of a rag and bone shop, effectively blows up, his body reducing to grease and smoke. According to John Carey's classic study of Dickens's imagination, Dickens "never missed a human carcass if he could help it."[1] But he also never missed the opportunity to take carcasses apart, to boil them down, blow them up, and turn them into base materials.

Dickens's Forensic Realism is, in a number of ways, a book about bodies in Dickens, especially the dead ones. As such it joins a legion of works that has appeared in the past fifty years or so with the aim of considering the

---

1. John Carey, *The Violent Effigy: A Study of Dickens's Imagination* (1973; London: Faber and Faber, 1991), 81.

author's preoccupation with the dead. Some of these studies have argued that Dickens's fictional corpses, in particular, indicate a life-long obsession with mortality,[2] while some see them as a product of the wider Victorian obsession with, and fetishization of, mourning;[3] others, meanwhile, have claimed that Dickens had "two primary fascinations with death: death as a cold, material fact, and death as a romantic escape from an unforgiving world."[4] What my book argues is that rather than offering a reconfiguration of death as something cherished, in the words of Miss Havisham, as a "sick fancy," or perceived, conversely, as a confirmation of the age's trivial commercialization, Dickens was attracted to the aesthetic, political, and philosophical potential of bodies and, much more, as forensic subjects. Because of television dramas and popular fiction, we all have some familiarity with the work of forensic science; indeed, the word *forensic* has become a byword for a penetrative form of analysis—the sort of investigation that is able to solve crimes with extraordinary skill. Consequently, the term is also associated with an exacting form of scientific realism, and *forensic realism* might seem, then, an odd idea to apply to the work of Dickens, particularly as he was an author so set against the kind of fact-based gospel preached by his own materialist Mr Gradgrind. In the nineteenth century, however, the field of forensic medicine was relatively new, and it meant something different to the popular view we have of it today; its

---

2. Carey notes that "Dickens's dead figures who subject the living to their alarmed and alarming gaze are made of wood and stone and metal and painted canvas as well as wax. The mingled terror and hilarity they cause harks back to Dickens's toddler days" (84). Harry Stone has observed, with reference to Dickens's writings about the Paris Morgue: "Dickens creates—he has no choice but to create—the vision that he perceives, a dark, insistent vision, a necessity-driven vision, the vision that haunts and torments him" (95). See Carey, *Violent Effigy*; and Harry Stone, *The Night Side of Dickens: Cannibalism, Passion, Necessity* (Columbus: The Ohio State University Press, 1994), 95.

3. For example, Philippe Ariés's idea on what he calls "the age of beautiful death" is one of the contexts in which Bianca Tredennick interprets Dickens as trying "to seize control over death" by making the material body an "art object, consumable good, or spectacular display" (73). Claire Wood has noted that "Charles Dickens's career offers an ideal framework through which to explore death commodification. [. . .] His work demonstrates a particular sensitivity to death's materiality and its occurrence within commercial contexts" (3). Andrew Sanders does not subscribe entirely to the belief that the Victorians beautified death, but he does see Dickens as "a man much preoccupied with mortality" (2) because he lived in an age where death, as an image and a reality, was everywhere (vii). See Bianca Tredennick, "Some Collections of Mortality: Dickens, the Paris Morgue and the Material Corpse," *Victorian Review* 36:1 (2010): 72–78; Claire Wood, *Dickens and the Business of Death* (Cambridge: Cambridge University Press, 2015); and Andrew Sanders, *Charles Dickens: Resurrectionist* (London: Macmillan, 1982). I regret that Wood's study was published too late for me to make a fuller engagement with it in these pages.

4. Daniel P. Scoggin, "A Speculative Resurrection: Death, Money, and the Vampiric Economy of *Our Mutual Friend*," *Victorian Literature and Culture* 30:1 (2002): 99–125 (107).

most dominant characteristic was that it embodied the coming together of conflicting modes of interpretation—particularly the legal and the medical. Bodies offer the most visible paradigm of how methods of interpretation became productively unstable when the notion of "the whole truth" was subjected to an intense tug-of-war between conflicting models of realism. It is this conflict, rather than any association with veridical perception, that I see as the most powerful aspect of Dickens's engagement with forensics.

Studies of fiction within the context of what might be called, in broad terms, the *forensic* or *detective* process have tended to use the work of Michel Foucault as a theoretical framework.[5] Such links have highlighted the ways in which disciplines associated with the control or care of the individual might develop into ideological coercions that the novel can reproduce, expose, and dismantle. In *Dickens's Forensic Realism*, my aim is to see in the complex set of conflicts that typify the forensic profession's interactions with its objects of study a culture obsessed with testing the hermeneutic processes involved in its most "basic" empirical ventures. My aim is not to reproduce work that has already been done by questioning how far these conflicts and discussions become subtle and complex forms of ideology that the Dickens novel was able to question. Rather, I aim to understand how the author's writings emerged from, and contributed to, a cultural reevaluation of what it meant to represent and interpret any given subject as a medico-legal "truth."

We know from the varied and inspiring range of scholarship on Dickens that the author's novels show that it is difficult, if not impossible, to throw the light of truth on anything with any confidence. His texts appear to interrogate the basic assertions of realism, both in a philosophical and a literary sense, and they make their importance manifest in their ability to question the very nature of how we know things. For some literary scholars, such equivocations anticipate the hermeneutic complexities of Modernism.[6] The poststructuralist view, led by J. Hillis Miller, has said

---

5. See, for instance, D. A. Miller, *The Novel and the Police* (Berkeley, CA, and London: University of California Press, 1988); Ronald R. Thomas, *Detective Fiction and the Rise of Forensic Science* (Cambridge: Cambridge University Press, 1999); and Andrew Mangham, *Violent Women and Sensation Fiction: Crime, Medicine and Victorian Popular Culture* (Basingstoke: Palgrave Macmillan, 2007).

6. Gillian Piggott, *Dickens and Benjamin: Moments of Revelation, Fragments of Modernity* (Hampshire: Ashgate, 2012), 211. Albert D. Hutter notes that "*Our Mutual Friend*'s 'transformation' and 'articulation' of a generalized and unstated preoccupation into a metaphor for social disintegration" highlights how his work "contributed directly to the perceptions and preoccupations of modern culture" (163). Sally Ledger mentions "Joseph Conrad's nihilistic fictional world that *Our Mutual Friend* anticipates by over thirty years" (376), a view that reproduces Audrey Jaffe's claim that "*Our Mutual Friend* is generally regarded as the most modern of Dickens's works

that the complexity of interpretation and methodological self-reflection is intrinsic to Dickens's language itself.[7] The games that his stories play with meaning and interpretation are "a play of language without beginning, and of extra-linguistic foundation,"[8] symptomatic of how language is ultimately "independent of the self, prior to the human."[9] John Bowen has suggested that this inability to pin down meaning goes some way toward explaining why the (un)dead had such a hold over Dickens's works: its disjointedness, weirdness, fragility, and plasticity appears paradigmatic of significations and distinctions that simply refuse to sit still.[10] *Dickens's Forensic Realism*

---

because of the absence of a prominent omniscient voice and a clear omniscient perspective" (91). See Albert D. Hutter, "Dismemberment and Articulation in *Our Mutual Friend*," *Dickens Studies Annual* (1983): 135–75; Sally Ledger, "Dickens, Natural History, and *Our Mutual Friend*," *Partial Answers* 9:12 (2001): 363–78; and Audrey Jaffe, "Omniscience in *Our Mutual Friend:* On Taking the Reader by Surprise," *The Journal of Narrative Technique* 17:1 (1987): 91–101.

7. Timothy Clark notes that the Dickens novel provides a kind of literature that is "a mode of language whose ambiguity is essential to it" (23). John Bowen adds:

> There is little we can take for granted in the genres, forms, or narratives of Dickens's early novels, for they enact one of the more sustained projects of textual experimentation in the language, one which seems to undo in the process so many of the distinctions—between popular and high culture, between fictional and non-fictional writing, between social and political thought, and, more radically still, between past and present, self and other, life and death. (3)

See J. Hillis Miller, *Charles Dickens: The World of his Novels* (Bloomington: Indiana University Press, 1958); J. Hillis Miller, "The Fiction of Realism: *Sketches by Boz, Oliver Twist,* and Cruikshank's Illustrations" (1971), repr. as "J. Hillis Miller on the Fiction of Realism," in *Realism*, ed. Lillian R. Furst (London and New York: Longman, 1992), 287–318; J. Hillis Miller, "Introduction," in *Bleak House,* ed. Norman Page (London: Penguin, 1971); John Schad, *The Reader in Dickensian Mirrors: Some New Language* (Basingstoke: Palgrave Macmillan, 1992); Christopher Morris, "The Bad Faith of Pip's Bad Faith: Deconstructing *Great Expectations*," in *Charles Dickens,* ed. Steven Connor, (Essex: Longman, 1996), 76–90; and Timothy Clark, "Dickens through Blanchot: The Nightmare Fascination of a World without Interiority," in *Dickens Refigured: Bodies, Desires and Other Histories,* ed. John Schad (Manchester: Manchester University Press, 1996), 22–38; and John Bowen, *Other Dickens: Pickwick to Chuzzlewit* (Oxford: Oxford University Press, 2000).

8. Hillis Miller, "The Fiction of Realism," 315.

9. Morris, "Bad Faith," 86.

10. Bowen notes, "Dickens's fiction is fascinated by what is dead but will not lie down, in things or people or people-things who cross or trouble the boundaries between what was, what is, and what may be living." Bowen, *Other Dickens,* 5. In *The Citizen's Body: Desire, Health, and the Social in Victorian England* (Columbus: The Ohio State University Press, 2007), Pamela K. Gilbert suggests that the body "is a key signifier" for Dickens. "Basic representative of a materiality that is malleable yet limited," the "un-self-contained body" is constantly under threat from "liquidity, garbage, filth, and waste" (9, 151). Gilbert discusses the body as a site of symbolic and material conflict between a perceived anatomical (and moral) unruliness, on the one hand, and a social desire for containment, order, and sanitization, on the other. Similarly, John Kucich has discussed the representation of death in Dickens as a means of reinstating moral order in *Excess and Restraint: The Novels of Charles Dickens* (Athens: University of Georgia Press, 1981). I have a similar method of viewing the body as a symbolic and material site of conflict, though my concern is with the

follows this line of thinking with the addition that the "disjointedness, weirdness, fragility, and plasticity" of Dickens's dead comes from a forensic preoccupation with death as a material process that both invites and resists interpretation.

Take, for instance, Dickens's famous description of his visit to the Paris Morgue in *All the Year Round* and, later, *The Uncommercial Traveller*:

> One Christmas Day, when I would rather have been anywhere else, I was attracted in, to see an old grey man lying all along on his cold bed, with a tap of water turned on over his grey hair, and running drip, drip, drip, down his wretched face until it got to the corner of his mouth, where it took a turn and made him look sly. [. . .] I was forced into the same dread place, to see a large dark man whose disfigurement by water was in a frightful manner, comic, and whose expression was that of a prize-fighter who had closed his eyelids under a heavy blow, but was going immediately to open them, shake his head, and "come up smiling."[11]

This is an extraordinary scene that prefigures a similar visit to the morgue which takes place in Emile Zola's *Thérèse Raquin* (1867). Historically, cadavers were laid out in the morgue near Notre Dame for the purpose of identification, yet the jovial carcasses in both Dickens and Zola appear to resist all processes of interpretation. In *Thérèse Raquin* the murderer Laurent visits the dead house in search for the man he has killed:

> One morning, he got a real fright. For some minutes, he had been looking at a drowned man, short in stature and horribly disfigured. The flesh of this body was so soft and decayed that the water running over it was taking it away bit by bit. The stream pouring on the face was making a hole to the left of the nose. Then, suddenly, the nose collapsed and the lips fell off, revealing white teeth. The drowned man's head broke into a laugh.[12]

Zola's account is clearly more "immediate" than Dickens's, yet it captures something of the latter's penchant for converting material horrors

---

epistemological rather than the ideological; I explore how the body became a symbol of the itinerant nature of "the whole truth" in law, medicine, and literature.

11. Charles Dickens, "Travelling Abroad," *All the Year Round* (7 April 1860), *Journalism* 4: 83–96 (88). Bianca Tredennick calls the "enigmatic smirking corpse" seen by Dickens in the Paris Morgue "a completely opaque image, resisting and mocking any effort to make it meaningful." Bodies, she adds, "invite and resist comprehension, as Dickens soon finds." Tredennick, "Some Collections," 79, 74.

12. Emile Zola, *Thérèse Raquin*, trans. Robin Buss (1867; London: Penguin, 2004), 72.

into comic absurdities. In both texts there is a pantomimic breach of the boundary between life and death: dead men are sly—they smile and laugh. Dickens returns to the theme in an *All the Year Round* article in which he recounts being a juryman in a coroner's inquiry:

> We were impanelled to inquire concerning the death of a very little mite of a child. It was the old miserable story. Whether the mother had committed the minor offence of concealing the birth, or whether she had committed the major offence of killing the child, was the question on which we were wanted. We must commit her on one of the two issues.
>
> The Inquest came off in the parish workhouse [. . . where] we went down stairs—led by the plotting Beadle—to view the body. From that day to this, the poor little figure on which that sounding legal appellation was bestowed, has lain in the same place, and with the same surroundings, to my thinking. In a kind of crypt devoted to the warehousing of the parochial coffins, and in the midst of a perfect Panorama of coffins of all sizes, it was stretched on a box; the mother had put it in her box—this box—almost as soon as it was born, and it had been presently found there. It had been opened, and neatly sewn up, and regarded from that point of view, it looked like a stuffed creature. It rested on a clean white cloth, with a surgical instrument or so at hand, and regarded from that point of view, it looked as if the cloth were "laid," and the Giant were coming to dinner.[13]

The words "poor little figure" put in mind the number of dead children we encounter in Dickens's works which are usually sad bundles of high sentimentality. However, he echoes an image in Jonathan Swift's "A Modest Proposal" (1729) where a "young healthy child" is noted as "a most delicious, nourishing, and wholesome food, whether *stewed, roasted, baked,* or *boiled,*"[14] in order to foreground his own preoccupation with the body as a *thing* that tells stories. A similar, though presumably less fantastic, concern is shared by his counterparts in the field of medicine, as is indicated in the way the baby's cadaver has been "opened, and neatly sewn up," and "a surgical instrument or so [is] at hand." As Dickens interprets the corpse as a thing of humor, pity, anger, and much more, so have forensic examiners been to collect *their* interpretations from the same package of skin and bone. Their

---

13. Charles Dickens, "Some Recollections of Mortality," *All the Year Round* (16 May 1863), *Journalism* 4: 218–28 (225–26).

14. Jonathan Swift, "A Modest Proposal for Preventing the Children of Poor People from being a Burthen on their Parents or the Country, and for making them Beneficial to the Public" (1729), in *Major Works,* ed. Angus Ross (Oxford: Oxford University Press, 2008), 492–99 (493–94).

search for meaning only complicates the process of interpretation. The medical process of autopsy represents the act of reading the body's clues, and yet this act of interpretation makes subsequent elucidations impossible. By the time the jury arrive to view the cadaver, the body has been read through and through by medical experts, and, for Dickens and his fellow jury members, the autopsy turns the *real* body into an intangible metaphor: it becomes a "stuffed creature" or a giant's repast; it misleads more than it enlightens.

In 1840 Dickens had described to Forster the impact the inquest had on his nerves:

> Whether it was the poor baby, or its poor mother, or the coffin, or my fellow-jurymen, or what not, I can't say, but last night I had a most violent attack of sickness and indigestion which not only prevented me from sleeping, but even from lying down. Accordingly Kate and I sat up through the dreary watches.[15]

It prefigures his narrator's reaction to seeing the large man laid out in the Paris Morgue in 1863: "O what this large man cost me in that bright city!" Dickens notes:

> It was very hot weather, and he was none the better for that, and I was much the worse. [. . .] I was in the full enjoyment of a delightful bath, when all in a moment I was seized with an unreasonable idea that the large dark body was floating straight at me.
>
> I was out of the river, and dressing instantly. In the shock I had taken some water into my mouth, and it turned me sick, for I fancied that the contamination of the creature was in it. [. . .]
>
> Of course I knew perfectly well that the large dark creature was stone dead, and that I should no more come upon him out of the place where I had seen him dead, than I should come upon the cathedral of Notre-Dame in an entirely new situation. What troubled me was the picture of the creature; and that had so curiously and strongly painted itself upon my brain, that I could not get rid of it until it was worn out.
>
> I noticed the peculiarities of this possession, while it was a real discomfort to me. That very day, at dinner, some morsel on my plate looked like a piece of him, and I was glad to get up and go out.[16]

---

15. John Forster, *The Life of Charles Dickens*, vol. 1 (1872–74; London: Chapman and Hall, 1876), 148.

16. Dickens, "Travelling Abroad," 88–90.

In one sense the narrator's obsession with the remembrance of the large man is about fixedness: like all obsessions the image remains with the narrator despite his best efforts to rid himself of it. Yet the physicality of the body also epitomizes fluidity and change by invoking images of decay, fragmentation, and dispersal. It also suggests that nothing can make sense anymore; if a dead man can accompany a member of the living around Paris, then Notre Dame might well be found at a different location one day.

The large man's body and its impact on the narrator's mind present an inversion of Dickens's psychosomatic reaction after the coroner's inquest. Whereas in the latter a vague, psychical sense of "I can't say" becomes a real, bilious experience, the large man's rotting remains become a collection of vague, psychical horrors. What haunts the visitor to the morgue after he has seen the large corpse is the "picture" of its actual matter; when he is swimming, it is the contamination of the body's chemical decay that troubles the narrator; and when he is eating, he imagines a physical morsel of it on his plate. The sketch "insists upon the refusal of matter to be taken leave of";[17] contrary to what we might expect from the author of Little Nell's saintly expiration, death is all about the grisly materiality of ending. What is particularly revealing, however, is the way a material cadaver leads to a set of immaterial fancies; the process of interacting with the physical remains has no less fantastic potential, it seems, than the sentimental martyrdom of a character like Nell.

In the 1840 inquest into the death of the child, Dickens notes, "We had the doctor who had made the examination, and the usual tests as to whether the child was born alive."[18] The doctor would almost certainly have used the hydrostatic test, which had been popularized by William Hunter in 1783 as a method of determining whether a child had lived outside of the womb. On 14 July of that year Hunter read a paper to the members of the Medical Society, "The Uncertainty of The Signs of Murder in the Case of Bastard Children." He published the talk as a tract the following year. Four years before the inquest in which Dickens served as a juryman, physician William Cummin wrote of Hunter's piece: "The judges quote it with implicit faith in its perfection: the bar study it, and cross-examine the crown witnesses on the difficulties which it suggests: and medical men probably will

---

17. Daniel Hack "'Sublimation Strange': Allegory and Authority in *Bleak House*," *ELH* 66 (1999): 129–56 (144). In his fine discussion of Mr Krook's spontaneous combustion, Hack notes that Dickens's "insistence on the textually of matter" (148) "functions as part of the novel's more general argument against the silencing or discrediting of individuals lacking what those in positions of authority deem sufficient cultural capital" (146).

18. Dickens, "Recollections," 227.

not find it safe to venture into the witness box without being familiarly acquainted with its contents."¹⁹ Considered one of the founding texts of medical jurisprudence, the short article by Hunter advocated the use of an ancient method of inferring whether a baby had lived or not:

> I come to the material question, viz. in suspicious cases, how far may we conclude that the child was born alive, and probably murdered by its mother, if the lungs swim in water? [. . .] If the air which is in them be that of respiration, the air-bubbles will hardly be visible to the naked eye; but if the air-bubbles be large, or if they run in lines along the fissures between the component lobuli of the lungs, the air is certainly emphysematous, and not air which had been taken in breathing.²⁰

To determine whether a baby's lungs contain the tiny air-bubbles that prove that he or she must have breathed independently (and therefore could not have been born dead), medical examiners were advised to place the organs in a bowl of water. If they sank, they contained no air. The test was seductively simple, yet, as Hunter indicated in the excerpt above, babies' lungs may contain air because of a pathological distention of the bronchial tissues (emphysema). The hydrostatic test was instructive, but it was no failsafe guide to the truth. This offers one possible explanation for why, in the inquest attended by Dickens, the medical expert provides vague and unsatisfactory evidence: "He was a timid muddle-headed doctor, and got confused and contradictory, and wouldn't say this, and couldn't answer for that."²¹ Luckily for the defendant, the inquest was presided over by Thomas Wakley, founder of the *Lancet* and staunch supporter of medical jurisprudence. According to Dickens, Wakley summed up the case in favor of the accused woman, and

> in private conversation after [it] was all over, [. . .] showed me his reasons as a trained surgeon, for perceiving it to be impossible that the child could, under the most favourable circumstances, have drawn many breaths, in the very doubtful case of its having ever breathed at all; this, owing to the discovery of some foreign matter in the windpipe, quite irreconcilable with many moments of life.²²

---

19. William Cummin, *The Proofs of Infanticide Considered: including Dr Hunter's Tract on Child Murder, with illustrative notes; and a Summary of the Present State of Medico-Legal Knowledge on that Subject* (London: Longman et al., 1836), v–vi.
20. William Hunter, "On the Uncertainty of the Signs of Murder in the Case of Bastard Children" (1784; London: J. Callow, 1818), 22.
21. Dickens, "Recollections," 227.
22. Ibid.

As in cases of emphysema, the foreign object in the windpipe is something that would have nullified the results of the hydrostatic test. To give Hunter his due, descriptions of the test were cautious from the start; there was always an acknowledgment that "unwanted" variables could get in the way of the results, and Hunter, like most other writers on the subject afterwards, expressed some caution in relying upon the experiment too much.

It is the argument of *Dickens's Forensic Realism* that Dickens's sense of the instability of narrative, perception, and interpretation learns a great deal from such medical equivocations. His awareness of the untrustworthiness of both appearances and materials stems in part from a forensic passion for finding answers in places where little could be relied upon to tell the truth. The analyzed body and its relationship with scenes and objects became, for Dickens, paradigmatic of his own wish to make sense of the changing and unstable energies of his world. Yet his was no passive appropriation of medical facts; he was aware of how medical jurisprudence relied upon opinion and professional interpretation, and, as such, the field needed to concede a human propensity to error. For example, during a lecture on medico-legal practice, delivered at the Royal College of Physicians in 1867, professor of clinical medicine J. Russell Reynolds said, "Science is dead when it does not grow, and its growth must remove old lines. It should not do so carelessly; it cannot progress unless it effects this carefully."[23] Accordingly, nineteenth-century forensics was a revisionist and a self-critical field. As we shall see in my first chapter, few textbooks were published without some sense of their need to correct certain errors and to provide a means of bridging embarrassing gaps in the discipline's coverage. Virtually all texts stressed the fact that the field was an incomplete, evolving science and that it was prone to error because it relied upon the interpretation of unfixed and fluctuating matter. It is such views that I see as informing Dickens's most self-reflective engagements with realism.

Part of chapter 1 will focus on how, as a new discipline, medical jurisprudence (the commonest name for forensics in the nineteenth century) saw a key part of its mission to be the replacement of old, "common sense" values with a more critical approach to the truth. According to most medical sources, the new science of forensics dealt with very unreliable materials and so benighted, antihermeneutic beliefs in the adage that "truth will out" could only fail to satisfy the demands of justice. Medical writings on death, in particular, showed a preoccupation with misleading "signs" and unstable clues,

---

23. J. Russell Reynolds, "Lumleian Lectures, Delivered before the Royal College of Surgeons," II, *British Medical Journal* (4 May 1867): 519–20 (519).

as well as with the trustworthiness of the interpretive strategies used for making sense of them. In *The Medical Aspects of Death*, a book that Dickens owned from 1852, the surgeon James Harrison noted how the medical establishment was finding ways of classifying and arranging postmortem clues:

> The *bodily changes* which immediately precede, and, in some sense, may be said to constitute death, deserve and repay consideration. It might seem, on a first attention, that the modes in which death takes place are so various, and the diseases to which the human frame is liable so numerous, that it would be impossible to reduce the subject to any simple and practical form of enquiry.
>
> It will be found, however, on a more intimate acquaintance, that much advantage may be gained by classification and arrangement, and a sort of analysis made which requires no forced construction, and no metaphysical nicety.[24]

The human body, particularly when dead, is a thing that represents no "simple," straightforward, or trustworthy narrative. Yet rather than despairing of any attempts to classify and arrange postmortem signs, Harrison, like many of his colleagues, was willing to accept uncertainty as an opportunity for bringing analytical awareness to the new powers of forensic science.

Another thing that differentiates Dickens's descriptions of the Paris Morgue from Zola's is its insistence on the *perspective* of interpretation. In *Thérèse Raquin*, as in just about all of Zola's novels, there is a solid separation between narrator and character. Zola enjoys a world in which the sagacity of his authorial voice embarrasses the fatal stupidity of characters like Laurent and Thérèse. In contrast, in "Travelling Abroad" Dickens writes about his own experiences of the morgue, and so there can be no authorial superiority like that we see in *Thérèse Raquin*. Yet the differences between Laurent's subjection and Dickens's determination to make sense of his narrator's horror capture forensic science's new insistence on evidence as understood best when it is filtered through the process of interpretation. Although in the Dickens piece the images of the dead house become instruments of psychological torture as they do in Zola, the mode of their description allows the text to underscore the analytical methods of the story itself: the narrator treats his horror as a mystery—a puzzle to be solved: "What troubled me was . . . I noticed the peculiarities of this

---

24. James Bower Harrison, *The Medical Aspects of Death, and the Medical Aspects of the Human Mind* (London: Longman et al., 1852), 41–42. Italics in original. Dickens's edition was signed "with the Author's Respects." See J. H. Stonehouse, ed., *Catalogue of the Library of Charles Dickens from Gadshill* (London: Piccadilly Fountain Press, 1935), 55.

possession, while it was a real discomfort to me." Zola's mortuary imagery supports a theory of Maurice Blanchot's that "when we are face to face with the things themselves—if we fix upon a face, the corner of a wall—[. . .] we abandon ourselves to what we see."[25] This appears to be the case for Laurent but not for Dickens, who cannot forget his own role as interpreter of the scene; *his* experiences and perceptions own up to the organizing principles of a narrational perspective.

My book suggests that Dickens is never able to abandon himself entirely to what he sees; or, to put it another way, in the act of seeing, noticing, and fact gathering, the observer-narrator never loses sight of him- or herself as an interpreting intermediary. As Richard H. Moye has noted, Dickens had an "awareness of his own interpretive bias."[26] Accordingly, the early works are pieces in which a naive-empiricist sense of the reality of things gets troubled by the sorts of questions that make the later works stand out as more in-depth explorations of the interpretive impulse. The later works have a better command of what Jacques Derrida termed the "breaches, divides [and] expropriat[ions of] the 'ideal' plenitude of self-presence of intention, of meaning, and, *a fortiori*, of all adequation between and meaning and saying."[27] Yet rather than say that Dickens was a man who had the ability to preempt the work of Derrida and other poststructuralists, I insist that he was a man very much of his time—a time, that is, when all strategies of interpretation were subjected to an intense cross-examination.

DICKENS AND SCIENCE

So how much did Dickens know about the period's developments in forensic medicine? We might tackle this question by looking at the broader

---

25. Maurice Blanchot, *The Space of Literature* (1955), quoted in Clark, "Dickens through Blanchot," 24.

26. Richard H. Moye, "Storied Realities: Language, Narrative and Historical Understanding," in *Contemporary Dickens*, ed. Eileen Gillooly and Deirdre David (Columbus: The Ohio University Press, 2009), 93–109. Moye adds: "Dickens's sense of the past and of written history was far from naïve, if highly problematic, and was keenly aware of historical narrative as interpretation (as opposed to a recitation of the facts as they actually happened)" (96). My book extends this point to more than just history; interpreter bias was something that Dickens saw as present in all acts of interpretation. One of the best accounts of Dickens's self-reflexivity is Juliet John's *Dickens's Villains: Melodrama, Character, Popular Culture* (Oxford: Oxford University Press, 2001), 122–40. John writes of *Oliver Twist* that "the most sophisticated layer of commentary depends, not on its exact representation of life, but on its self-referential, textual investigation of the ideological and moral complexity of the relationship between life and fiction" (129).

27. Jacques Derrida, *Limited, Inc* (1988), quoted in Suzy Anger, *Victorian Interpretation* (Ithaca, NY, and London: Cornell University Press, 2005), 9.

subject of "Dickens and Science," a topic that has attracted a modest flurry of critical attention in recent years and, as noted by Ben Winyard and Holly Furneaux, "remains a provocative combination, in which attitudes about the division and relationship between high and low culture, authorised and unofficial epistemologies, and intellectual and popular ways of knowing are still contested."[28] Winyard and Furneaux highlight how in 1839 Dickens was visited by George Henry Lewes, who was "appalled to find in the young writer's library just a standard set of books and presentation copies"; he (Lewes) believed that Dickens "remained completely outside philosophy, science, and the higher literature."[29] Two years after Dickens's death Lewes had had no change of heart: "He never was and never would have been a student," he wrote in the *Fortnightly Review*. "Compared with that of Fielding or Thackeray, his was merely an *animal* intelligence, *i.e.*, restricted to perceptions."[30] In 1849 Harriet Martineau complained about Dickens's "vigorous erroneousness about matters of science,"[31] and a number of modern critical opinions seem to have agreed. It is not the aim of *Dickens's Forensic Realism* to suggest that these interpretations have been incorrect, though some of them have been expressed with more force than is merited by the evidence.[32] Although I have used up a fair amount of space, in this study, focusing on what the author was likely to have read and whom he was likely to have known, I have not been motivated by the idea of writing a book that is limited by biographical links. Nor has my aim been to supplement the work that has been done in suggesting how Dickens preempted many of the labels we now have for medical conditions. Instead,

---

28. Ben Winyard and Holly Furneaux, "Dickens, Science and the Victorian Literary Imagination," in *19: Interdisciplinary Studies in the Long Nineteenth Century* 10 (2010), www.19.bbk.ac.uk [accessed October 2015].

29. Peter Ackroyd, *Dickens* (1990; London: Vintage, 1999), 312.

30. George Henry Lewes, "Dickens in Relation to Criticism," *Fortnightly Review* (1 February 1872): 141–54 (151). Italics in original.

31. Quoted in Sally Ledger, *Dickens and the Popular Radical Imagination* (Cambridge: Cambridge University Press, 2007), 103.

32. K. J. Fielding has been most prolific in suggesting that Dickens's knowledge of science has been exaggerated by contemporary readers. Along with Shu Fang Lai, he noted in 1999 that "Dickens was not particularly well informed about the latest advances in science, and it is ludicrous to suppose that he was or could have been" (206). Andrew Sanders's more measured view is that Dickens's "grasp of the steadily advancing scientific thought of his time probably went no further than that of an intelligent general reader" (165); this view is supported by Jude V. Nixon. See K. J. Fielding, "Dickens and Science?" *Dickens Quarterly* 13:4 (1996): 200–216; K. J. Fielding and Shu Fang Lai, "Dickens's Science, Evolution and 'The Death of the Sun,'" in *Dickens, Europe and the New Worlds,* ed. Anny Sadrin (London: Macmillan, 1999), 200–211; Andrew Sanders, *Authors in Context: Charles Dickens* (Oxford: Oxford University Press, 2003); and Jude V. Nixon, "'Lost in the Vast Worlds of Wonder': Dickens and Science," *Dickens Studies Annual* 35 (2005): 267–333.

I have been inspired by the idea of writing a book that agrees with George Levine's view that "it would have been impossible for anyone, no less someone as imaginatively alive as Dickens, to have written without absorbing into his language something of the way science had been changing it."[33] A number of high-profile court cases, many of which will be discussed in the chapters that follow, featured what became known as "expert" medical evidence. In 1831 Dickens produced a shorthand account of one of these: the trial of John Bishop, Thomas Williams, and James May. The three men were put on trial for the murder of a teenage boy whose cadaver they had sold to the anatomists at King's College, London. Some such indictments are mentioned in Dickens's novels directly; others had a less overt influence on the shape and texture of his writing. Thanks to popular journalism, the field in which young Dickens served his novitiate,[34] crimes against the body became fodder for the reading public, and reports of medical experts giving their opinions on anatomical or circumstantial evidence reached the doormats and breakfast tables of millions of households every day. We see in the work of Dickens, a man who certainly did not have the scientific interests of an author like George Eliot, just how ubiquitous, subtle and powerful these ideas became.[35] Along with John Parham, I believe that a

---

33. George Levine, *Darwin and the Novelists: Patterns of Science in Victorian Fiction* (Chicago: University of Chicago Press, 1988), 121.

34. On the influence of journalism on Dickens's fictional writings see Kathryn Chittick, "Dickens and Parliamentary Reporting in the 1830s," *Victorian Periodicals Review* 21 (1988): 151–60; Matthew Bevis, "Temporizing Dickens," *The Review of English Studies* 52:206 (2001): 171–91; and John M. L. Drew, *Dickens the Journalist* (Basingstoke: Palgrave Macmillan, 2003).

35. Contrary to much of the scholarship that has been produced on Dickens and science, I will not be claiming that the novels set an "emotional" or a "fanciful" tone against the empirical strategies of science. Toshikatsu Murayama noted in 2002 that "the literary imagination maintains [a] privileged access to truth by claiming that scientific eyes can see only shallow surface and never reach inner truth" (408). Brooke D. Taylor adds that "empirical analysis must be tempered by finer emotion feeling; otherwise significant avenues of understanding are crippled or even destroyed" (173). John R. Reed suggests that Dickens "wanted to emphasize the human capacity to imagine. He wanted to heighten human experience through fancy" (106). Winyard and Furneaux contrast Dickens with George Eliot, concluding "Dickens championed a democratically accessible science that resembled fiction in its ability to stir the imagination, produce incredible narratives and bind together a reading public. For George Eliot, however, science could mould fiction by offering it a method posited on the steady accretion of facts and details and the precise and objective representation of reality." Most recently, Katherina Boehm claims that "emotional involvement rather than analytical detachment characterized Dickens's response to many popular scientific cultures of his day"; "his other appeals to literature as a realm of non-empirical 'evidence' hint at his desire to maintain the possibility of an intuitive, emotive knowledge that exists alongside the materialist knowledge of professional medicine" (8, 36). Such polarization of science and sentiment has been a common interpretation of Dickens's work. The seeming conflict between "fact" and "fancy" in *Hard Times* (1854) offers evidence of Dickens's seeming dislike of any form of thinking that may not be identified as improved by "fancy." Yet Dickens's brief mention of science in that novel was a parody

legitimization for an analysis of Dickens and medicine "can be found if we examine more closely his place in the complex crosscurrents between culture and science."[36]

My first chapter lays out how a central part of forensic investigation was a discussion of what comprises the best interpretation of evidence. Relying on scientific approaches to questions of law, forensic medicine opposed a predominating, traditional belief in self-evident moral judgments. When scientific induction entered the legal arena, it brought with it a new version of the maxim "murder will out"; truth will come to the surface, men of science suggested, but only after the material facts have been interpreted by an expert. To critics of this new method, most of them traditional legal figures, science was guilty of suppressing the voice of "common sense" with noncommittal statements like those used by Dickens's muddle-headed doctor. Such objections are why, I argue, the forensic profession approached its key areas of focus with a healthy surveillance of both its abilities and its limitations.

Chapter 2 is dedicated to the fantasy of absolute certainty, and it shows how despite the fact that *forensic* became a byword for penetrative modes

---

of the kind of hard-line positivism he had come up against in G. H. Lewes's criticism of Krook's spontaneous combustion in *Bleak House* (discussed in chapter 3). It should not, I argue, be seen as typical of Dickens's engagements with scientific ideas throughout his oeuvre. My thoughts are more in tune with those of Adelene Buckland, who writes in her excellent essay on Dickens, geology, and visual culture that the author "seeks objective, scientific, and accurate observation of the natural world" and "attempts to retain the pleasures of superstition and spectacle through a poetic vision of [. . .] science" (681). Buckland's thoughtful book *Novel Science* adds that "a precise analysis of the visual and material cultures through which Dickens engaged with nineteenth-century science reveals that his interest in its developments was far from "nugatory" (273). See Toshikatsu Murayama, "A Professional Contest over the Body: Quackery and Respectable Medicine in *Martin Chuzzlewit*," *Victorian Literature and Culture* 30.2 (2002): 403–19; Brooke D. Taylor, "Spontaneous Combustion: When 'Fact' Confirms Feeling in *Bleak House*," *Dickens Quarterly* 27:3 (September 2010): 171–84; John R. Reed, *Dickens's Hyperrealism* (Columbus: The Ohio State University Press, 2010); Winyard and Furneaux, "Dickens, Science and the Victorian Literary Imagination"; Katharina Boehm, *Charles Dickens and the Sciences of Childhood: Popular Medicine, Child Health and Victorian Culture* (Basingstoke: Palgrave Macmillan, 2013); Adelene Buckland, "'The Poetry of Science': Charles Dickens, Geology, and Visual and Material Culture in Victorian London," *Victorian Literature and Culture* 35 (2007): 679–94; and Adelene Buckland, *Novel Science: Fiction and the Invention of Nineteenth-Century Geology* (Chicago: University of Chicago Press, 2013).

36. John Parham, "Dickens in the City: Science, Technology, Ecology in the Novels of Charles Dickens," in *19: Interdisciplinary Studies in the Long Nineteenth Century* 10 (2010), www.19.bbk.ac.uk [accessed October 2015]. Parham's insightful reading uses Bruno Latour's idea that technical science must be offered cultural translation if it is to have any useful application to the "betterment of society." Dickens, Parham contests, "is consistent with Latour's paradigm" because he "translated what he knew about these concepts into the language and shape of his own 'poetic science.' That translation offered a conception of science different from but equally legitimate to a more literal understanding." See also Bruno Latour, *Science in Action* (Milton Keynes: Open University Press, 1987).

of perception, medical jurisprudence emerged unsure of what might qualify as "the whole truth." As old beliefs qualified as the kinds of assumptions that the new field would seek to unsettle, so too did the sorts of claims of certainty that were espoused by other more material disciplines such as chemistry—a field which forensics would often interact with. The excellent research of Amanda Anderson, George Levine, and Lorraine Daston and Peter Galison has, in varying ways, demonstrated how a predominant aim of science, in the nineteenth century, was the quest for complete "detachment" or "self-abnegation."[37] What I argue in chapter 2 is that forensic medicine

---

37. See Amanda Anderson, *The Powers of Distance: Cosmopolitanism and the Cultivation of Detachment* (Princeton, NJ: Princeton University Press, 2001); George Levine, *Dying to Know: Scientific Epistemology and Narrative in Victorian England* (Chicago and London: University of Chicago Press, 2002); and Lorraine Daston and Peter Galison, *Objectivity* (2007; New York: Zone Books, 2010). Anderson observes:

> An ideal of critical distance, itself deriving from the project of Enlightenment, lies behind many Victorian aesthetic and intellectual projects, including the emergent human sciences and allied projects of social reform; various ideals of cosmopolitanism and disinterestedness; literary forms such as omniscient realism and dramatic monologue; and the prevalent project of *Bildung*, or the self-reflexive cultivation of character, which animated much of Victorian ethics and aesthetics from John Stuart Mill to Matthew Arnold and beyond. (4)

Levine notes that "the power to observe accurately becomes a moral as well as an epistemological virtue—it requires 'patient industry,' 'honest receptivity,' and 'the sacrifice of self' [. . .] Epistemology here has many of the characteristics of narrative" (5). Daston and Galison add:

> To be objective is to aspire to knowledge that bears no trace of the knower—knowledge unmarked by prejudice or skill, fantasy or judgement, wishing or striving. Objectivity is blind sight, seeing without interference, interpretation or intelligence. [. . .] Scattered instances of scientific objectivity in word and deed started to appear in the 1830s and 1840s, but they did not thicken into a swarm until the 1860s and 1870s. (17, 49)

On the relationship between medicine and realism, Lawrence Rothfield notes that "medicine enjoys by far the closest and most long-standing association with the issues of mimesis and knowledge so crucial to critical conceptions of realism," and "there would seem ample reason to examine medicine [. . .] as involving the quasi-poetic elaboration of something like a style, point of view, or mode of representation that conveys truth-value—as a constitutive element of the realistic novel and its allied genres" (12, 14). More recently, Meegan Kennedy has noted:

> Clinical methods of observation and representation offered writers some useful and powerful strategies, conveying a sense of rigorous scrutiny, careful description and narration, and professional knowledge. It is evident how useful these could be for novelists facing what Peter Brooks has called the "descriptive imperative" of the nineteenth-century novel, since physicians used these methods to meet the same imperative in medicine. (1–2)

See Lawrence Rothfield, *Vital Signs: Medical Realism in Nineteenth-Century Fiction* (Princeton, NJ: Princeton University Press, 1992); and Meegan Kennedy, *Revising the Clinic: Vision and*

bucked the trend by insisting upon the presence of human intellection as an organizing principle. With its legal dimension, medical jurisprudence had to hang on to the idea that there was a supreme principle of good that was linked to an absolutely unattainable standard of truth "embodied" in the idea of God. Dickens is often omitted from studies of realism or is seen as a sentimental "alternative" to such modes of writing, because he has such an obvious attachment to sentimental scenes and grotesque and satirical characters which, in realist terms, appear exaggerated, idiosyncratic, and incredible. What I suggest in chapter 2 is that Dickens's works explored and satirized the quest for absolute truth and that his own style of writing, far from being of no interest to students of realism, appropriates the methodological questions discussed in forensic medicine as a means of testing the skills of interpretation that realism implicitly relied upon. It is in this chapter that I consider the two novels that I believe show the most obvious interest in objective and subjective means of knowing: *Oliver Twist* and *Our Mutual Friend*. Considering these two novels in relation to the specific context of medicine's discussion of objectivity and "truth-to-nature" enables us to reconsider what interpretive strategies we have come to associate with realism and to recast Dickens as central to this discussion.

My explorations of the complex intersections between conflict and interpretation in chapters 1 and 2 lay the ground for a consideration in chapters 3 and 4 of the two "tangible" areas of forensic expertise: bodies and collateral evidence. As I have already noted, medical jurisprudence relied upon a perceived ability to understand evidence that may or may not be written on the body; supplementary to this was the skill of reading anatomy through physical clues like weapons left at a scene, suicide notes, and footprints. (Although not an obvious focus for medicine, these "things" were collateral *to* the body—they made sense of anatomy and were given meaning by it.) Chapter 3 concentrates on the works that appear to have a clear interest in the links between "realistic" representation and corporeal symbolism: the early journalism and *Bleak House*. Though the theme evolves, these texts have in common an interest in the city as a forensic subject. The appropriation of forensic ideas is both thematic and formal: "thematic" in the sense that images and ideas are transplanted from medical discourses in order to represent a compelling and faithful account of London; and "formal" in the sense that Dickens draws on the forensic reconfiguration of the body as a "text" that might contain as many questions as

---

Representation in Victorian Medical Narrative and the Novel (Columbus: The Ohio State University Press, 2010).

it does answers. What this affords the early sketches and *Bleak House* is a self-judging, playful, and enigmatic representation of the city—a form of realism, in other words, that is more complex and discursive than any attempt to capture the subject as faithfully as possible.

Criticism that has dismissed Dickens's realism by judging it against a fixed idea of what "realism" is should be challenged, then, by looking at the self-scrutinizing strategies of medical jurisprudence as an alternative, more flexible definition of what the mode might consist of. Indeed, in chapter 4, I explore how Dickens's determination to situate the focus of medical attention (the body) in context—to scrutinize its signs among the scenes and objects that may or may not give it meaning—reveals a preoccupation with the unfixed nature of evidence. Although they are very different novels in many ways, *The Pickwick Papers* and *Great Expectations* share an interest in the meanings of the objects that people (and their bodies) come into contact with. Details make up a vital part of Dickens's realism, as we shall see; and, drawing on the forensic idea that circumstantial evidence, like anatomical clues, can be misleading as well as revealing, the novels suggest that reading signs self-distrustfully is a fundamental part of a good interpretation. To borrow the words of Bill Brown, author of *A Sense of Things* (2003), "These are texts that [. . .] ask why and how we use objects to make meaning," and although there are clear "phenomenological parities between understandings and methods of object relations and material science,"[38] the "thingness" of the Dickens novel draws on medical jurisprudence in order to question the very nature of interpretation.

The recent surge of interest in "thing theory" has been of some interest to me in considering the relationship between narrative, forensic evidence, and interpretation. In *The Ideas of Things* (2006) Elaine Freedgood expresses the intellectual conundrum faced by literary critics who wish to interpret the objects that litter nineteenth-century realism. Such a venture, she says, "involves bearing in mind that the 'literal is, in most contexts, metaphorical,' so that the idea that things might be taken literally suggests a longing or an aspiration rather than a method."[39] Freedgood's method is recuperative ("the object is investigated in terms of its own properties and history and then refigured alongside and athwart the novel's manifest or dominant narrative—the one that concerns its subjects"[40]), yet it is also aware of how

---

38. Bill Brown, *A Sense of Things: The Object Matter of American Literature* (Chicago: University of Chicago Press, 2003), 4. Winyard and Furneaux, "Dickens, Science and the Victorian Literary Imagination."

39. Elaine Freedgood, *The Ideas in Things: Fugitive Meaning in the Victorian Novel* (Chicago: University of Chicago Press, 2006), 5.

40. Ibid., 12.

the process of interpretation requires the reader to evaluate his or her own role in the process. With reference to Jaggers's injunction that Pip "take nothing on looks; take everything on evidence," she notes:

> The apparent *opposition* Jaggers invokes between the superficial (what we see) and the deep (what can count as evidence) describes instead a disorienting *sequence* in the process of reading realism, and one in which the reader must decide, many times per page, on the possible weight of meaning an object might be able—or be intended—to support.[41]

Where I differ from this view is in my insistence that the interpretive anxiety is not a new anxiety, felt only by those of us who have had the benefits of literary theory, but that nineteenth-century medical jurisprudence and the Dickens novel asked the hermeneutic, epistemic, and philosophical questions attached to the "fugitive meanings" of "things" with equal complexity. In a revealing reading, Freedgood draws on the excellent reading of *Sketches by Boz* (1836) by J. Hillis Miller, noting the latter's recognition of how

> certain household items [. . .] should *not* be interpreted. He notes that a pewter pot and a beer-chiller don't "start to life." [. . .] "We," [Boz] admits, are not in a "romantic humour; and although we tried very hard to invest the furniture with vitality, it remained perfectly unmoved, obstinate and sullen."[42]

Outlining Miller's view that the decision not to anthropomorphize certain objects signifies the text's acknowledgment of its own artificiality (an interesting and telling tension with its journalistic objectives), Freedgood argues that "the force of history" will give these objects "a life of their own. The history of pewter in the nineteenth century—its place in early metal recycling, for example—might render the pewter pot in *Sketches* resonant."[43] The problem with this interpretation, for me, is that it misses how the furniture is already resonant. What is important about the representation of the pewter pot is how Dickens negotiates his own position as an interpreter who may or may not invest his "things" with the meanings that are represented in personification. It all depends, as Boz admits in the quote made by Hillis Miller, on his "romantic humour." Dickens's "things," like

---

41. Ibid., 19. Italics in original.
42. Ibid., 16.
43. Ibid., 16–17.

forensic evidences, are all about questioning the role of interpretation in the telling of any given story. While I do not disagree with the view that a great deal might be learned by appreciating the historical context of the things in the Dickens text, I insist that the intelligent self-scrutiny properly associated with this sort of interpretation is as present in the medico-legal and literary worlds of the nineteenth century as it is in twenty-first-century literary criticism.

To return to the subject with which I began, the unstable nature of bodies and their surroundings in Dickens owes much to the ideas and strategies of forensic science, and, like that new and fascinating discipline, his writings became engaged in a long study of representation. We cannot assign to Dickens any studies of epistemology that might sit alongside J. S. Mill and Auguste Comte, but we can view his works as the unique and fertile product of an age in which discussions about the relationship between clues and alleged truths, and evidences and answers, prompted complex, interdisciplinary discussions of what we know and how we know it.

CHAPTER 1

CONTEXTS
Common Sense, Medicine, Law

JOSEPH SELLIS

On 31 May 1810 the Duke of Cumberland, fifth son of George III and Queen Charlotte, decided to go to bed about one o'clock in the morning. About an hour later he was awoken by what he thought was a bat flying about his head but which he soon found out to be an intruder attacking him with a sword. After receiving a severe blow to the head, the royal tried to defend himself "with his naked arms, which were much cut in various parts; and in the struggle while getting out of bed, he received a further wound in the thick part of the thigh."[1] The duke's attacker, seeming to find himself resisted more than he expected, ran away while the duke called out to his valet, "NEALE, NEALE, *I am murdered! I am murdered!*" According to *The Morning Post*:

> NEALE, who was sleeping in the adjoining room, got up instantly; and the Duke informed him of the particulars, and said the murderers were still in his bed-room. *NEALE* armed himself with a poker, and he and his Royal Highness proceeded along the passage; [...] *NEALE* stepped upon the sword with which the Duke had been attacked, and which had been sharpened for the purpose.[2]

---

1. Unsigned, "Horrid Attempt to Assassinate H.R.H. The Duke of Cumberland," *The Morning Post*, 1 June 1810, 3.
2. Ibid.

The duke and Neale called for help at the door of one of the royal's pages, an Italian man named Joseph Sellis. This man was "heard opening a drawer, in which probably was a razor; for when discovered, he was found to have cut his throat in such a manner, as nearly to have severed his head from the body."[3] From this it was ascertained that Sellis must have been the man who attacked the duke; he had, it was suggested, hidden himself in his master's water closet until the duke fell asleep. The next day *The Morning Post* made the most it could of the particulars by embellishing their ugliest aspects:

> Whatever the motive may have been, the crime is greatly aggravated by the blackest ingratitude. The assassin, who has a wife and four small children, has experienced countless instances of the kindness and condescension of his Royal Highness [. . .]. The monster took the advantage of this indulgence, and converted it into an engine to accomplish his sanguinary purpose. [. . .] At two o'clock, [he] sallied from his lurking place, and entered his Master's bed-chamber with his sword [. . .] in one hand, and a dark lanthorn in the other, and finding his intended victim asleep, he thrust his sword through his bed-clothes, which penetrated the Duke's neck and providentially awoke him: immediately on extricating the sword, he made two cuts, which laid open the pericranium in two places. [The Duke got out of bed . . .] SELLIS pursued him, and renewing his blows, cut his Royal Highness's left arm in several places, and two of his fingers nearly off, by drawing the sabre through his hand. The Duke likewise received several wounds in his loins and thigh in retreating. [. . .] SELLIS, stung with the compunctions of a guilty conscience, or dreading the punishment due to the crime, retired to the antechamber, where [. . .] with that hand which he had imbrued in his master's blood, he [terminated] his own existence, by almost severing his head from his body.[4]

Worthy of the kind of gothic and crime-laden literature that was being sold by peddlers and street-corner vendors at the time, the *Post*'s account is an example of how much work the most attenuated facts can be made to do. This journalist made more of the duke's injuries than was likely to have been the case, and he chose to interpret the "facts" in a way that told a dark and conservative story. Although the duke's wounds were reportedly so extensive that they made George III faint when he saw them, there is no evidence to suggest that he received anything more than an insignificant

---

3. Ibid.
4. Ibid.

head laceration and minor cuts to his hands and thigh. Whether Sellis was ungrateful, monstrous, or even guilty of the deed in the first place was hotly contested by many commentators, some of whom saw a more complex scandal at the heart of the Italian's death.

On the night of the attack the duke was treated by a number of well-known physicians, including Sir Everard Home—a figure who was well known to the medical establishment as brother-in-law to the celebrity surgeons John and William Hunter.[5] He had been appointed Sergeant Surgeon to the King in 1808. Outlining the scene of Sellis's death at the inquest he said:

> I visited the Duke of Cumberland upon his being wounded, and found my way from the great hall to his apartment by the traces of blood, which were left on the passages and staircase, and found him on the bed, still bleeding, his shirt deluged with blood. [...] The cap, scalp, and scull, were obliquely divided, so that the pulsations of the arteries of the brain were distinguished. While dressing this and the other wounds, report was brought that Sellis was wounded, if not murdered; his Royal Highness desired me to go to him, as I had declared his Royal Highness out of immediate danger. [...] I went to [Sellis's] apartment, found the body lying on his side, on the bed, without his coat and neckcloth, the throat cut so effectually, that he could not have survived above a minute or two; the length and the direction of the wounds were such as left no doubt of its being given by his own hand. Any struggle would have made it irregular.[6]

The Law Magazine declared itself satisfied with Home's interpretation of the evidence: "What can be more conclusive than the inferences that naturally present themselves?" it asked. "This question ought, indeed, to be set at rest by Sir E. Home's declaration, and an admirable lesson is thus furnished on the importance of medical investigation in cases of difficulty and doubt."[7] The magazine's outline agreed that "the length and the direction of [Sellis's] wounds were such as *left no doubt*" that the Italian had killed himself, which, all things considered, is not a medical investigation. Professional experience of long standing, which Home had, seemed to make

---

5. It was claimed by several medical men that Home plagiarized John Hunter's work and burned much of the latter's documents in order to hide the evidence of his charlatanism.

6. Quoted in Unsigned, *The Trial of Josiah Phillips for a Libel of The Duke of Cumberland* (London: J. Hatchard, 1833), 4.

7. Unsigned, "Medical Jurisprudence," *The Law Magazine* 1 (1830): 506–27 (520). Italics in original.

his "investigations" a simple matter of confirming obvious appearances as opposed to offering a more rigorous scrutiny of the scene and the body. As a number of commentators were quick to point out, Home's findings were decidedly "unscientific," which highlights how his methods clashed with a new, emerging vision of how suspicious deaths ought to be dealt with. Evincing nothing of the "sound and rational" analysis that had famed the Hunters,[8] Home reported himself satisfied with the "obvious" nature of the Italian's death. The coroner's jury took a short amount of time to find that Sellis had attempted to assassinate the duke and that, being frustrated in his efforts, he had taken a razor to his own throat. They returned a verdict of *felo de se*, and three days later the man's cadaver was interred at a crossroads in London.

This final act of superstition—replicating how alleged witches and vampires were once dealt with—crystallizes how much of the investigation of Sellis's death was old-fashioned and driven by outdated beliefs. Suspicious or aggravating "facts" seem to have fallen into place rather easily: it was implied that Sellis was quarrelsome; his victim was a member of royalty; and—most incriminating of all—the would-be assassin was a foreigner. It told a ready-made tale which *The Morning Post* seemed delighted to sum up as follows:

> Upon this subject, we shall for the present add but one reflection; but we hope it will ring in the ears of Englishmen like the thunder of Heaven. [. . .] Englishmen, you have too much at stake to allow you to suffer, without unceasing remonstrance, the continuance of this danger. [. . .] Demand the expulsion from the families of your Legislators and Protectors of all these vermin [foreigners]—send them out of the country—let the bread of

---

8. According to Roy Porter:

> John Hunter was an indefatigable experimentalist. Addressing topics such as inflammation, shock and disorders of the vascular system, his main treatises [. . .] contributed to surgery's emergence from a manual craft into a scientific discipline involving physiological investigation. [. . .] As in France where surgeons vied with physicians for professional distinction, in Britain Hunter was seen to embody surgery's claim to be the true basis of experimental physiology and, through the cultivation of anatomy, the model of medical instruction and research.

See Roy Porter, *The Greatest Benefit to Mankind: A Medical History of Humanity from Antiquity to the Present* (1997; London: HarperCollins, 1999), 280–81. One early historian of medicine noted that "Hunter [. . .] perceived that medicine was in its infancy, and he undertook the stupendous task of revolutionizing ancient methods of study and launching science anew upon sound and rational lines." James Gregory Mumford, *Surgical Memoirs and Other Essays* (New York: Moffat and Yard, 1908), 60.

England be eaten by her own children, and the persons of your great men be guarded by her own sons!⁹

Lady Anne Hamilton, a figure who, as we shall see, played no small part in the sequel to the Sellis affair, criticized *The Morning Post* as a "Tory Organ," and she certainly had some justification.[10] Every detail the newspaper chose to embellish led to a right-wing conclusion: the duke was a heroic victim, and his page was a base foreign parasite who had hidden among the mess of the water closet in order to slay a figure at the center of the British Court.

COMMON SENSE

In the "Tory Organ," prejudice masqueraded itself as "common sense," which is a familiar enough strategy in rightist arguments; yet what seems more surprising, given the fact that science had been familiar with Francis Bacon's doctrine of the idols for almost two centuries, was the way Everard Home's "scientific" evidence relied upon assumption. His views exposed him to a barrage of criticism from less conservative figures as well as from those who had a more modern idea of what constituted a scientific investigation. Yet a charitable interpretation of the doctor's evidence would suggest that it was not uncharacteristic of the traditional ways of thinking about crime. Before the nineteenth century, crime scene investigations would have been a matter for legal clarification rather than medical opinion, and, as Jan-Melissa Schramm argues in her excellent book *Testimony and Advocacy in Victorian Law, Literature and Theology* (2000), traditional thinking among lawyers assumed that facts could speak for themselves. It was, she contends, "an anti-hermeneutic model that could not be sustained in the more critical culture of the nineteenth century, where new definitions of evidence complicated the moral compasses of fiction, law and theology."[11] On the face of it, mythic conceptions of the self-evident fact proved the ancient maxim "truth will out,"[12] or, in the words of William

---

9. Ibid.
10. Anne Hamilton, *Secret History of the Court of England from the Accession of George the Third to the Death of George the Fourth* (1832; London: John Dicks, 1883), 65.
11. Jan-Melissa Schramm, *Testimony and Advocacy in Victorian Law, Literature and Theology* (Cambridge: Cambridge University Press, 2000).
12. In *The Merchant of Venice* Lancelot says, "Truth will come to light; murder cannot be hid long. [. . .] In the end truth will out" (2.2.74–76). Chaucer wrote in The Nun's Priest's Tale that "mordre wol out, that we see day by day" and "Though it abide a yeer or two or three. Mordre wol out: this is my conclusioun" (*The Canterbury Tales*, 1.232, 236–37).

Paley, "Circumstances cannot lie."[13] Roger Smith notes in *Trial by Medicine* (1981) that before the nineteenth century, "the law's approach to miscreants was entrenched, it appeared natural (devoted to 'natural justice') and self evident."[14] As Mrs Bumble puts it in *Oliver Twist* (1837–38), "There are those who will lie dead for twelve thousand years to come, or twelve million, for anything you or I know, who will tell strange tales at last."[15] This was an old pattern of thinking derived from a belief in natural principles of right and wrong. "True law," wrote Cicero, "is right reason in agreement with Nature; it is of universal application, unchanging and everlasting [. . .]. We cannot be freed from its obligations by Senate or People, and we need not look outside ourselves for an expounder or interpreter of it."[16] "No man can be ignorant of the laws within him," added the eighteenth-century jurist and philosopher Gaetano Filangieri:

> They are not the ambiguous results of the maxims of moralists, nor of the barren meditation of philosophers. They are the dictates of that principle of universal reason, of that *moral sense of the heart* which the Author of nature has impressed on all the individuals of our species, as the living measure of justice and honesty, and which speaks to all men the same language, and prescribes in all ages the same laws.[17]

Natural law suggested that inferences and "gut feelings" could be trusted, mainly because "facts" in investigations appeal to a universal sense of "plain truth." It was not the same as believing that the law could be relaxed into a belief that crimes cause their own detection, but rather that each man's intellectual hardwiring made him capable of making correct judgments without the need to consult any opinion that would come to be identified as "expert." The belief was an enduring one and something, moreover, that forensic experts of the nineteenth century would do battle with time after time in order to justify the importance of their science. Following the conviction of William Palmer for the murder of John Parsons Cook in 1856,

---

13. Quoted in George Augustus Sala, "Notes on Circumstantial Evidence," *Temple Bar* 1 (1861): 91–98 (91). Sala says that this is a comment made with "less wisdom than was [Paley's] wont" (ibid.).

14. Roger Smith, *Trial by Medicine: Insanity and Responsibility in Victorian Trials* (Edinburgh: Edinburgh University Press, 1981), 67.

15. Charles Dickens, *Oliver Twist*, ed. Stephen Gill (1837–38; Oxford: Oxford University Press, 1999), 299.

16. Quoted in J. W. Harris, *Legal Philosophies* (London: Butterworths, 1980), 7–8.

17. Quoted in Anon., *The Origin, Science, and End of Moral Truth; or, An Exposition of the Inward Principle of Christianity* (London: C. J. G. and F. Rivington, 1831), 169. Italics in original.

for instance, *The Illustrated Times* stipulated that evidence in court of law should be "plain and popular to twelve average citizens of respectability." "If allowed to degenerate into scientific 'pedantry,'" summarizes Ian Burney, "truth, justice, and public safety would count among Palmer's victims."[18]

Notions of a "common sense," of "plain truth," would find their most systematic application in the practice of common law, as we shall note, yet it is also true that the school of commonsense philosophy, originating mainly in Scottish writings of the eighteenth century, provided one of the period's most persuasive vocabularies for enforcing the idea that understanding "the whole truth" was a universal human ability. "Some philosophers," wrote James Beattie in his *Essay on the Nature and Immutability of Truth* (1770), "have given the name of *Common Sense* to that faculty by which we perceive self-evident truth":

> In the science of body, glorious discoveries have been made by a right use of reason. When men are once satisfied to take things as they find them; when they believe Nature upon her bare declaration, without suspecting her of any design to impose upon them; when their utmost ambition is to be her servants and interpreters; then, and not till then, will philosophy prosper.[19]

Thomas Reid, Scotland's foremost philosopher of common sense, asked, in more measured terms, about the same "science of human nature":

> What is all we know of mechanics, astronomy, and optics, but connections established by nature, and discovered by experience or observation, and consequences deduced from them? All the knowledge we have in agriculture, gardening, chemistry, and medicine, is built upon the same foundation. And if ever our philosophy concerning the human mind is carried as far as to deserve the name of science, which ought never to be despaired of, it must be by observing facts, reducing them to general rules, and drawing just conclusions from them.[20]

T. E. Webb was wrong to write in an 1860 installment of *Fraser's Magazine* that Reid's "appeal to common sense [is] little more than an appeal to

---

18. Ian Burney, *Poison, Detection and the Victorian Imagination* (Manchester: Manchester University Press, 2006), 133–34.

19. James Beattie, *An Essay on the Nature and Immutability of Truth: In Opposition to Sophistry and Scepticism* (1770; Philadelphia: Solomon Wieatt, 1809), 34.

20. Thomas Reid, *An Inquiry into the Human Mind on the Principles of Common Sense* (1764; Edinburgh: Bell and Bradfute, 1801), 112.

vulgar prejudice."[21] The Scot's argument was that the mind's faculties had to be "mature" before any "sense" could become a common one: "When men's faculties are ripe," he wrote with reference to moral sense, "the first principles of morals, into which all moral reasoning may be resolved, are perceived intuitively, and in a manner more analogous to the perceptions of sense, than to the conclusions of democratic reasoning."[22] As one anonymous author put it in *The Origin, Science, and End of Moral Truth* (1831):

> The knowledge of moral obligation, as well as the knowledge of things useful and things hurtful, is *got* and *attained* by sensation, conscientiousness, observation, experience, information, memory, reflection, and reason; means of knowledge which are open to all men, and which gradually form our plain common sense and understanding.[23]

Both Reid and this author were indebted to the philosophies of Locke and Hume: they saw *experience*, rather than nature, as equipping one with common sense. "Let us accustom ourselves to try every opinion by the touchstone of fact and experience," Reid suggested. Such is "the voice of God, and no fiction of human imagination."[24]

COMMON LAW

William Blackstone's monumental *Commentaries on the Laws of England* (1765–69) suggested that it was the responsibility of the law courts to convert common sense, this "voice of God," into practical decree. Although he had some reservations about the binding potential of precedent, Blackstone considered tradition "the first ground and chief corner stone of the laws of England" and "one of the characteristic marks of English liberty." For him, judge-made law is a paradigm of august tradition and English common sense:

> How are these [legal] customs or maxims to be known, and by whom is their validity determined? The answer is, by the judges in the several courts of justice. They are the depository of the laws; the living oracles, who

---

21. T. E. Webb, "The Metaphysician: A Retrospect," *Fraser's Magazine* 41 (1860): 503–17 (504).
22. Thomas Reid, *Essays on the Powers of the Human Mind* (1785; London: Thomas Tegg, 1827), 355.
23. Anon., *Origin*, 14. Italics in original.
24. Reid, *Essays*, 23.

must decide in all cases of doubt, and who are bound by an oath to decide according to the law of the land. The knowledge of that law is derived from experience and study; from the *"viginti annorum lucubrationes,"* which Fortescue mentions; and from being long personally accustomed to the judicial decisions of their predecessors. And indeed these judicial decisions are the principal and the most authoritative evidence, that can be given, of the existence of such a custom as shall form a part of the common law. [. . .] For it is an established rule to abide by former precedents, where the same points come again in litigation; as well to keep the scale of justice even and steady, and not liable to waver with every new judge's opinion [. . .] he being sworn to determine, not according to his own private judgement, but according to the known laws and customs of the land [. . .]. The doctrine of the law then is this: that precedents and rules must be followed, unless flatly absurd or unjust.[25]

In the early nineteenth century, *Commentaries* was viewed as "an era in legal literature"[26] because of the way it interpreted the knotty precedents of the eighteenth-century legal system. A particularly rosy portrait was offered of the ancient method of enforcing and modifying law through the experiences of the courts. Alongside government legislation, legal precedent maintained that every judicial decision would lay down a principle that all future indictments of a similar nature would do well to follow. The specific way in which that principle was obeyed was subject to the interpretation of the judge in each case, yet any modifications would add a further layer to the record of arraignments, and so, the theory went, the law would become more "finessed" the more it was practiced. One example of the common law in action is the trial of Daniel McNaughten in 1843 for the murder of Edward Drummond and the attempted assassination of Robert Peel. Resulting in an acquittal on the grounds of insanity, the case led to the legal rule (now defunct) that a defendant should be considered unaccountable of his or her actions if it can be proven that he or she was unable to tell right from wrong at the time of the deed. The rule was contested hotly by psychology specialists who claimed that in many cases featuring diminished responsibility, the defendant knew that he or she was doing wrong but that he or she was powerless to resist the impulse. The "musty rule of the judges," noted one correspondent to the *British Medical*

---

25. William Blackstone, *Commentaries on the Laws of England,* 3 vols. (1765–69; London: Sweet, Pheney, Maxwell, Steven and Sons, 1829), vol. 1, 68–70.
26. Unsigned, "Life of Sir William Blackstone," *The Law Magazine* 15 (1836): 292–315 (306).

Journal, "confounds *knowing* with *willing*. Of what use is my knowing, if I cannot help doing a thing? Will knowledge restrain me?"[27]

Such objections were in part a response to the understanding that precedents bound where they ought to have guided. Although precedential reasoning had been a part of European courts since antiquity, it was, according to Neil Duxbury, the nineteenth century that introduced the concept of the *binding* precedent, or *stare decisis* ("to stand by things decided"): J. Parke observed in 1833 that "for the sake of attaining uniformity, consistency and certainty," rules derived from precedents must, unless they are "plainly unreasonable and inconvenient," be applied "to all cases which arise."[28] Parke was willing to admit that past judgments could be "unreasonable" and "inconvenient" and that subsequent cases might offer a "new combination of circumstances," yet he also held the not-unpopular view that decisions from the past help to keep judgments on a straight course. The judge is "sworn to determine, not according to his own private judgement," Blackstone said, "but according to the known laws and customs of the land." As late as 1905, professor of law A. V. Dicey supported the idea by writing, "Beliefs are not necessarily erroneous because they are out of date; there are such things as ancient truths as well as ancient prejudices."[29] Dicey's own opinion was not exactly erroneous, but it was out of date. Those who had any faith in common law in the nineteenth century were likely to stress the *interpretability* of its record rather than any connection with "ancient truths." What had gone out of fashion was the view that the book of judicature could be applied blindly—without any critical hesitation, that is, over the patterns that were used to link "similar" cases. In 1861 jurist and historian Henry Sumner Maine noted, "English lawyers of the last century were probably too acute to be blinded by the paradoxical commonplace that English law was the perfection of human reason, but they acted as if they believed it for want of any other principle to proceed upon."[30]

Faith in judges as "living oracles" was exactly the kind of thinking that troubled commentators who feared that judges might be too sheeplike and uncritical in following to the letter the pronouncements of their predecessors. As early as 1678 John Bunyan wrote in *The Pilgrim's Progress*, "Custom,

---

27. F. T. Poncia, "Law v. Medical Science," *British Medical Journal* (4 April 1863): 360. Italics in original.

28. Quoted in Neil Duxbury, *The Nature and Authority of Precedent* (Cambridge: Cambridge University Press, 2008), 18.

29. A. V. Dicey, *Lectures on the Relation between Law and Public Opinion in England during the Nineteenth Century* (1905; London: Macmillan, 1924), 369.

30. Henry Sumner Maine, *Ancient Law: Its Connection with the Early History of Society, and its Relation to Modern Ideas* (London: John Murray, 1861), 78–79.

it being of so long standing, as above a thousand years, would doubtless now be admitted as a thing legal, by any Impartial Judge."³¹ Such is the basis upon which one of the pilgrims is executed:

> I think meet to instruct you into our Law [says the judge to the jury].
> There was an Act made in the days of *Pharaoh* the Great, Servant to our Prince, That lest those of a contrary Religion should multiply and grow too strong for him, their Males should be thrown into the River. There was also an Act made in the days of *Nebuchadnezzar* the Great [. . .] That whoever should not fall down and worship his golden Image, should be thrown into a fiery Furnace. [. . .] Now the substance of these laws this Rebel has broken, not only in thought, (which is not to be born) but also in word and deed; which must therefore needs be intolerable. [. . .]
> They therefore brought [the pilgrim] out, to do with him according to their Law; and first they Scourged him, then they Buffetted him, then they Lanced his flesh with Knives; after that they Stoned him with Stones, then prickt him with their Swords, and last of all they burned him to Ashes at the Stake.³²

In the arch tones of Jonathan Swift, Lemuel Gulliver reports half a century later:

> It is a Maxim among [the] Lawyers, that whatever hath been done before, may legally be done again: And therefore they take special Care to record all the Decisions formerly made against common Justice and the general Reason of Mankind. These, under the Name of *Precedents*, they produce as Authorities [. . .] and the Judges never fail of decreeing accordingly.³³

Defendants wrongly convicted in the time of McNaughten might have fared a little better than Bunyan's pilgrim, but it was their lives at stake nonetheless. Common law had justified "the most iniquitous Opinions,"³⁴ according to Swift. The legal philosopher John Austin said of Blackstone: "He truckled to the sinister interests and to the mischievous prejudices of power; and he flattered the overweening conceit of their national or

---

31. John Bunyan, *The Pilgrim's Progress*, ed. W. R. Owens (1678; Oxford: Oxford University Press, 2003), 40.
32. Ibid., 94–95.
33. Jonathan Swift, *Gulliver's Travels*, ed. Claude Rawson and Ian Higgins (1726; Oxford: Oxford University Press, 2005), 232.
34. Ibid., 232.

peculiar institutions."[35] And in *The Comic Blackstone* (1844) Gilbert à Beckett wrote:

> The judges decide what is a custom and what it not. They, in fact, make the law by saying what it means; which, as it scarcely ever means what it says, opens the door to much variety. "Variety is charming," according to the proverb; and the study of the law must, on this authority, be regarded as one of the most fascinating of preoccupations.[36]

It was on this ground of infinite variety that Blackstone would also find opposition from a number of legal authors, including Jeremy Bentham, Austin, and James Fitzjames Stephen, who believed that all laws and reforms should be defined by *state-created* laws rather than common practice.[37] It is Dickens's *Bleak House* (1852–53), however, that leaves us with one of the period's most damning pictures of common law. The novel is well known to have little faith in the machinations of the legal system, especially the Court of Chancery which by mid century had become so riddled with technical procedure that it soaked up money and energy and provided little in the way of justice in return.[38] According to Mr Krook, his shop is given "the ill name of Chancery" because he "can't abear to part with anything once lay hold of [. . .] or to alter anything, or to have any sweeping, nor scouring, nor cleaning, nor repairing going on about me."[39] Set up by William the Conqueror in 1067, "the labyrinthic vaults of the Court of Chancery," as Charles Knight termed the real court in *Household Words*,[40] were intended to add a "moral gloss" to the existing system of legislative and precedential law by appealing to *aequitas naturalis*, that is, the natural law of equity. Such notions of natural law began to look outdated when set against the seemingly objective powers of statute, as well as the rhetorical

---

35. John Austin, *Lectures on Jurisprudence; or The Philosophy of Positive Law*, 2 vols. (1861; London: John Murray, 1873), vol. 1, 71.

36. Gilbert Abbott à Beckett, *The Comic Blackstone* (London: Punch, 1844): 10.

37. See Duxbury, *Precedent*, 39; Gerald J. Postema, *Bentham and the Common Law Tradition* (Oxford: Oxford University Press, 1986); and Ayelet Ben-Yishai, in *Common Precedents: The Presentness of the Past in Victorian Law and Fiction* (New York: Oxford University Press, 2013).

38. Pamela K. Gilbert calls the Chancery in *Bleak House* "an institution that substitutes endless verbosity and formality for any real engagement between individuals and that therefore, instead of conferring benefits on its clients like a good social institution, turns vampiric and sucks them dry, like Mr Vholes." Pamela K. Gilbert, *The Citizen's Body: Desire, Health and the Social in Victorian England* (Columbus: The Ohio State University Press, 2007), 144.

39. Charles Dickens, *Bleak House*, ed. Andrew Sanders, (1852–53; London: J. M. Dent, 1994), 49. Subsequent references to this edition will be given in the text.

40. Charles Knight, "The Law," *Household Words* 2 (1850): 407–8 (408).

strategies of counsel and expert witnesses in the indictments themselves. In *Bleak House* Dickens associates Chancery with the system of precedent and the Blackstonean notion of judges as "living oracles": "It appears to me," he wrote in *Household Words* in 1850, "as if there were too much talk and too much law—as if some grains of truth were started overboard into a tempestuous sea of chaff"[41]—a view that is certainly reproduced in the portrait of Chancery in the choking London fog:

> On such an afternoon the various solicitors in the cause, some two or three of whom have inherited it from their fathers, who made a fortune by it, ought to be—as are they not?—ranged in a line, in a long matted well (but you might look in vain for truth at the bottom of it) between the registrar's red table and the silk gowns, with bills, cross-bills, answers, rejoinders, injunctions, affidavits, issues, references to masters, masters' reports, mountains of costly nonsense, piled before them. Well may the court be dim, with wasting candles here and there; well may the fog hang heavy in it, as if it would never get out; well may the stained-glass windows lose their colour and admit no light of day into the place; well may the uninitiated from the streets, who peep in through the glass panes in the door, be deterred from entrance by its owlish aspect and by the drawl, languidly echoing to the roof from the padded dais where the Lord High Chancellor looks into the lantern that has no light in it and where the attendant wigs are all stuck in a fog-bank! (4)

Associated with Chancery, the fog joins the piles of affidavits, papers, and bills to symbolize the gradual obfuscation of legal procedure with the "inheritance" of precedent. "The Court of Chancery," adds Dickens, is a thing of "precedent and usage; [an] oversleeping Rip Van Winkle [..., which] has played at strange games through a deal of thundery weather" (8); "the forensic wisdom of ages," he adds (meaning *forensic* in the Latin sense "of the forum," that is "of the law"), "has interposed a million obstacles to the transaction of the commonest business of life" (125). Such was a common complaint in Dickens's circle. In his satirical version of Blackstone's *Commentaries,* Dickens's friend À Beckett wrote:

> If a man has the misfortune to fall into a cellar by an oversight of his own, he may wait a long time before equity can get him out of it. [. . .] If a man

---

41. Charles Dickens, "The Ghost of Art," *Household Words* (20 July 1850); *Journalism* 2, 257–64 (259).

has the tooth-ache, equity has no specific way of relief, except, perhaps, extraction—for Chancery will take the bread from the mouth, and may, therefore, as well extract the tooth from the jaw, for the latter without the former is superfluous.[42]

In an 1856 installment of *Household Words*, Henry Morley added:

> We add heap to heap confusedly, and mingle living laws with dead. [. . .] We labour under written and unwritten law, common law and customs, and distinct systems of legislation for England, Scotland, and Ireland; [. . .] to remedy this evil, we have another tribunal for the restraining of the first, and maintaining the balance of equity by means of a machinery most cumbrous and iniquitous of all.[43]

On the estrangement that develops between Richard Carstone and his guardian on the subject of Jarndyce *v.* Jarndyce, Dickens writes:

> Chancery, which knows no wisdom but in Precedent, is very rich in such Precedents; and why should one be different from ten thousand? [. . .] But injustice breeds injustice; the fighting with shadows and being defeated by them, necessitates the setting up of substances to combat; from the impalatable suit which no man alive can understand, the time for that being long gone by, it has become a gloomy relief to turn to the palpable figure of the friend who would have saved him from this ruin, and make *him* his enemy. (504–5)

That the Court of Chancery is a failure and a costly drain on the vital energies of men like Carstone and Gridley is one thing, but this passage also gives a sense of the epistemological problems that precedent placed at the center of the legal method. Wisdom is gained through a history of arraignments, says the old system, and in the terms of William Blackstone, the gravity of forefathers ought to guard against arbitrary judgments. Yet Dickens was critical of the view that one case might stand for a hypothetical ten thousand of a similar nature. With his inherited gout and love of outmoded titles, honors, and values, the conservative relic Sir Leicester Dedlock represents this kind of thinking which, in the novel, becomes infectious: "Sir Leicester has no objection to an interminable Chancery suit. It is a slow,

---

42. À Beckett, *Comic Blackstone*, 14.
43. Henry Morley, "Law and Order," *Household Words* 13 (1856): 241–45 (241).

expensive, British, constitutional kind of thing. [. . .] And he is upon the whole of a fixed opinion." He "appears to have a stately liking for the legal repetitions and prolixities, as ranging along the national bulwarks" (13–14). His lawyer Tulkinghorn best personifies these archaisms of law:

> Here, in a large house, formerly a house of state, lives Mr Tulkinghorn. It is let off in sets of chambers now, and in those shrunken fragments of its greatness, lawyers lie like maggots in nuts. But its roomy staircases, passages, and antechambers still remain; and even its painted ceilings, where Allegory, in Roman helmet and celestial linen, sprawls among balustrades and pillars, flowers, clouds, and big-legged boys, and makes the head ache—as would seem to be Allegory's object always, more or less. Here, among his many boxes labelled with transcendent names, lives Mr Tulkinghorn, when not speechlessly at home in country-houses where the great ones of the earth are bored to death. Here he is to-day, quiet at his table. An oyster of the old school whom nobody can open.
>
> Like as he is to look at, so is his apartment in the dusk of the present afternoon. Rusty, out of date, withdrawing from attention, able to afford it. Heavy, broad-backed, old-fashioned, mahogany-and-horsehair chairs, not easily lifted; obsolete tables with spindle-legs and dusty baize covers; presentation prints of the holders of great titles in the last generation or the last but one, environ him. A thick and dingy Turkey-carpet muffles the floor where he sits, attended by two candles in old-fashioned silver candlesticks that give a very insufficient light to his large room. The titles on the backs of his books have retired into the binding; everything that can have a lock has got one; no key is visible. (121)

What Tulkinghorn represents, like Chancery, is law "of the old school"; that is, law before the new methods of science and other forms of interpretive rhetoric supplemented its rusty ideas of *aequitas naturalis*. I see nothing of "terrifyingly modern agency" in him, as Lauren Goodlad does.[44] He dresses like a man from the eighteenth century, and the way he becomes a repository for the stories and scandals of elite families echoes how the common law collects tales on the assumption that they might be useful at a later point. Everything that surrounds the lawyer is "old-fashioned," "obsolete," or "broken." Dust or rust settles on all of his things: locks, like old laws, have outlived their usefulness. The idea, indeed, of locks with no

---

44. Lauren M. E. Goodlad, *Victorian Literature and the Victorian State: Character and Governance in a Liberal Society* (Baltimore, MD, and London: Johns Hopkins University Press, 2003), 105.

keys signals Tulkinghorn's impotence in the modern world, and his antiquated candlesticks, giving "insufficient light," testify to a deep-set dimness shared by Blackstone's dwindling disciples. Goodlad proposes that "Tulkinghorn's accumulation of 'secrets' represents a modern tendency, the power of expert."[45] Although Tulkinghorn's outwitting of Lady Dedlock shows some cunning, his inability to read the character of Hortense as adeptly as the more expertly forensic Inspector Bucket (a plot we will return to in the third chapter) is what costs him most dearly. *Bleak House* is not skeptical of modern expertise, in fact, but dismissive of the kind of thinking that Tulkinghorn represents: old-fashioned assumption.

COMMON LITERATURE

The twin influences of natural law and the words of "canonized forefathers" can be said to have influenced the act of telling stories for as long as that practice has existed. Indeed, there is something to be said for viewing the legal construction of precedent as a form of belief in stories as determining the nature, and providing an example of, the workings of natural law. Turning to Dickens's juvenile reading, for example, we see how popular fiction of the early nineteenth century, based unashamedly on old wives' tales and inherited legends, was preoccupied with the solemn concept of "poetic" justice. Journals like *The Terrific Register* made natural law their central theme; their features, based on "true" yet well-traveled accounts, were designed to offer salutary and retributive lessons on the "fact" that truth will eventually come to light in order to convict the guilty and exonerate the innocent. Young Dickens was an avid reader of the *Register*:

> I used, when I was at school, to take in the *Terrific Register*, making myself unspeakably miserable, and frightening my very wits out of my head, for the small charge of a penny weekly; which considering that there was an illustration to every number, in which there was always a pool of blood, and at least one body, was cheap.[46]

Entertainment was the primary objective of the *Register*, and it capitalized fully on the gore and melodrama of "real" stories. Yet the publication also responded to a broader cultural understanding of the links between

---

45. Ibid., 107.
46. Forster, *Life*, 48.

experience and interpretation as more ambiguous than the Blackstones of that world were willing to admit. The *Register* was in circulation around the time *Blackwood's Edinburgh Magazine* was established in 1817. Although its Tory counterpart aimed for a different level of readership altogether, the *Register* shared the aim of creating "a realistic terror through precision of descriptive detail."[47] According to Harvey Peter Sucksmith, "objects which arouse horror" in *Blackwood's* "are described [therein] with a meticulously scientific accuracy and the sensations of horror are analysed with an almost medical thoroughness."[48] The traditional gothic tale, he adds, "generally arouse[d] a purely romantic terror through vague suggestion," while the tales of horror in *Blackwood's* used a frightening mimesis that amounted to "a revolutionary technique."[49] Edgar Allan Poe famously said of the same magazine that "the impressions produced were wrought in a legitimate sphere of action, and constituted a legitimate although sometimes an exaggerated interest."[50]

Serialized as a cheap weekly then printed in volume form in 1825, the *Register* followed suit (without, it should be noted, the kind of discursive sophistication to be found in *Blackwood's*). It achieved its most chilling effects by claiming that its uncanny and disturbing stories were grounded in "a legitimate sphere of action." The two things that each of its stories had in common were that they were all factual (allegedly) and that they had been written as a means of proving that, sooner or later, the truth will come to light. The preface to the volume edition of 1825 stated that "as we should be sorry to have it supposed that we had no motive superior to the exciting of curiosity, or the enlisting of the passions for mere selfish purposes, we shall point out the moral tendency of the work, to those (if there be any such), to whom it is not apparent."[51] The full title of the publication, *The Terrific Register; or, Records of Crimes, Judgements, Providences, and Calamities*, makes it sound like a written-out version of the common law as it had been defined in Blackstone's *Commentaries*. The preface continues:

> Satisfied that the real welfare of mankind ought to be the object of all our labours, we were persuaded that by selecting from the histories of

---

47. Harvey Peter Sucksmith, "The Secret of Immediacy: Dickens' Debt to the Tale of Terror in *Blackwood's*," *Nineteenth-Century Fiction* 26:2 (1971): 145–57 (146).
48. Ibid.
49. Ibid., 146.
50. Quoted in ibid., 147.
51. *The Terrific Register; or, Records of Crimes, Judgements, Providences, and Calamities*, 2 vols. (London: Sherwood, Jones and Company, 1825), vol. 1, i. This quotation, like all subsequent quotations, is from the volume reprint of the journal.

individuals and of empires, instances of suffering, induced by human folly, and of crime, perpetrated by human depravity, we should excite that sympathy, and arouse that indignation which are essential to the end we had in view. [. . .] The instances we have given of the surprising discoveries of crime, even after a long lapse of years, teaches the depraved that there is no safety in their pursuits. [. . .] There is one always in their council, whose scrutinizing eye penetrates the darkest dens of sin, and who in his good time makes known those hidden mysteries, which "appal the guilty and make mad the free." This fact is particularly striking in cases of murder, and from the narratives we have given, we come to this deduction, that however the deed may be surrounded by mystic circumvolutions, it "will out and speak with the most miraculous organ."[52]

What is significant about the preface is the way it negotiates a relationship between natural justice and narrative. Like numerous other contributions to the periodical, it testifies to the "fact" that sooner or later "truth will out," yet its vision of the journal's role in enforcing that belief through narration supports a legal model of justice as working best when it works through testimony.

Around the book's title in the frontispiece to the volume edition (figure 1.1) we see a range of weapons, tempestuous seas, falling castles, broken columns, and human figures in varying transports of panic and despair. Below the publisher's details there sits a grisly collection of objects on a Catherine Wheel, including a severed hand that holds a dagger by the point and, on the left, a truncated foot poking out from underneath some drapery. An axe, a chain, a poison chalice, and a burning faggot all nod to the theme of crime and punishment, which is dealt out by no unsparing a hand in the magazine. What is perhaps most significant, however, is the pictorial representation of the *Register* itself—pointed to by a skeletal hand and opened at one of the pages containing the running story "God's Revenge Against Murder." At first glance, this seems to be a sobering reminder that "truth will out": God will have his revenge and justice will be done. Yet the image's prominent display of both the *Register* and the objects relating to crime and punishment suggests that "truth" and "justice" require the mediation of evidence or testimony in order to be understood and fulfilled, respectively. The "things" on the frontispiece, in other words, indicate tantalizingly that there are stories behind them. They promise meanings beyond

---

52. Ibid., i, iii.

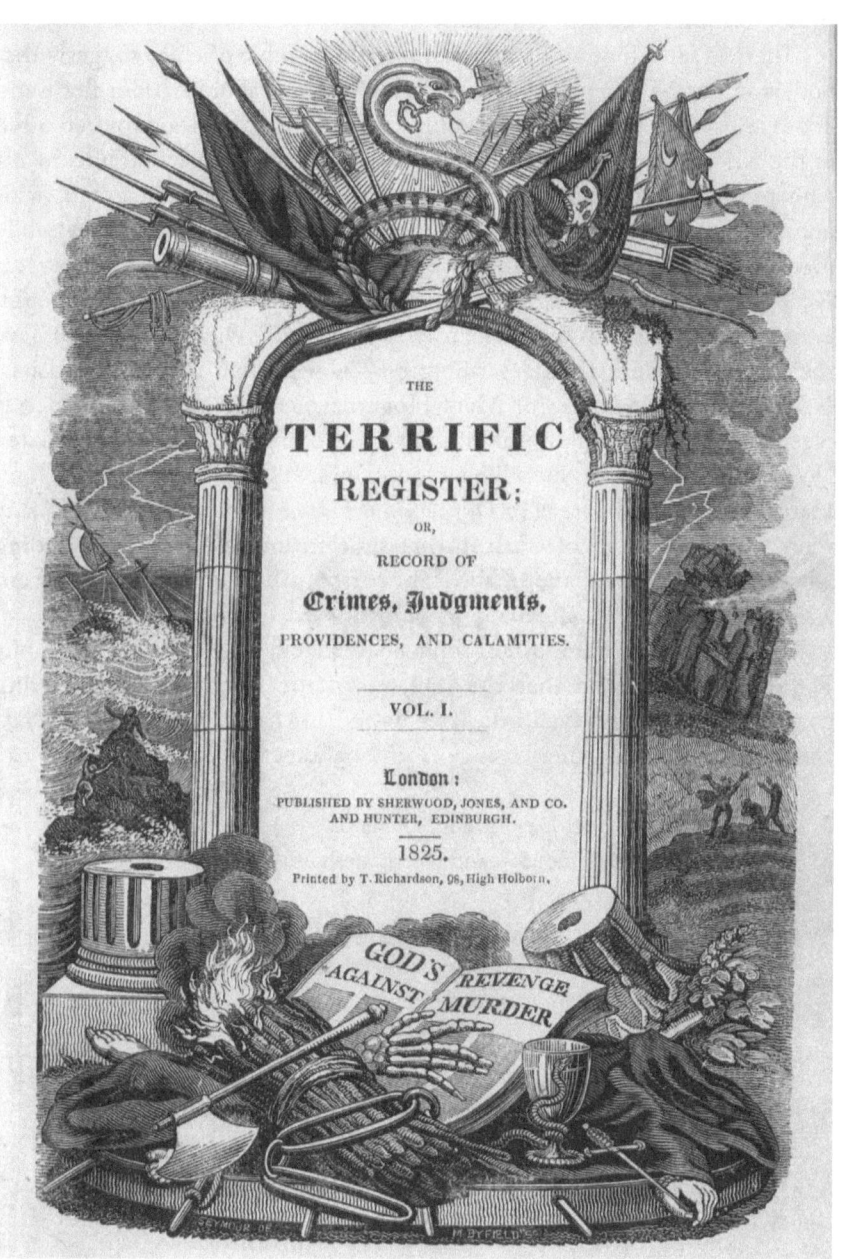

FIGURE 1.1. Frontispiece to *The Terrific Register*

their immediate representation, and it is the function of the text to outline those meanings through its narratives.

That we see a foot and a hand among this jumble of clues suggests that bodies might be receptive to the same process of illumination: flesh and bones tell stories too. Such is certainly supported by the idea, explored often in the *Register*, that criminals betray their own guilt by reacting uncontrollably to the sight of their victims' bodies or that cadavers bleed, groan, or sit up when in the presence of their murderers. By 1854 journalist and erstwhile man of medicine Henry Morley wrote of the phenomena in *Household Words* with a clear idea of it as nonsense: "A murdered man, it was thought, even if buried, bleeds when his murderer walks by."[53] Dickens seems to have the subject in mind when describing his feelings about the death of Little Nell, which reminds him of Mary Hogarth's death in 1837: "Old wounds bleed afresh when I only think of the way of doing it," he wrote to Forster. "What the actual doing it will be, God knows."[54] On the discovery of John Harmon's supposed corpse in *Our Mutual Friend* (1864–65), he notes: "Pity there was not a word of truth in that superstition about bodies bleeding when touched by the hand of the right person"; the truth is "you never got a sign out of bodies," not in any straightforward sense anyway.[55]

The authors of an important forensic textbook, John Paris and Anthony Fonblanque, lamented that the "fallacy" of the spontaneously bleeding corpse had "extended even into later days." In *Medical Jurisprudence* (1823) they quoted the following passage from Shakespeare's *Richard III*:

> O gentlemen, see, see! Dead Henry's wounds
> Ope their congealèd mouths, and bleed afresh.—
> Blush, blush, thou lump of foul deformity,
> For 'tis thy presence that ex-hales this blood
> From cold and empty veins where no blood dwells.
> Thy deed, inhuman and unnatural,
> Provokes this deluge supernatural.[56]

Shakespeare's dramas had an obvious commitment to the dramatic spectacle of murder "coming out": the freshly bleeding cadaver is just one

---

53. Henry Morley, "Man as a Monster," *Household Words* 9 (1854): 409–14 (412).

54. Charles Dickens, letter to John Forster, 8 January 1841, *Letters* 2, 181–82 (182).

55. Charles Dickens, *Our Mutual Friend*, ed. Stephen Poole (1864–65; London: Penguin, 1997), 35.

56. John Paris and Anthony Fonblanque, *Medical Jurisprudence*, 3 vols. (London: W. Phillips, 1823), vol. 3, 20. The *Richard III* quote is from I.2.55–61.

step away from the livid ghost of a murdered man appearing to catch the conscience of his killer. In *The Terrific Register*, however, this same idea is presented as a seeming fact and as a literal embodiment of the view that justice gets done when corpses tell stories. In "Touching a Dead Body," for example, the history of the custom is outlined as follows:

> Christernus the Second, then king [of Denmark], to find out [a] homicide, caused [the potential perpetrators] all to come together in the room; and standing round about the dead corpse, he commanded that they should one after another lay their right hand on the slain gentleman's right breast, swearing that they had not killed him [. . .]; as soon as [one man] laid his hand on his breast, the blood gushed forth in great abundance, both out of his wound and nostrils, so that, urged by this evident accusation, he confessed the murder, and by the king's own sentence, was immediately beheaded. Hereupon arose that practice (which [was] ordinary in many places) of finding out unknown murderers, which by the admirable power of God, are for the most part revealed, either by the bleeding of the corpse, or the opening of its eyes, or some other extraordinary sign.[57]

An example is provided of a dead traveler's hand being cut off and hung in a prison:

> About ten years after the murderer coming upon some occasion into the prison, the hand that had been for a long time dry, began to drop blood upon the table that stood underneath it; which the gaoler beholding, stayed the fellow, and gave notice of it to the magistrates; who examining him, the murderer confessed his guilt, and submitted himself to the rigour of the law, which was inflicted on him, as he well deserved.[58]

Everything turns out well in this story. The man confesses; he submits to his sentence, which the law furnishes; and, most importantly, he gets what he deserves. Justice happens so neatly because the severed hand betrays the "truth" so prominently. Like any other type of clue, such as a bloody footprint or a hidden dagger, the freshly bleeding wound points to guilt, but what is particularly fascinating about the latter is the way it reinstates agency: it gives life back to the dead in order that it might implicate the killers. It is a gothic tableau that underscores how, in the *Register*, natural

---

57. Unsigned, "Touching a Dead Body," *The Terrific Register*, vol. 1, 253.
58. Ibid.

law is actively powerful, and anything approaching "forensic" interpretation is, by implication, surplus to requirements. Christernus II seeks to "find out [a] homicide," yet he does nothing to ferret out the "truth." Instead, all of the actions belong to the perpetrator and the victim: it is the former who lays his hands on the dead man (a symbolic act that would be performed later by forensic examiners), and it is the corpse that bleeds accommodatingly.

In another of the *Register*'s tales, "Surprising Discovery of a Murder," a Dutch surgeon by the name of Van Helmont murders his friend so that he may rob him. He is not the early modern chemist and physician Jan Baptist van Helmont who, as the father of pneumatic chemistry, shows a great deal more intelligence than the *Register*'s doctor of the same name. This latter individual dissects the body of the man he slays in order to get rid of it, and he then throws the remains into a river. A fortnight later the remains are discovered and are "exposed [. . .] on [a] quay."[59] Walking past the disembodied limbs, the murderer remarks, rather foolishly, that "it must have been dissected by some expert anatomist; adding that he could hardly have done better himself."[60] Something in his tone attracts suspicion: "He was accordingly taken up [. . .] and carried before a magistrate, who, upon examining him, found strong reasons to think him guilty of the murder, and accordingly committed him to prison." When the surgeon's home is investigated, police find the murdered man's clothing and a servant who admits to having "smelt a strong stench like that of a dead corpse, which came from her master's closet." When he is convicted and sentenced to death, the surgeon admits that "he had in the same manner murdered and dissected two of his wives, and thrown their bodies into the river."[61] A Bluebeard for the chirurgical age, Van Helmont becomes reassuringly tormented by his guilt before being executed:

> During his confinement in gaol, between the sentence and execution, his dreams were replete with horror; he thought that those he had murdered appeared to him every night, and threatened him with eternal misery; insomuch that when the day of his execution came, he looked upon death as a deliverance from the horrors of a guilty conscience.[62]

The story may be viewed as anticipating the characterizations of Bill Sikes and Fagin, particularly how they are torn by their respective fears and guilt

---

59. Unsigned, "Surprising Discovery of a Murder," *The Terrific Register*, vol. 1, 787–88 (788).
60. Ibid.
61. Ibid.
62. Ibid.

after Nancy is killed. Yet "Surprising Discovery" also endorses a traditional view that, left to its own devices, guilt will implicate itself. Legal officials have to do virtually nothing to capture Van Helmont: The body proclaims its presence with a bad smell, and it then emerges from the river. The surgeon cannot resist incriminating himself in both this murder and that of his two wives. Truth will come to light, it seems, even while investigators rest.

In another of the *Register*'s tales, featured just eight pages before, the relationship between anatomy and truth is entirely different. The magazine included a number of stories in which people had been buried alive. Such stories followed, more often than not, the thematic drift of the journal's focus on the extraordinary and supernatural, and they reproduced the same kind of traditional link between evidence and justice that we see in the story of Van Helmont. But in "Coming to Life," the same subject is dealt with from the perspective of a couple of doctors, namely, Edward Baynard and George Cheyne. Their story concerns Colonel Townsend, "a gentleman of honour and integrity," who was able to put himself into a state that resembled death. The *Register* lifts the tale straight out of the pages of Cheyne's *The English Malady* (1733). It is an interesting appropriation in this context because of the contrast it makes both with "Surprising Discovery" and various other stories of natural justice. Told from the point of view of the doctors rather than that of the "victim" or any unspecialized witness, the story appears to contravene everything the *Register* stands for by presenting a series of clues without allowing them to work toward a reassuringly appropriate conclusion. Cheyne narrates:

> I found his pulse sink gradually, till at last I could not feel any, by the most exact and nice touch. Dr. Baynard could not feel the least motion in his heart, nor Mr. Skrine the least soil of breath on the bright mirror he held to his mouth: then each of us, by turns, examined his arm, heart, and breath, but could not, by the nicest scrutiny, discover the least symptom of life in him.[63]

Colonel Townsend dies (for certain) soon afterwards, and he is given an autopsy by the same doctors. Observe how inconsistent the tone of the following passage is with the other, melodramatic passages in the *Register*:

> Next day he was opened (as he had ordered); his body was the soundest and best made I had every seen; his lungs were fair, large and sound, his

---

63. Unsigned, "Coming to Life," *The Terrific Register*, vol. 1, 779–780 (780).

heart big and strong, and his intestines sweet and clean; his stomach was of a due proportion, the coat sound and thick, and the villous member entire. But when we came to examine the kidneys, though the left was sound and of a just size, the right was about four times as big, distended like a blown bladder, and yielding as if full of pap; he having often passed a weyish liquor during his illness. Upon examining the kidney we found it quite full of white chalky matter, like plaster of Paris, and all the fleshy substance dissolved and worn away, by what I called a nephritic cancer.[64]

"Coming to Life" represents a different way of telling stories: distinct to the discourses of medical science, it outlines the facts as they had occurred and expects the reader's interpretation to carry the burden of truth. So whereas in the stories of freshly bleeding corpses and the demon surgeon Van Helmont, evidence is active and interpretation passive, the story of Colonel Townsend presents the opposite: the body stays dead and requires experts to interpret its evidence. Conclusions are based on sensory experience: what the doctors see, touch, and hear, in particular, are crucial to their elucidations. The concluding sentence is "I have narrated the facts as I saw and observed them deliberately and distinctly, and shall leave to the philosophic reader to make what inference he thinks fit; the truth of the material circumstances I will warrant."[65]

This seeming inconsistency across the pages of the *Register* is evidence, of course, of the ragbag nature of the journal's editorial policy. Yet we ought to notice how the inconsistency, like the Sellis case, signals a conflict between ideas of natural justice and the emergence of science as a prominent way of interpreting the relationship between bodies and truth. When scientific induction entered the world of crime investigation early in the nineteenth century, it brought with it a new interpretation of the maxim "truth will out." Truth may come to the surface, men of science suggested, but only after the material facts have been interpreted by an expert. According to George Augustus Sala, science now rejected a world in which "'common sense' will prevail, and not uncommon penetration."[66] Schramm argues that "to concede that facts were complex rather than self-evident was to open the way for legal and literary feats of analysis and rhetorical power." Facts, she adds, "were increasingly seen as multi-faceted and open to professional interpretation."[67] Scientific testimony was exactly the kind

---

64. Ibid.
65. Ibid.
66. Sala, "Circumstantial Evidence," 93.
67. Schramm, *Testimony and Advocacy*, 21.

of expert maneuvering that constituted "feats of analysis and rhetorical power." Indeed, the belief in facts as having numerous possible interpretations was the driving force behind much early research on medical jurisprudence. The new science's inbuilt distrust of signs and evidence contrasted with the more traditional modes of interpretation where "things" frequently told an obvious truth. In an essay entitled 'Objectivity and the Escape from Perspective' (1992), Lorraine Daston suggests that "by the mid-nineteenth century, [. . . it was believed that] mechanical objectivity opposed interpretation."[68] There developed an opposition between "the aperspectival objectivity attributed to late nineteenth-century science" and the "subjectivity of individual idiosyncrasies, which substituted for the individual interests and 'situations' analysed by the eighteenth-century moral perspectivists."[69] In the conflicted naissance of medical jurisprudence, we see what seems to be a mirror image of this view. Set against the "hands-off" approach of allowing truth to emerge by itself was a new, "hands-on" approach that involved mapping and organizing evidence as a means of providing an interpretation. While it is true that nineteenth-century medicine would frequently insist on a "transcendence of individual idiosyncrasies" in the pursuit of science,[70] traditional "common-sense" logic was being challenged by the new clinicians who, with a microscope in their kit, offered a secular vision of *analysis* as the way to justice. William A. Guy, professor of forensic medicine at King's College Hospital in London, summed up the point rather neatly:

> Industrious observation [. . .] is the first requisite; but it must be observation, in the true, and not in the vulgar sense of that word—not in the sense of a mere passive exercise of the senses, but as the union of thought and perception; of thought electing an object, maturing a plan, guarding against every source of error, inventing instruments, improving methods, arranging and classifying the facts collected, and lastly, submitting them to a searching analysis. The simple employment of the senses in not observation, nor is the frequent exercise of them experience; it is in the true sense of these terms that the one is the parent of the science, and the other of the art, of medicine.[71]

---

68. Lorraine Daston, "Objectivity and the Escape from Perspective," *Social Studies of Science* 22:4 (1992): 597–618 (607).
69. Ibid.
70. Ibid.
71. William A. Guy, "Introductory Lecture, delivered at King's College," *Provincial Medical Journal and Retrospect of the Medical Sciences* 5 (1842): 23–32 (30).

The story of Colonel Townsend was resurrected in the pages of Dickens's journal *All the Year Round* for the article "Medical Nuts to Crack" (1861). "Many a tough riddle is put to the doctor in a court of law," this piece begins, "and the professional witness is expected with his facts and opinions, to show the cause of death, or to fix crime upon the guilty."[72] To indicate how "sometimes there is the riddle of apparent death to solve,"[73] the author cites the case of Townsend and focuses, unlike *The Terrific Register*, upon the colonel's ability to suspend his vital functions:

> Doctor Cheyne writes thus of the colonel's exhibition of his power. "He told us he had sent for us to give him some account of an odd sensation he had for some time observed and felt in himself, which was, that composing himself, he could die or expire when he pleased, and yet, by an effort or somehow, he could come to life again, which, it seems, he had sometimes tried before he sent for us. [. . .] While I held his right hand, Dr. Baynard laid his hand on his heart, and Mr. Skrine held a clean looking-glass to his mouth. I found his pulse sink gradually, till at last I could not feel any by the most exact and nice touch. Dr. Baynard could not feel the least motion in his heart, nor Mr. Skrine discern the least soil of breath on the bright mirror he held to his mouth. Then each of us by turns examined his arm, heart, and breath, but could not by the nicest scrutiny discover the least symptom of life in him. This continued about half an hour. As we were going away (thinking him dead) we observed some motion about the body, and upon examination found his pulse and the motion of his heart gradually returning; he began to breathe gently and speak softly."[74]

What *All the Year Round* demonstrates is that while the Townsend story stresses the need for interpretation as an alternative to the maxim "truth will out," it also highlights the complex semiotic riddles that faced medical examiners.

MEDICAL JURISPRUDENCE

Forensic medicine emerged parallel to the rise of both physiology and laboratory medicine and insisted, as they did, upon the importance of thinking

---

72. Unsigned, "Medical Nuts to Crack," *All the Year Round* (6 July 1861): 358–60 (358).
73. Ibid., 360.
74. Ibid.

carefully and self-distrustfully about the evidence of one's own senses.[75] It was a spirit that suited the Enlightenment ideals that had come to dominate scientific research,[76] as well as the new focus on individual responsibility that said, in contrast to the principles of "natural law," that a man was "free to go to the bad [epistemologically speaking] as well as to the good."[77] In 1789, the year of revolution, François Chaussier, anatomist at the Academy of Dijon, published an important memoir on aspects of medicine that he believed to be useful during legal investigations. He gave a course of lectures on the same subject, stressing the importance of the interpretive strategies of empirical science as opposed to blind "natural law." He also "enforced the necessity of the careful personal examination, by the medical man, in all cases of violence, as blows and wounds; and pointed out the precautions he should adopt in such visits. He gave admirable models of reports, and shewed the attention which was necessary to arrive at truth."[78] His dedication to systematic and painstaking analysis laid the foundation for a new phase of clinical rigor in medico-legal history that matched what was occurring in medicine more generally. As Meegan Kennedy has noted:

> During the late eighteenth and early nineteenth centuries, a new kind of medicine arose around the clinic. Patients received a standard daily ritual examination, and patients with similar diseases could be observed over time and compared. Historians since Foucault have chronicled the effects rippling outward from Paris: the rise of hospital medicine; the burgeoning spirit of research bringing new medical treatments, instruments, and statistics; the formalization of medical training; and, most important, the birth of a science of pathology based on the cold gaze of the autopsy, regularly confirming or denying diagnosis after death.[79]

---

75. "This is the period," writes Foucault, "that marks the suzerainty of the gaze, since in the same perceptual field, following the same continuities or the same breaks, experience reads at a glance the visible lesions of the organism and the coherence of pathological forms; the illness is articulated exactly on the body and its logical distribution is carried out at once in terms of anatomical masses." Michel Foucault, *Naissance de la Clinique*, trans. A. M. Sheridan as *The Birth of the Clinic* (1863; London and New York: Routledge, 2007), 2.

76. "For Enlightenment naturalists," note Daston and Galison, "to see like a naturalist required more than just sharp senses: a capacious memory, the ability to analyse and synthesize impressions, as well as the patience and taken to extract the typical from the storehouse of natural particulars, were all key qualifications." Daston and Galison, "Objectivity," 58.

77. Isiah Berlin, "The Romantic Revolution: A Crisis in the History of Modern Thought" (1960), in *The Sense of Reality: Studies in Ideas and their History*, ed. Henry Hardy (London: Chatto and Windus, 1996), 169–93 (176).

78. Michael Ryan, *A Manual of Medical Jurisprudence and State Medicine* (London: Sherwood, Gilbert and Piper, 1836), xxxi.

79. Kennedy, *Revising the Clinic*, 55.

Seven years after Chaussier's lectures, the anatomist and coroner François-Emmanuel Fodéré wrote the *Traite de Medicine Legale, et d'Hygiene Publique* (1796). It was enlarged and revised in 1813, after which no work had such an impact on the field of medical jurisprudence. Fully indebted to Chaussier, it is "universally allowed," noted one devotee in 1836, "to be the most valuable systematic treatise in the French language; it evinces great research, learning, judgement, and ability."[80] When Dickens sought to validate his representation of spontaneous combustion in *Bleak House*, Fodéré's was one of the sources he turned to for support. The reputation of the Frenchman's textbook was irrefutable. Beginning with a long and thoughtful introduction on the responsibilities and requirements of the forensic examiner, the massive *Traite* offered, in three substantial volumes, a guide to the kind of work that would be necessary in medico-legal investigations. Such included the examination of wounds, burns, suspected poisonings, signs of childbirth, "monsters" (deformities), supposed instances of spontaneous combustion, somnambulism, insanity, and a great deal more. "I have spared nought," suggested Fodéré in the preface, "in the discovery of crime, or the manifestation of innocence. I have invoked upon each point all the efforts that the human mind has made for the perfecting of the healing art, and for reducing to practice the *beau ideal* of justice that we form to ourselves."[81] It is a preface that highlights the enormity of the task that forensic specialists seemed to set themselves: they wished to introduce the best scientific practices into the law courts and make justice a matter of clinical procedure. It was an ambitious project borne out of the interlocking energies of science and revolutionary spirit during the late eighteenth century, when lofty principles of fairness and justice seemed to require the precision of science rather than the benighted prejudices of any "canonized forefathers." What we see in the medical works that followed Fodéré's is a like commitment to satisfying the high demands of justice through a scientific belief in a measurable truth.

Virtually every author of these later books expressed some indebtedness to their French predecessors, yet few drew as indelible a link between their own ideas and Fodéré as Mathieu Orfila's *Treatise on Poisons* (1814) and Theodric Romeyn Beck's *Elements of Medical Jurisprudence* (1823). Orfila was a native of Spain who graduated from a Paris medical course in 1811. He later became professor of legal medicine and published a work that

---

80. Ryan, *Manual*, xxxii.

81. François-Emmanuel Fodéré, *Traite de Medicine Legale, et d'Hygiene Publique* (1796), quoted in John Gordon Smith, *The Principles of Forensic Medicine, Systematically Arranged and Applied to British Practice* (London: Thomas and George Underwood, 1821), xx.

was considered to be the founding text of toxicology. The advertisement to the English translation of *Treatise on Poisons* (1815) noted that "M. Orfila has undoubtedly rendered a great service to Science, by opening the way to the study of this department of Medical Jurisprudence, hitherto little understood, and rarely cultivated, notwithstanding its importance to the Practitioners of Medicine."[82] Beck, one of Orfila's main disciples, wrote in his *Elements* that the *Treatise on Poisons* was

> copious, beyond all former treatises, in original experiments, and it has done much to increase our knowledge of the action and the tests of individual poisons. The career of Orfila, so splendidly commenced, has been successfully and ardently pursued; and his lectures on Legal Medicine, his word on Juridical Disinterments, and his numerous essays on detached subjects, have all served to improve and advance his favourite science.[83]

Beck's own *Elements*, another of the works that Dickens referenced when defending the combustion of Krook, was no insignificant contribution to the field either. Published in New York, where Beck worked as a physician, the book was the first notable American contribution to forensics. Two editions of the text were printed in London soon after, and the work attracted the attention of the medical establishment on both sides of the Atlantic. One reviewer called it "remarkable for the extent of research it displays, the minuteness of detail, and the luminous arrangement of facts and observations which are to be found on every page," adding that

> the work before us possesses decidedly sterling merit, and ought to find its way into the library of every medical practitioner in the kingdom. The notes of the editor are frequently curious and valuable, and the whole production is, in our opinion, decidedly superior to any other that has yet appeared on the subject of medical jurisprudence.[84]

What constantly reappear in such commendations are references to scientific rigor. Against what might be viewed as a rather frothy, traditional belief in natural justice was placed the immensity of Fodéré's, Orfila's and Beck's "laborious researches." Unlike previous works, however, Beck's

---

82. Mathieu P. Orfila, *A General System of Toxicology, or, A Treatise on Poisons* (London: E. Cox and Son, 1815), iii.
83. Theodric Romeyn Beck, *Elements of Medical Jurisprudence* (1823; London: Longman et al., 1842), xv.
84. Unsigned review of Beck, *Elements*, *The Lancet* (12 February 1825): 172–88 (180).

textbook confined itself to questions of medical jurisprudence, and it excluded wider-ranging discussions of sanitation and contagious disease. The topics he covered included how the body of a person "found dead" should be examined, including how to interpret wounds, examine poisons, ascertain the perpetration of infanticide, determine whether rape has been committed, and diagnose insanity.

Despite the great advances that Britain had made in a vast range of other sciences, including medicine, the country's contributions to forensic medicine were virtually nil until the publication of George Male's *Epitome of Juridical or Forensic Medicine* in 1816. Samuel Farr, a physician to the Bristol Infirmary, had published a text titled *Elements of Medical Jurisprudence* in 1788, but it was considered by many to be a rather "imperfect production" based on outdated methods.[85] Thomas Percival's *Medical Ethics* (1803) was originally intended to be called *Medical Jurisprudence,* but the author's friends advised him rightly that such a title did not suit a book that was about how a medical man ought to conduct himself in a range of situations, including hospital rounds and home visits. Male's *Epitome* was, then, according to his colleague John Forsyth, "the first original English work of any magnitude or value on Medical Jurisprudence," and it had "been instrumental in a great measure in directing the public mind to this science in Great Britain."[86] Male, a physician at the General Hospital in Birmingham, was "the father of the science [of medical jurisprudence] in Britain and Ireland."[87] His great contribution was in making his subject accessible to professionals who did not necessarily view forensics as vital to their training. His short book of 199 pages was aimed at lawyers as well as doctors, and it was divided into the topics of poisoning, violent crime, "sexual misconduct," and insanity. "My object," Male said, "has been, not to write a system, but to extract from the best authorities those remarks which appear to be worthy the attention of my readers, and compress them into a form most convenient for speedy consultation."[88] It stressed the need for every legal and medical expert to familiarize himself with forensic questions.

A professorship in medical jurisprudence was created at the University of Edinburgh in 1807. Around the time that Chaussier was running his course on forensics in Dijon, Andrew Duncan, the energetic professor of the Institutes of Medicine, gave a series of lectures on the same subject in

---

85. Ryan, *Manual,* xxxvii.
86. John Forsyth, *A Synopsis of Modern Medical Jurisprudence* (London: W. Benning, 1829), xiii.
87. Ryan, *Manual,* xxxvii.
88. George Male, *An Epitome of Juridical or Forensic Medicine; for the use of Medical Men, Coroners and Barristers* (London: Underwood, 1816), 4.

Edinburgh. The course's success led to the first chair in the subject being instituted, and it was Duncan's son, also named Andrew, who later took the position. Courses on medical jurisprudence all over Britain followed, each stressing how the subject formed an important part of medical education. In 1821 Dickens's future acquaintance John Elliotson taught "State Medicine" (a term that he used to describe medical jurisprudence) at Grainger's Theatre in Southwark—just a few steps from where the forlorn young Dickens would pass on his way to Warren's Blacking Factory.[89] Michael Ryan delivered lectures on medical jurisprudence at the Westminster School of Medicine in 1821, and John Gordon Smith, a surgeon who had served in the Twelfth Lancers at Waterloo, presided over a course at the Westminster Hospital and the University of London.

In 1821 Smith used his lectures as the basis for the important *Principles of Forensic Medicine*, a book that stressed the expert role of the forensic scientist. It was a "celebrated" exposition of the duties, responsibilities, and expectations of the medical examiner in cases of suspected crime. The book ran through three editions in the subsequent six years, followed by the *Analysis of Medical Evidence* (1825) and *Hints for the Examination of Medical Witness* (1829), each showcasing the perceived talents of medical expertise in cases of law. When the office of coroner came up in London in the early 1830s, Smith canvassed for the position but lost. He "was so much mortified by his defeat that he soon afterwards gave way to drinking and irregular habits, which greatly impaired his constitution, involved him in pecuniary difficulties, and ultimately brought him to [the Fleet] prison, where he gradually sunk and expired."[90]

Smith's melancholy fate is a far cry from the glittering successes of other practitioners in his field. In 1822 the chair at Edinburgh was taken up by Robert Christison, a man whose name became synonymous with toxicology and expert medical evidence. As a man of some celebrity, he attended a dinner in Dickens's honor in 1841. Dickens wrote about him and the other medical men present: "I felt it was very remarkable to see such a number of grey-headed men gathered about my brown flowing locks; and it struck most of those who were present very forcibly."[91] The venerable Christison

---

89. On the relationship between Dickens and Elliotson, see Fred Kaplan, *Dickens and Mesmerism: The Hidden Springs of Fiction* (Princeton, NJ: Princeton University Press, 1975), 26–27; and Steven Connor, "All I Believed Is True: Dickens under the Influence," in *19: Interdisciplinary Studies of the Long Nineteenth Century* 10 (2010), www.19.bbk.ac.uk [accessed October 2015].

90. Unsigned, "Coroner's Inquest on Dr. Gordon Smith," *The Morning Post* (17 September 1833): 3.

91. Charles Dickens, letter to John Forster, 30 June 1841, *Letters* 2, 313–18 (315).

had risen to fame after testifying in the case against Burke and Hare, the notorious "Resurrection Men" who had committed seventeen murders in order to supply Edinburgh Medical College with cadavers to dissect. A year later he published *A Treatise on Poisons* (1829), which synthesized existing toxicological knowledge with new insights into the effects of substances that were readily available to most nineteenth-century households. Writing in *The British Medical Journal* in 1951, Sydney Smith noted:

> A contemporary account says of him that, "as a witness, he was remarkable for a lucid precision of statement, which left no shadow of doubt in the mind of the Court, Counsel, or Jury, as to his views. Another noteworthy characteristic was the candour and impartiality he invariably displayed." He remains one of the great figures in whom the University of Edinburgh will always take a great and legitimate pride.[92]

In the trial of Robert Reid, outlined in chapter 2, Christison's attainments would be brought into question as part of the ongoing discussions over the trustworthiness of medical jurisprudence's methods, yet it is certain that he made a reputation out of being lucid, precise, and impartial.

Although forensic science aimed to bring two august disciplines—law and medicine—together, it was in the provinces of the latter that the field took root and flourished. Most writers on the subject were doctors rather than lawyers, yet there were some noteworthy exceptions such as when John Paris, a Fellow of the Royal College of Physicians, teamed up with Anthony Fonblanque, barrister at law, to write the three-volume *Medical Jurisprudence*. The textbook aimed to educate medical men on matters of legal practice and precedent. How often, it waxed, may medical witnesses "refute a groundless accusation, remove a causeless fear, and prevent a public exposure, by forming and demonstrating correct views of the subject? How often too may he aid the oppressed, defeat the guilty, and protect the innocent, by a knowledge of the legal remedies against fraud and coercion?"[93]

Paris and Fonblanque's partnership provided a rather rosy picture of law and medicine as having common objectives, yet their amicable coalition was an exception to the rule. Lawyer Joseph Chitty's 1834 *Practical Treatise on Medical Jurisprudence* sought to instruct legal professionals on how to deal with expert medical witnesses. A note of the full title of the

---

92. Sydney Smith, "The History and Development of Forensic Medicine," *British Medical Journal* (24 March 1951): 599–607 (605). For an excellent account of the contribution of Christison to toxicology, see Burney, *Poison*, 78–116.

93. Paris and Fonblanque, *Medical Jurisprudence*, vol. 1, xlix.

work will provide as full a description to the work as anything else: *A Practical Treatise on Medical Jurisprudence, with so much of the Anatomy, Physiology, Pathology, and the Practice of Medicine and Surgery, as are essential to be known by Members of Parliament, Lawyers, Coroners, Magistrates, Officers in the Army and Navy, and Private Gentleman, and all the Laws relating to Medical Practitioners, with Explanatory Plates.* The title hints at the fact that legal professionals would need to have some command over scientific information for when their wits would be pitted against those of expert medical witnesses. The very fact that this book—for lawyers by a lawyer—was felt to be a necessary contribution to a busy market of forensic publications suggests that law and medicine did not always speak the same language. The main source of contention between experts, however, was a difference in values rather than in terminologies. Although the jargon employed by each profession would pose the occasional problem in court proceedings, as we shall see, it was around the perceived differences in how one might define "the truth" that most hostilities developed.

In 1831 the Society of Apothecaries stipulated that all candidates for its license should have attended a three-month course on medical jurisprudence. The policy had the effect of "increasing the number of lectureships in medical jurisprudence attached to metropolitan institutions of medical education."[94] One lectureship created as a result was at Guy's Hospital, and its first incumbent was Alfred Swaine Taylor. Three years later the position was made into a professorship, and Taylor took the promotion. His name will appear often in this study because he became the period's foremost practitioner and theorist of medical jurisprudence. Not only did his writings dominate the field from the 1830s onwards, but he also became a regular witness in the period's criminal indictments. In 1836 he published his *Elements of Medical Jurisprudence*, which he saw as filling a sizable gap in medical knowledge:

> It has long been an acknowledged fact, that no branch of literature is so deficient in this country, as that of Medical Jurisprudence. A few treatises only have as yet appeared, and these, partly from a want of practical application in the details, and partly in consequence of the medico-legal illustrations being drawn from old and recondite sources, have not succeeded to any great extent, in preparing the British medical practitioner for those duties which he is occasionally called upon to perform.[95]

---

94. Burney, *Poison*, 42.
95. Alfred Swaine Taylor, quoted in Beck, *Elements*, iii.

Taylor's criticisms of preceding textbooks centered on what he saw as a seeming lack of evidence from real case studies. Just as the law was feeling the need to learn more about medicine, medicine needed to introduce more practical law into its discourses. Taylor's *Elements* begins, then, with a chapter titled "Medico-Legal Questions and Cases," which is set out as follows:

> *Under what circumstances are notes or memoranda admitted in evidence?*
>
> Trial of Sir A. G. Kinloch. Edinburgh, 1795 ....
>   .... Page 15
> Trial of Wright. Norwich Association. 1833: before Mr. Baron Bolland ...
>   .... 16[96]

What the decision to focus on individual arraignments demonstrates is that Taylor believed his field to be improved by a more open-minded understanding of the law's bearing on certain medical questions. He had a thorough acquaintance with real cases as well as the usual textbook knowledge, and his works signaled the importance of expert accounts in the study of forensics.[97] *Elements* was followed by the *Manual of Medical Jurisprudence* (1844), *Medical Jurisprudence* (1845), *On Poisons* (1848), and the two-volume magnum opus *Principles and Practice of Medical Jurisprudence* (1865).

We will pause here in our history of forensic medicine because other important developments occurred during the years in which Dickens was writing, and it is my intention to discuss those developments, especially the ones that emerged from real indictments in the criminal courtrooms, alongside the novels themselves. However, a useful way to proceed, for the purposes of what remains of this chapter, is to consider how the Joseph Sellis story fared in the new climate of the 1830s, a time when ideas and approaches connected to crime scenes and dead bodies had been revolutionized by forensic science.

JOSEPH SELLIS: SEQUEL

To recapitulate, Everard Home's views on the violent death of Joseph Sellis proved conclusively, for him and for others, that Sellis had committed suicide. The wound, in particular, was literally a cut and dried "fact" because

---

96. Ibid., xv.
97. Ibid., iii.

the incision was done evenly, which means it must have been done by the determined hand of a suicide rather than the desperate hand of an assassin. The evidence, Home said, "left no doubt of its being [done] by his own hand."[98] Yet considering both Home's links to the Hunters and the various developments in forensic medicine which had come about over the preceding twenty years or so, it is hardly surprising that other commentators (medical and otherwise) began to suspect that Home had failed in his duties as a man of science; the idea of clues having "left no doubt" was glaringly out of touch with the emerging theories of forensic medicine, which suggested that even the most salient facts are—and should be—open to doubt.

It was in the 1830s that the duke himself prosecuted the young publisher Joseph Phillips for printing a book which suggested that the royal had murdered the Italian because he had witnessed his master sodomizing a valet. The book in question was *The Authentic Records of the Court of England* (1832). It was written anonymously, but later sources reveal it to have been authored by Lady Anne Hamilton, former lady-in-waiting to Cumberland's sister-in-law (the princess who was to become Queen Caroline). Lady Hamilton's section on the Sellis affair was brief but damning. In the poem "England in 1819" Percy Bysshe Shelley captured the common view that George III's sons were "the dregs of their dull race," and Hamilton's portrait of Cumberland hardly challenged the poet. The duke's name, she wrote, "has proved a stain upon the kingdom in which he was born. Sensibility and virtue are strangers to his breast, while cruelty and the baser passions [have] perfect control over his imagination and actions. His countenance [is] indeed an index to his mind; as it is scarcely possible that more horrible features could be associated in one human being."[99] Her libel said that Sellis's death

> was said to have been the result of malice on the part of the Duke's valet, named Sellis; but as faithful historians, we give the particulars of these authenticated facts. [...] A short period before this dreadful catastrophe, the Duke had been surprised in an improper and unnatural situation with this Neale by the other servant, Sellis, and exposure was expected. A brother of the Duke had also received accommodation in the same very suitable apartments, and had by that act disqualified himself from any public expression upon the case, or opportunity to punish an aggressor.[100]

---

98. Quoted in Unsigned, *The Trial of Josiah Phillips*, 4.
99. Ibid., 3.
100. Ibid., 2.

Lady Hamilton included the testimony of another of the duke's servants who, being instructed to summon the Italian on the night of the duke's "attack," saw what he describes here:

> I went to Sellis's door, and upon opening it, the most horrific scene presented itself. Sellis was lying perfectly straight in the bed, the head raised up against the head-board, and nearly severed from the body; his hands were lying quite straight on each side of him; and upon examination, I saw him weltering in blood, it having covered the under part of the body. [. . .] A razor covered in blood was lying at a distance from his body, but too far off to have been used by himself, or to have been thrown there by him in such a mutilated condition, as it was very apparent death must have been immediate after such an act. [. . .] During the time the Duke's wounds were being dressed, the deponent believes Neale was absent, in obedience to arrangement, and was employed in laying Sellis's body in the form in which it was discovered, as it was an utter impossibility that a self-murderer could have so disposed of himself.
>
> Deponent further observes, that Lord Ellenborough undertook to manage this affair, by arranging the proceedings for the inquest, and also that every witness was previously examined by him. Also that the first jury being unanimously dissatisfied with the evidence adduced, as they were not permitted to see the body in an undressed state, positively refused to return a verdict; in consequence of which they were dismissed and a second jury summoned and impannelled.[101]

As well as the disagreements with Everard Home over small details, this witness denied that the medical evidence demonstrated beyond all reasonable doubt that Sellis had killed himself. In fact, since 1810 commentators had been suggesting that the razor was too far away from Sellis's corpse for the Italian to have inflicted the injury upon himself, and, more importantly, in cutting his *own* throat, Sellis could not have done so almost to the point of decapitation.

In 1815 Dickens's future illustrator George Cruikshank created a satirical image based on the Duke of Cumberland's unsuccessful application to the House of Commons for additional income (figure 1.2). It features Lord Cochrane shooting a canon at the duke, saying, among other things, "No, No, we'll have no Petitions here—do you think we are not up to your hoaxing, Cadging tricks?" A ghostly representation of the ghost of Joseph

---

101. Ibid., 6.

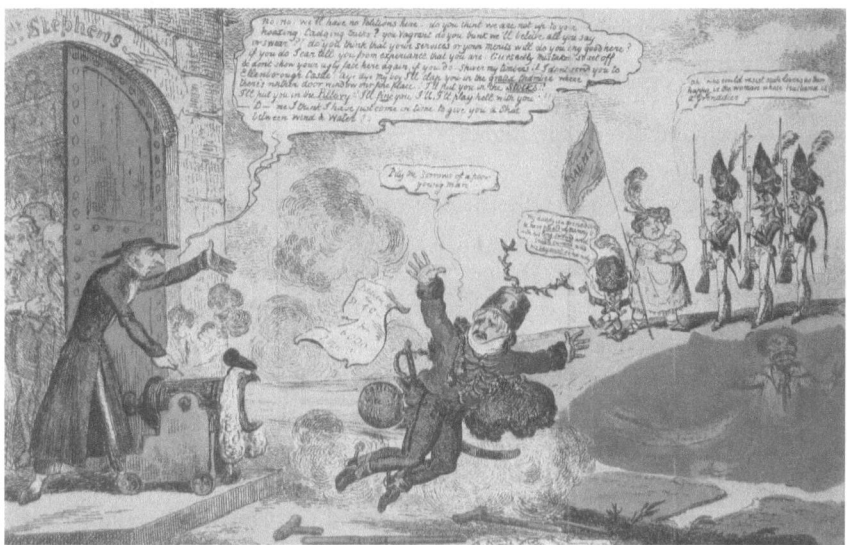

FIGURE 1.2. George Cruikshank, "A Financial Survey of Cumberland" (1815)

Sellis, beside the duke on the right, can be seen beneath a daub of dark paint. He wears a nightshirt and his throat is cut. Holding a razor he says: "Is this a razor which I see before me? Thou can'st not say, I did it." Cruikshank obliterated the reference in fear of being prosecuted. He was right to take the precaution, for when Hamilton and Phillips joined forces to allege that the duke had murdered Sellis in order to hide a scandalous rendezvous with his valet, Cumberland responded with force: "[I] doth hereby most solemnly and positively swear and declare," he said, "that the whole and every part of the said charge or insinuation is a most scandalous, wicked, and malicious falsehood."[102] His suit against Phillips was a success.

Undeterred, and with her name still untarnished by the affair, Lady Anne Hamilton wrote another book, this time attaching her name to the title page, and reaffirming her accusations against the duke. The publisher, William Stevenson, saw fit to keep the book off the presses until 1840. *The Secret History of the Court of England* claimed that it was motivated by a quest for the truth. "Readers," Hamilton writes in her preface,

> will have their attention turned to the truths submitted to them and the end in view. *That end* is for the advancement of the best interests of society;

---

102. Ibid., 14.

to unite more closely each member in the bonds of friendship and amity; and to expose the *hidden causes* which for so long a period have been barriers to concord, unity, and happiness.

"May God defend the Right."[103]

In the passage where she tells the story of Sellis, she notes:

> In a former work of ours, called "The Authentic Records of the Court of England," we gave an account of the extraordinary and mysterious murder of one Sellis, a servant of the Duke of Cumberland [. . .]. In that account we did what we conceived to be our duty as historians—we spoke the TRUTH. The truth, however, it appears, is not always to be spoken, for his Royal Highness instantly commenced a *persecution* against us for a "malicious libel." We are no cowards in regimentals, nor did we make our statement with a view of slandering the royal pensioner. We would have willingly contended with his Royal Highness in a court of law if he had had the courage to have met us on fair grounds. [. . .] If the Duke of Cumberland, however, imagines he can *intimidate* us from speaking the truth OUT OF COURT, he has mistaken us. We are not, as we said in our first work, to be prevented from doing whatever we conceive to be our duty.[104]

Hamilton then criticizes *The Morning Post* for its partisan reporting of the scandal:

> That we may not be accused of partiality, we take the report of this judicial proceeding from that Tory organ, the *Morning Post,* which, it will be observed, deals out its abuse with no unsparing hand on the poor murdered man, whom it calls by the charitable appellation of *villain,* and sundry other hard names, which had better suited the well-known characters of other persons, who acted a prominent part in this foul business.[105]

What these passages suggest, on a broad level, is that different parties had different methods of approaching the idea of truth and that the search for answers in some medico-legal contexts of the nineteenth century was a venture distorted by politics. In his book on the history of the inquest between 1830 and 1926, Ian Burney suggests, with excellent evidence, that the increased presence of specialist, medical knowledge in the coroner's

---

103. Hamilton, *Secret History,* viii.
104. Ibid., 65.
105. Ibid. Italics in original.

court was a result of the influence of reformist and radical politics of the early part of the century: "A new compound vision of the inquest—as a medically driven tribunal guarding the interest of the people—emerged out of an intense reformist activity during the first half of the nineteenth century, activity that constituted a singular movement of convergence in radical medicine and politics."[106] This view is certainly upheld by the arguments of Lady Hamilton which set the image of an imposing truth against the pandering right-wing politics of *The Morning Post*. What appears to have emerged in the intervening years between Home's original evidence and the commentaries of Lady Hamilton is a distrust of neatly sewn plots. Adelene Buckland has argued that in the new science of geology there was a similar wariness associated, by men of science, with well-rounded narratives: "Nineteenth-century geologists," she writes, "suggested that there may well be a 'plot' but that geologists did not yet have enough information to reveal it, leaving plots implicit or unarticulated, or threading narratives together in episodic or deliberately disjointed fashion."[107] Like experts in forensic medicine, Lady Hamilton had no such aversion to plot; as we have seen, she told a sensational story of her own in regard to the Sellis affair. What she and the medical jurists were interested in, however, was the *means* of going about telling stories. The new method of questioning self-evident truth wanted justice to be done and deserts appropriately delivered, yet Lady Hamilton disliked the idea of a plot being sewn up too easily. What she recognized in the Tory Organ's method of processing the truth was how privilege, prejudice, and fusty traditional thinking worked together to provide an identikit plot to suit the establishment's notions of state, rank, and privilege. The picture of the Italian lurking in the shadows until the vulnerable duke fell asleep presented not truth simply (or at all) but an approach that pleased those in power. Hamilton had a different, more modern, concept of how facts should be processed. Her preface and her open dismissal of the duke show that, for her, interpretation should be fettered by no partisanship; it should be weighed down by no politicking and clouded by no regard for royals, ranks, or legal representations. A maxim that was often noted in the period's forensic texts and that would have delighted Lady Hamilton is "Do not let any authority, however

---

106. Ian Burney, *Bodies of Evidence: Medicine and the Politics of the English Inquest, 1830–1926* (Baltimore, MD, and London: Johns Hopkins University Press, 2000), 52.

107. Adelene Buckland, *Novel Science: Fiction and the Invention of Nineteenth-Century Geology* (Chicago: University of Chicago Press, 2013), 20–21. Buckland finds excellent evidence of geological images of "dark and disturbing ruptures" (275) having an influence on the form and design of the nineteenth-century novel.

eminent, shake you on simple matters of fact."[108] That Hamilton accepts the wisdom of such a view is clear in the comments she makes on the medical evidence of Everard Home. She begins with the rather explosive "fact" that the evidence of other expert witnesses had been suppressed:

> One or two other professional persons *did* examine the body of poor Sellis; and, *if they had been allowed to give their opinion*, would assuredly have convinced every honest man of the *impossibility* of Sellis being his *own* murderer. One of these, Dr. Carpue, has frequently been heart to say that "The head of Sellis *was nearly severed from his body and that even the joint was cut through!*" Dr. Carpue has also stated that "no man could have the power to hold an instrument in his hand to *cut* ONE-EIGHTH of the depth of the wound in the throat of Sellis!"[109]

In the case of Joseph Sellis's death, a convenient interpretation had been favored over what Hamilton saw as "real truth." Carpue's evidence showed that the evidence was capable of telling more than one story; the wound *did* leave doubts:

> "Mr. Home soon returned, and said there was no doubt the man had killed himself!" Oh, talented man, who could perceive at a glance that "the man had killed himself!" Dr. Carpue must never more pretend to a knowledge of surgery when his opinion can be set aside by a single glance of a man of such eminence in his profession as Mr. Home! As to the joint in his neck being cut through, Mr. Home easily accounted for it. What! a man cut his own head off [. . .]?
> [. . .] Sir Everard's description of the matter, however, is only calculated to involve it in still greater mystery and contradiction.[110]

Hamilton implies that the examination was not scientific enough: it was based on an ill-judged confidence in Home's ability to read facts quickly and on his willingness to take the same facts at face value; he probably shared the Tory Organ's conservative notion that a British prince's word is more trustworthy than the testimony of a foreigner's cadaver. A review of Beck's *Elements of Medical Jurisprudence* in *The Lancet*, however, makes it

---

108. R. J. Kinkead, "Introductory Address to the Courser of Lectures on Medical Jurisprudence," *The Lancet* (8 March 1879): 325–27 (327).
109. Hamilton, *Secret History*, 73. Italics in original.
110. Ibid., 76–77, 79.

clear that in the early century such peremptory interpretations were being superseded by a more forensic approach:

> Respecting the necessity of a general examination of the body of a person found dead, a curious opinion of a northern professor is quoted [. . .]:
>
>> "When," said he, in his lectures, you find any appearance sufficient to account for death, rest satisfied with that, and inquire no further; as further examination will only tend to embarrass your evidence, and render it contradictory." [. . .]
>
> In other words, do not proceed too far, or your testimony may be less positive when called upon to give your opinion in a court of justice.[111]

In 1836 Alfred Swaine Taylor returned to the Sellis affair in his *Elements of Medical Jurisprudence*. He believed that "the man who attacked the Duke, was his servant Sellis, and [. . .] from the general and circumstantial evidence, there does not appear to be any reason to doubt, that the wound on Sellis's throat, was inflicted by himself."[112] Yet he was also disappointed with Home's means of processing the evidence. His opinion is worth citing at length because it contains the medical and logical apparatuses for querying Home's methods:

> The part of the report which more especially calls for attention, is that wherein Sir Everard states, that the *length* and *direction* of the wound were such as *left no doubt* of its having been suicidal. It would be well if the medical jurist could determine these doubtful questions relative to homicide or suicide by so simple a test. Let the length and direction of such a wound in the throat be what they may, they can never afford more than a very slight presumption of its origin: and it is difficult to conceive of any case in which suicides of this description, to meet with every variety in the length and direction of the wounds. But we find it added, that any struggle would have made the wound *irregular*; a statement which leads of course to the implication that regularity in such a wound, is sufficient to remove a suspicion of homicide; and, it is a singular illustration, of the influence of this opinion, that the able counsel who supported the criminal

---

111. Unsigned review of Beck, *Elements*, 173.
112. Taylor, *Elements*, 349–50.

information, on the part of the Duke in the [civil] trial [. . .] should have repeatedly dwelt on this statement, which medico-legally speaking, appears to be the weakest portion of Sir Everard's declaration. Regularity in a fatal incised wound of the throat is far from being universally seen, in cases of suicide: where there is considerable resolution and firmness of purpose, the wound may be regular; but there are many whose hands tremble, and who, probably from the flow of blood, lose the power of holding the instrument firmly, before the incision through the soft parts can be completed; in such, the wound, must necessarily be irregular. Is it not possible, moreover, that a regular wound of the throat may be inflicted by a murderer? And is it necessary that, in all cases of murder, the victim should struggle while a mortal wound is being inflicted?

To attempt to maintain either of these positions would be equal to opposing what the most common observation will establish; and I cannot, therefore, agree in the commendatory view of Dr. Smith, that Sir Everard Home's declaration "furnishes an admirable lesson on the importance of medical investigation in cases of doubt and difficulty." If medical reports are to contain such sweeping inferences from such feeble data, they will certainly rather embarrass, than assist the course of justice.[113]

Like Lady Hamilton, Taylor sees the main problem with Home's evidence to be his "sweeping inferences," or the indications that he had trusted too much in perceived "common sense." In the new scientific culture of medical jurisprudence, a field to which Taylor certainly belonged, practitioners were instructed never to assume that appearances may be trusted or that good would come out by its own accord. "Man runs after truth as the only nourishment which can satisfy him," said *The Portfolio*, one of the monthly rags that Dickens read alongside *The Terrific Register*, but he must "distrust appearances" and "seek for truth under their disguise."[114] The sequel to the Sellis affair, situated as it was, more firmly within the new climate of medical jurisprudence, presented a picture of "truth" as open to interpretation. The emerging focus on the possibility and the value of clinical analysis equipped Lady Hamilton and some medical experts with the ammunition they needed to question the more benighted methods of Home. What the new system of scientific labor rejected, specifically, was what David Carroll calls "the unexamined premise, those absolutes of every kind which have been simply handed down, like old clothes, and with them the belief in

---

113. Ibid., 352–53.
114. Unsigned, "Truth," *The Portfolio*, 31.

watertight systems of thought."[115] In 1867 J. Russell Reynolds said in a thoughtful address to the Royal College of Physicians:

> The law-court is the exponent of that which was agreed upon in times gone by. [...] The lawyer is governed by a precedent that may be wrong; the expert witness is directed by facts that he knows to be true. The one says the line between innocence and guilt, between sanity and insanity, lies here; the other that the line lies yonder, or does not exist at all. [...] Society suffers from the errors of the past, and its present wrongs cannot be redressed by the slow growth of legal precedent.[116]

CONFLICT

Represented by the expert medical witness, a public figure whose job it was to update the "old clothes" method of relying on dogmatic assumptions by insisting on rigorous interpretation, the new analytical approach was never entirely confident when it came to "facts" known "to be true." Nor did it aim to be. Litigious combat between lawyers and doctors—of which we will consider a couple of examples below—formed one of the key incentives for medical men to self-critically consider the viability of their methods before laying their opinions before the public. A number of studies of recent years have demonstrated how the emergence of the expert medical witness led to some dramatic tensions between legal and medical opinion. "There were deep differences between medical legal discourse," writes Roger Smith, and "alternative legal and medical 'truth' existed." What was "at stake in the presentation of competing witness narratives," adds Schramm, "is a claim to the reconstruction of 'reality' itself."[117] The one thing law and medicine could agree on was that truth was central to safeguarding the nation's moral well-being. In an 1834 review of Joseph Chitty's *Practical Treatise on Medical Jurisprudence*, *The Legal Observer* conceded that biological facts were an important part of understanding the behavior of men and women:

> Practical lawyers are not in the habit of considering, that the nature and operation of the functions and organs,—the living aggregate of which constitute a human being,—form an essential part of their study; but it cannot

---

115. David Carroll, *George Eliot and the Conflict of Interpretations: A Reading of the Novels* (Cambridge: Cambridge University Press, 1992), 11.
116. Reynolds, "Lumleian Lectures," 519–20.
117. Smith, *Trial by Medicine*, 77; and Schramm, *Testimony and Advocacy*, 1.

be disputed that it is as necessary to the lawyer as the physician, to make himself master of the nature and peculiarities of the intellectual faculties and moral feelings, as well as the animal propensities of mankind, inasmuch as it is out of the workings of these faculties, feelings and propensities, and the consequences to which their exercise or indulgence naturally lead, that he is called upon to labour in his vocation.[118]

Yet the statement has some telling ambiguities. On the one hand, it implies that medicine and law share the same interests: they are both concerned with the "nature and peculiarities of the intellectual faculties and moral feelings." Therefore, making oneself master of such will make one a better lawyer as well as a better physician. Yet it is possible to hear subtle echoes of how medicine and the law were competing for intellectual authority over the process of interpretation. The suggestion that lawyers should become acquainted with anatomical minutiae is a barely disguised intimation that they ought to have as much control over the facts as their medical cousins. An article titled "The Sciences, in their Relation to the Practice of the Law" (1835) in *The Legal Observer* noted that "the law is jealous of all rivals; [. . .] she demands the undivided affection of her adherents. "The lady of the Common Law," says the old maxim 'must needs lie alone.'"[119]

In other legal sources, more overt in defaming scientific intervention, the argument emerged that science was incapable of reading questions of law with the sort of "common-sense" skill that lawyers could bring to any given case. Such a view is what fueled many heated exchanges between legal and medical men in court. In 1867 the Bristol surgeon J. A. Symonds delivered a lecture to the British Medical Association in which he related what "on one occasion passed between a most eminent member of the legal profession" and himself. The incident took place, "not in court of law, [but] at a [. . .] lecture on certain points of the English language, delivered at the Bristol Institution, by the Rev. J. Earle." The "eminent member of the legal profession" ushered a vote of thanks for the reverend, adding that "those spoke best, and with most clearness and precision, who thought least of the effect which what they were saying would produce upon their hearers; and he declared that it was the want of such unconsciousness that made medical witnesses the worst of all witnesses in courts of law."[120] Now, these remarks were uttered with "playful

---

118. Unsigned review of J. Chitty, *Practical Treatise*, 243–45 (243).

119. Unsigned, "The Sciences, in their Relation to the Practice of the Law," *The Legal Observer* 9 (1835): 449–51 (449).

120. J. A. Symonds, "On Medical Evidence in Relation to State Medicine," *British Medical Journal* (2 September 1865): 227–30 (227).

malice," according to Symonds, because "many of his [the lawyer's] medical friends were present."[121] Nevertheless, Symonds stood up and

> ventured to say that, whatever psychological or philological truth there might be in the remark [...], my learned friend had omitted to mention the chief cause of the disadvantageous figure made by medical witnesses, which was, that they had to speak of things about which their audience, including the simple-minded jurors, the quick-witted gentlemen at the bar, and even the august occupants of the bench, were profoundly ignorant; and, moreover, that such witnesses had to translate as they were speaking, to put aside the language in which their professional knowledge and ideas most naturally flowed, and to accommodate what they had to say not only to the uninstructed understanding of their hearers, but also to the vernacular language; that, in the course of this process, much might be lost both of force and accuracy; and that the process required some presence of mind, especially under cross-examination, which mental quality was not likely to be aided by a severe injunction from the bench to give a plain answer to a plain question, or by an ironical petition from counsel that the witness should for the time being disencumber himself of his superfluous leaning, and condescend to the language of ordinary mortals.[122]

There was some heat in this exchange, to be sure, yet it was positively convivial compared to some of the century's battles between doctors and lawyers. *The Legal Observer* noted in 1831:

> It is not a little surprising, that so intelligent and respectable a class of men as the medical profession should make so poor a figure in the witness-box. In our own experience, we have known so many gentlemen of this profession "break down," as it is called, that we have a great distrust of this kind of evidence.[123]

This writer then includes an example that he hopes will embarrass the medical profession but that, to most clear eyes, reflects badly on legal participants as well:

> Mr. Simmons, a surgeon of Manchester, is undergoing a cross examination by Mr. Hamer [in an inquest]. "I think," says Mr. S., "I am more capable

---

121. Ibid.
122. Ibid., 227–28.
123. Unsigned, "Medical Evidence," *The Legal Observer* 1 (1831): 245–47 (245).

of forming a correct opinion on the subject than Mr. Cox." "The jury, Sir," replies Mr. H., "will no doubt duly appreciate the value of that self-opinion." *Mr. Ashworth.*—Really, Mr. Coroner, I must interpose to protect the witness from this sort of attack. *Witness*—Oh! Mr. Ashworth, let me go on, I will teach him surgery; I am anxious for a little more discussion; he is not the first lawyer I have taught surgery. *Mr. Hamer.*—Perhaps not; but notwithstanding the opinion you entertain of your own skill, I should be very sorry to be under your hands.

Simmons wonders, with no irony, whether the lawyer would have had the equal audacity to "bring down [. . .] Sir Everard Home, and the other leading members of the faculty." We can imagine the well-founded rejoinder that Hamer might have had up his sleeve, but he never got to say it because the coroner ended the bickering with "I have exhausted all my patience."[124]

In the *Association Medical Journal* of 1856, J. G. Davey, another Bristol surgeon, complained bitterly about his experience of one cross-examining lawyer:

> Mr. Sergeant Wilkins's love of mischief, and his other peculiarities as a practising barrister, some of you may have also experienced. I can see him now, as he rose from his seat to question me, his massive solid form encompassed by its silken robes, and his large and broad head surmounted by that eccentric and ancient sheep-skin—or something very like it, by which his class is recognised. [. . .] The man of iron will, large intellect, and firm if not high resolves. [. . .] You [would] not fail to perceive how entirely gratuitous and foreign to the inquiry on hand, was the course pursued by the gentleman named.[125]

Other commentators noted how ironic it was that so equivocal a discipline like the law should take umbrage over the vacillations in the testimonies of medical experts. In his introduction to an 1879 course of lectures on medical jurisprudence, Irish obstetrician R. J. Kinkead said:

> We find judges themselves, and counsel differing as to the meaning of the laws and statutes of the land, framed by men of like understanding with themselves; is it wonderful that men who have to interpret the laws, unwritten and often imperfectly understood, framed by an infinite intelligence,

---

124. Ibid.
125. J. G. Davey, "On Medical Evidence," 1074–77 (1076); 1089–92.

the face of ever-varying phenomena—is it wonderful, I say, that we, whose intelligence is finite, should differ as to their interpretations?"[126]

What is particularly interesting about these conflicts is how they were converted by medical men into indications that they themselves needed to take extra care in their analyses in order that they be well armed when it came to witness-box warfare. In 1817 John Haslam, physician and writer of a number of works on insanity, told his readers that as medical witnesses, they should expect, and work hard to resist, "the blandishments of eloquence, and the subtle underminings of cross-examination." He added that "the lawyer's object is the interest of his employer, and for the fulfilment of his duty, he is frequently compelled to report to a severity of investigation, which perplexes the theories, but more frequently kindles the irritable feelings of the medical practitioner."[127] In his lectures on medical jurisprudence in 1837 Alexander Thomson told his medical students, "Your evidence, in such cases, becomes an object of general criticism: it is delivered in public, and will be scrutinised with severity; and little favour will be shown in animadverting upon its defects."[128] According to Alfred Swaine Taylor, writing in 1865:

> The witness will be closely questioned as to his qualifications, the time during which he has been engaged in practice, the accuracy of his judgment, his general professional knowledge, and his special experience in reference to the matter in issue, the number of cases he has seen, &c. Straightforward answers should be given to all these questions.[129]

Taylor was himself subjected to heavy questioning during the trial of William Palmer in 1856. When queried on his knowledge regarding the effects of strychnine, he was forced to admit that he had never seen a case for himself. "Having overreached his limited knowledge of strychnine," Burney surmises, "Taylor had found himself upon a legal stage where he had to defend his personal and professional reputation at the expense of his own science."[130] Yet, based on what we have been discussing above, it may be suggested that the act of defending one's professional qualifications did

---

126. Kinkead, "Introductory Address," 326–27.
127. John Haslam, "Medical Jurisprudence as it relates to Insanity" (1817), quoted in Forsyth, *Synopsis*, 30.
128. Alexander Thomson, "Lectures on Medical Jurisprudence: Lecture 1," *The Lancet* (8 August 1836): 65–70.
129. Taylor, *Principles*, vol. 1, 23.
130. Burney, *Poison*, 142.

not seem to entail a maneuver that went against the science of forensic experts. Indeed, medical jurisprudence was forged out of conflict. From the very start it used a language that was defensive and self-critical because it needed to respond to the traditional, legal preference for parables and precedents over analysis and discussion.

But this is only half the story. Added to the adversarial nature of medical jurisprudence was the moral burden of the "the whole truth," which medicine inherited from the law and which made the discipline unique among sciences. In addition to the various research pressures that faced colleagues in the more laboratory-based sciences, for example, the medical jurist did not have the luxury of "pushing aside the church and religion as authority in knowledge."[131] The concept of moral truth, embodied most obviously in the concept of God, was important to forensic scientists because the legal aspects of their work required them to work with a standard of truth that had a moral as well as an empirical weight. My next chapter will suggest that in conceding the existence of a higher truth, forensic experts were able to become self-critical in a way that allowed them to develop strategies and vocabularies for questioning their own representational structures.

---

131. Levine, *Dying to Know*, 4.

CHAPTER 2

THE WHOLE TRUTH
Oliver Twist and *Our Mutual Friend*

In Stephen Williams's *Catechism of Medical Jurisprudence* (1835), there is envisaged a world where forensic interpretations might emulate the powers of God:

> Disentangled from the web with which worldly caprice, credulity, and empiricism, are ever seeking to embarrass the more ordinary path of her labours, [medicine] at once bursts forth, in all the pride and strength of undeniable facts and endless resources, and her disciples are enabled proudly to present additional claims upon the respect of the learned, the confidence of the oppressed, and the gratitude of the public. In the exercise of his art as a medical jurist, how exalted and honourable is the occupation of the physician. There is scarcely a circle of natural science, upon the boundaries of which he does not impinge, in some point of his extensive orbit, and on which he does not shed additional rays of knowledge and of light. It is when thus called on, he develops the vast resources, and hidden stores which have for ages been accumulating in the sanctuary of his tutelary divinity, and following his precept and his example, offers them as a safeguard to innocence, and a shield to the oppressed.[1]

Williams's references to God, though elaborate, are not atypical of nineteenth-century forensic discourses. Medical jurisprudence was not

---
1. Williams, *Catechism*, 43–44.

perceived to just be doing the work of God; in texts like these it was also seen to be working *like* God. The facts within its range were "undeniable," Williams says; its resources are "endless," and, like the Deity, it had disciples and an omniscient command of knowledge. On this last point Williams is not representative of the more measured views held by many of his colleagues. A greater number of medical jurists actually saw their work as undertaken firmly within the bounds of *human*, rather than *godly*, experience and believed that it was important for them to see their science as an *approximation* of absolute knowledge. References to God were usually an admission of a higher truth to which man's interpretations only aspired. Medical jurisprudence took its cue from the larger developments in the field of medicine on this topic. In 1834, for instance, the surgeon Ezekiel Webb published a book titled *The Philosophy of Medicine*. The text's major claim was that medicine ought to be a purely inductive science and that it should "exercise [its powers] through appropriate observation and experiment, for discovering the beautiful associations of material substances, composing many of the things and beings of creation within [our] reach for investigation."[2] Skills of "observation and experiment" ought to be undertaken, in other words, with a sense of how there is a more "perfect" standard of truth beyond the human "reach for investigation." As Suzy Anger notes in her fine book *Victorian Interpretation* (2005), some nineteenth-century sciences "accepted that our forms of representing reality are always provisional, that science does not get certainty with its stories, and that we are limited by the power of our representational systems."[3] Medicine, I add, utilized a theory of higher truth as a means of exploring and seeking to better the limited nature of its "representational systems." As early as 1772 John Gregory noted in his *Lectures on the Duties and Qualifications of a Physician* that the medical man is a sort of philosopher who

> from a more enlarged experience, and more accurate observation, does not easily trust to appearances; he is aware of the various sources of deception, and therefore examines every minute and latent circumstance, before he ventures to form a judgment and the difficulty of ascertaining, with precision, the exact familiarity of cases, makes the true philosopher extremely skeptical in drawing conclusions of what will happen, and what has happened.[4]

---

2. Ezekiel Webb, *The Philosophy of Medicine* (New York: Printed for the author, 1834), xxii, xvi.

3. Anger, *Victorian Interpretation*, 88.

4. Gregory, *Lectures*, 117–18.

The key word here is *skeptical*; it signals a philosopher's reluctance to take any "fact" for granted—not because some higher power is playing tricks, potentially, with the order of one's understanding—but because human perceptions cannot be wholly accurate or complete.

In *The Powers of Distance* (2001) Amanda Anderson discusses how the quest for objectivity or "detachment" was a concern shared by a number of intellectual areas in the nineteenth century. The pervasive "aim to objectify facets of human existence so as to better understand, criticise and at times transform them," she writes, was a self-reflexive venture:

> There [were] procedural and educational questions about how ideal forms of detachment might best be cultivated; there [were] philosophical questions about whether such procedures produce reliable forms of knowledge or valuable forms of art; there [were] psychological and cultural questions about whether individuals are even capable of transcending their interests, their pasts, and their racial heritage; and there [were] moral and political questions about whether forms of cultivated detachment uniformity promote the well-being or overall progress of individuals, communities or nations.[5]

The psychological and cultural question of whether individuals are capable of transcending their human subjectivities is what my assessment of medical jurisprudence is concerned with. It was a key question for science, as George Levine has observed in *Dying to Know: Scientific Epistemology and Narrative in Victorian England*: "After about 1830 [...] for nineteenth-century scientists, the responsibility to be 'objective,' to gain access to objects of knowledge and thus allow the facts to speak for themselves, took priority over fullness of understanding."[6] Medical texts of the period contain some acknowledgment of an objective standard of truth, but it is also claimed that the subjectivity of human experience and "the inescapable presence of the interpreting self"[7] will always get in the way.

One of the most prominent expressions of the view of medical knowledge as an *approximate* truth may be found in Claude Bernard's *Experimental Medicine* (1865), one of the founding texts of the field that we now call *medical research*. With respect to "living bodies," the French physiologist writes, "absolute truth" is difficult to attain:

---

5. Anderson, *Powers*, 4–5.
6. Levine, *Dying to Know*, 3.
7. Ibid.

> Man behaves as if he were destined to reach this absolute knowledge; and the incessant *why* which he puts to nature proves it. [. . .] Our feelings lead us at first to believe that absolute truth must lie within our realm; but study takes from us, little by little, these chimerical conceits. Science has just the privilege of teaching us what we do not know, by replacing feeling with reason and experience and clearly showing us the present boundaries of our knowledge. [. . .] To sum up, if our feeling constantly puts the question *why*, our reason shows us that only the question *how* is within our range.[8]

We can understand the cogs, Bernard insists, but we can never know the whole machinery. Physician and psychologist John Abercrombie appeared to have agreed. He wrote much earlier on what he called "the uncertainties of medicine"[9] in his *Inquiries into the Intellectual Powers and the Investigation of Truth* (1830), a book that Dickens owned at the time of his death:[10]

> It is humbling to the pride of human reason, but it is not the less true, that the highest acquirement ever made by the most exalted genius of man has been only to trace a part, and a very small part, of that order which the Deity has established in his works. When we endeavour to pry into the causes of this order, we perceive the operation of powers which lie far beyond the reach of our limited faculties. They who have made the highest advances in true science will be the first to confess how limited these faculties are, and how small a part we comprehend of the ways of the Almighty Creator.[11]

In "Progress: Its Law and Cause" (1857) Herbert Spencer would express something very similar. It is the scientist who "alone *knows* that under all things, there lies an impenetrable mystery."[12] Unlike Abercrombie, who saw this "impenetrable mystery" as the "ways of the Almighty Creator," Spencer held agnostic values that led him to include God in the list of things that we can have no certain knowledge of.

At mid century Spencer was part of a "group of closely-linked Victorian thinkers" that included George Henry Lewes, John Stuart Mill, and

---

8. Claude Bernard, *Introduction à l'Étude de la Médecine Expérimentale*, trans. Henry Copley Greene as *An Introduction to the Study of Experimental Medicine* (1865; New York, Dover Publishing, 1957), 81–82.

9. John Abercrombie, *Inquiries into the Intellectual Powers and the Investigation of Truth* (1830; Edinburgh: Waugh and Innes, 1831), 388.

10. Stonehouse, *Catalogue*, 5.

11. Abercrombie, *Inquiries*, 22–23.

12. Herbert Spencer, "Progress: Its Law and Cause" (1857), quoted in Carroll, *George Eliot*, 17.

Auguste Comte, all keen to "create synthetic philosophies based on the methods of the physical sciences."[13] It was out of this scientific climate that *Medicinische Logik* (1852), a study by the German physician Friedrich Oesterlen, emerged. Translated and published as *Medical Logic* in 1855, the text argued:

> There is scarcely any department of human knowledge in which the number of established truths and facts, which no one doubts or attempts to shake, is so small; in no other field are our rules of action so uncertain and disputed as in medicine, the noblest and most important of all arts. [. . .] We sometimes find a rashness, or even presumption in the hypotheses, and a bitterness between the disputants, such as do [no credit to] departments where a scientifically established, and, consequently, calm insight, has taken the place of mere opinion and subjective, *a priori*, conjecture.[14]

The idea of a "scientifically established," "calm insight" replacing "subjective, *a priori*, conjecture," might seem like a very "un-German" view, given that country's traditional confidence in the importance of a priori intellection, but what Oesterlen meant to attack was subjective *conjecture*—the kind of "evidence" where perceptions of any given subject seem to have been conditioned by a preformed opinion. Everard Home's "analysis" of the Sellis crime scene, discussed in the previous chapter, furnishes a good example. Jonathan Smith's study of Baconian science and the nineteenth-century literary imagination observes that the idea of investigator bias, or dogmatic thinking, was a popular point of discussion among scientific and literary thinkers.[15] What the Sellis controversy and other cases in the period suggest is that the same topic became part of medical jurisprudence and that it found its way there more by necessity than by design. Arguments over assumptive evidence, which usually took place in the courtroom, but also filled columns and correspondence pages in newspapers and medical journals, led forensic medicine to develop strategies of self-criticism in both its verbal evidence and its written discourses. Borne out of a conflict with legal traditionalists and the perceived need to challenge ideas of self-evident truth, forensic medicine often resisted the urge to be satisfied with a language of absolute "certainty." Take, for instance, the 1835 trial of Robert Reid for the murder of his wife. It is an early and important case in which

---

13. Carroll, *George Eliot*, 15.
14. Oesterlen, *Medicinische Logik (Medical Logic)*, 6.
15. Jonathan Smith, *Fact and Feeling: Baconian Science and the Nineteenth-Century Literary Imagination* (Madison: University of Wisconsin Press, 1994).

the parameters of disagreement between the law and medicine seem to get laid out and which highlights the strategies of self-reflection that came to typify the forensic method, much to the annoyance of lawyers with a firm belief in the "whole truth."

ROBERT REID

According to one witness, Robert Reid was heard to tell his wife, on the night she died, to "lie about or he would haul her atour [*sic*] the bed and choke her."[16] The following day, Elizabeth Reid was found dead, her body "sitting on the floor by the side of the bed, nearly naked, with a portion of the bedclothes wrapt around the lower part of her body; the head erect, but inclined a little backward and to one side, with the back of the hand on the bed."[17] According to Alfred Swaine Taylor's *Principles and Practice of Medical Jurisprudence* (1865):

> This extraordinary posture was presumed by all who saw it and by the medical witnesses for the prosecution, to be such that the deceased could not have assumed it herself in the act of dying; and this was rendered still less probable when it was considered that the cervical vertebræ were fractured. And one of them was displaced, so that the she had probably died a violent and very sudden death.[18]

The second piece of incriminating evidence was discovered by the surgeon who performed the postmortem examination. Mr Williams found dark marks (bruises apparently) on the victim's neck, on her back, and behind one ear, all of which indicated that she must have experienced several blows from a blunt instrument. When the "murder" scene was searched, an axe was discovered in the fire grate, and prosecutors claimed that the defendant must have used the blunt end of it to kill his wife. Additionally, a number of witnesses testified to the fact that Reid was an unpleasant and a brutal man who had been violent toward Elizabeth. He was overheard making "a declaration of satisfaction at being released from his wife" and heartlessly expressed his "regret at not having treated [her] worse than he

---

16. Unsigned, *Remarks on the Trial of Robert Reid for the Murder of His Wife, before the High Court of Judiciary at Edinburgh* (Edinburgh: John Carfrae and Son, 1835), 4.
17. Taylor, *Medical Jurisprudence*, vol. 1, 71.
18. Ibid.

had done."[19] Elizabeth's own brother testified that Robert had "palsified" his wife with his constant violence and neglect.[20]

The evidence against Reid, then, seemed cast-iron. He was arrested and he made a confession:

> Joseph M'Cally, baron officer of Pathhead, apprehended the prisoner at Dysart, on board a steamer, on his return from Edinburgh. He showed surprise, and asked, "What is't? What is't?" Witness advised him to tell the truth, and it would be better for him, upon which the prisoner said, "Well, I did kill her." Witness asked if "it was with your axe?" to which Reid replied, "Aye."[21]

It seems remarkable, given the weight of evidence against the defendant, that he was eventually acquitted.

At the trial Robert Christison was called to give his expert opinion. Although he agreed with Williams's view on the whole, he was careful to avoid making any direct inferences based on the anatomical evidence:

> Professor Christison.—Had heard the evidence, and had formed the opinion that the blackness *might have been* the effect of a blow before death, or extracted after death; or perhaps violence used after it. A blow struck obliquely *might have produced* it, and the vertebrae *might have been* fractured by a blow from a heavy blunt instrument without breaking the skin; such a blow would cause instant death. Has known a dead body sensibly warm to the hand even at the distance of 24 hours after death; but the heat usually leaves long before that period. The body must have been placed in the situation in which it was found by the witnesses. The quantity of blood that flowed was a very material point in the case, as tending to show that the injury was inflicted during life, and that blood could not have been discharged by any dissection of the jugular vein made by Mr Williams. Coagulated flood would flow if not supported, although it was a sort of gelatinous. The injury produced in this case was very uncommon, and could not be caused by a person falling from their own height, otherwise it would be quite common.[22]

---

19. John Fletcher, *Remarks on the Trial of Robert Reid for the Murder of His Wife, before the High Court of Judiciary at Edinburgh* (Edinburgh: John Carfrae and Son, 1835), 43, 44.
20. Unsigned, "High Court of Judiciary," 4.
21. Ibid.
22. Ibid.

At this point in his career Christison was professor of medicine and therapeutics. He had written his masterful *On Poisons* in 1829, and he knew, like many of his professional colleagues, that the appearances of anatomies could be misleading as often as they were revealing. His testimony, therefore, reads like a clever exercise in diagnostic prevarication: evidence *might* indicate this, he says, or it *might* produce that. Any facts are based carefully on previous experience rather than on a promise of the whole truth: injuries like Elizabeth Reid's are "uncommon," for example, rather than "probable" or "improbable."

Despite such subtleties, Christison became tainted, by association, with the evidence of Williams, a man who showed nothing of the former's theoretical sophistication and was guilty of forming his opinions based on unexamined assumptions. According to physiologist John Fletcher, Williams was a charlatan and a fraud. Aiming a shot at Christison, he noted "how any well-informed Medical Witness could sit by to hear such arrant nonsense, and still hold to any opinion founded upon the evidence of the man who could utter it, is [. . .] unaccountable."[23] In Fletcher's published tract, titled *Remarks on the Trial of Robert Reid* (1835), he said that the "medical evidence for the Crown" had been "disgraceful in the extreme."[24] Elizabeth was, he showed, prone to fits of catalepsy, and it is odd, therefore, that neither Williams nor Christison considered that she may have broken her neck during an awkward fall. Her "bruises" were likely to have been livor—the natural blackening that occurs after death. Williams's postmortem examination took place "*thirty one hours* after [the] alleged injury"; "there can [. . .] be little rational doubt," then, "that the discoloration now under consideration resulted from the dead process of *Livor*, and not from the living process of *Ecchymosis*."[25]

Fletcher was willing to concede that Robert Reid was "a low, drunken fellow" and that the evidence looked bad for him, but the most aggravating "fact" was how "the foundation of the whole edifice against the Prisoner was the "bare word" of one "expert" whose qualifications were a fabrication. Williams was "at once morally unqualified, and legally unauthorized to speak to any medical questions whatever." He was "grossly ignorant and unblushingly false" and had nothing of the professional subtlety that a trained expert like Christison was able to bring to the case.[26] "What will the public think," he added,

---

23. Ibid., 29–30.
24. Ibid., 4.
25. Ibid., 18, 21. Italics in original.
26. Ibid., 53.

when told that WILLIAMS is no surgeon at all—that he never had a diploma from the Royal College, or, as he called it, "the Body" of Surgeons of London—that he SWORE WHAT WAS FALSE, first in stating that he had such a diploma, and again in stating that he had not been cited (which he was three several times) to produce it—and that Reid was in danger of being sacrificed on the presentations of a man who was not only unauthorized to give any evidence at all in this case, but who was obviously no more competent to describe the appearances presented on the dissections a dead body than a street porter?[27]

Although Williams's testimony is an extreme example of faulty medical evidence, Fletcher's angry denunciation highlights that what ought to be prized most of all in medical evidence is an expert ability to dig deeper than basic, surface appearances. Williams, like any street porter, will not have the specialist ability to realize that he cannot answer for anything with the kind of certainty he claimed to have had. The most striking error is the one that confuses livor for bruising—a mistake that any layman would make but that no professional ought to make, knowing full well how bodies present a system of signs that mislead as often as they instruct.

At the time of Reid's trial, juries were instructed, as they are today, that they must agree to a "guilty" verdict only when there is "no reasonable doubt" that the defendant had done the crime. As George Male wrote in his *Epitome of Juridical or Forensic Medicine* (1816), "It is better that many guilty men escape, than one innocent man suffer."[28] It is ironic that the failure in the medical evidence in the Reid case was caused by Williams himself showing no reasonable doubt. He had made hasty assumptions based on a badly skilled analysis he had undertaken on the victim's body.

Despite the fact that the law demanded a lack of "reasonable doubt" from jurymen, such uncertainty became the bread and butter of medical jurisprudence, and this was the root of a number of conflicts with the law, which believed, in contrast, that doubt was the enemy of justice. The medical discipline's job was to assist the legal profession in searching for a conviction based on its version of "no reasonable doubt," but, for itself, forensics embraced the idea of a healthy skepticism brought about by careful reasoning. James Edmunds, a correspondent in the *British Medical Journal*, commented on problems like the Williams evidence in 1863:

---

27. Ibid., 23.
28. Male, *Epitome*, 10.

The cure of [the] sore place is in our hands. Let us carefully scrutinise the conduct of those who appear in the witness box; and, when we see a man presumptuously condemning those who have a right to think differently, or prostituting his science for a one-sided advocacy, in place of a humble exposition of simple truth, or aping omniscience with his own narrow dogmatism, then note that man, and, quite apart from any spirit of trades-unionism, let the Association meet for the purpose of marking their sense of such conduct; and, whether the fault be presumption, ignorance, carelessness in the performance of so important a duty, or anything even less venial, let us act out the fair inference that such an one is unfit for our noble profession, and avoid meeting him in practice.[29]

Edmunds's idea of blacklisting rogue individuals is an exaggerated example of medicine's determination to keep its regulation within its own ranks. Like Fletcher, Edmunds was dismayed by the lack of self-awareness, in some experts, in thinking that they cannot be wrong. It is, he says, "narrow dogmatism" and, worse still, an "aping of omniscience." Yet a by-product of Edmunds's attack on his profession's worst offenders is a picture of forensic medicine at its best: careful, self-critical, and "noble." Aping omniscience is a transgression precisely because it goes against the critical strategy of juxtaposing "the whole truth" with approximate human truth in order to promote a careful, self-watchful system of science.

APPROXIMATE TRUTH

The turn against perceived ideals of objective induction in the nineteenth century—a shift outlined by Smith in *Fact and Feeling* (1994)[30]—gave a vital relevance to Oesterlen's *Medicinische Logik*. In accordance with what figures such as William Whewell and John Herschel were saying about science, Oesterlen believed that what he termed "subjective aid" was an unavoidable part of the work of medicine:

> We must, it is said, observe and describe all the phenomena and processes of health and disease, according to their actual appearance, without any

---

29. James Edmunds, "Medical Advocates," *British Medical Journal* (2 May 1863): 465.
30. On William Whewell, for instance, Smith notes that there was a commitment to a "philosophy that included necessary truths and fundamental ideas" and that the "empirical exercise in fact-collecting, generating theory without the mediation for the mind, could only be, as it was for [Stanley] Jevons, a half truth." Smith, *Fact and Feeling*, 20.

subjective aid, whether in the conception or interpretation of them, or in the comparison and classification of them with others. And this must be carried out with a resolute independence of all theoretical views, and without allowing ourselves to be influenced by any dogma, preconception, or peculiar mental tendency; as if this were in any way possible for man in the present state of his intellectual being![31]

We may remove "our view of the actual state of things," he added, no more "than we can strip off our skin."[32] Immanuel Kant once said that "out of the crooked timber of humanity no straight thing was ever made."[33] This may seem like a pessimistic outlook for medical jurisprudence; its perceived function, after all, was to assist in the protection of the nation's morals by providing evidence of where their ethical code had been violated. If such investigations were always to be sullied by the thumbprint of human practice, then what hope might there be of getting at "the whole truth"? As indicated by the note from James Edmunds above, the best forensic experts were able to turn this potential shortcoming into a strength. We are flawed and fallible, their argument suggested, but this should not dissuade us from striving to be otherwise. Michael Ryan's *Manual of Medical Jurisprudence and State Medicine* (1836) is just one among many texts from the period to suggest that medical jurisprudence has much to gain from incubating the watchful strategies that come from acknowledging one's interpretation to be imperfect:

> Illness requires us to implore the Deity for assistance and relief, and humbles pride. The seeds of art, the wonderful cures, and the powers of remedies, are in the hands of God. He has beneficently supplied various remedies, and pronounces with our tongues, the fate, life and death, of man. Whence, we see the dignity of medicine, and what reverence is due to the Divine Author of it.[34]

Such passages negate the hackneyed view that science was (and is) "a materialistic, anti-human force," believing itself to be "the only thing that matters."[35] Usually part of a larger project that aims to advocate the value of

---

31. Oesterlen, *Medicinische Logik (Medical Logic)*, 13, 16.
32. Ibid., 361.
33. Immanuel Kant, *Gesammelte Schriften* (1784), quoted in Isiah Berlin, "The Romantic Revolution: A Crisis in the History of Modern Thought" (1960), in *The Sense of Reality: Studies in Ideas and their History*, ed. Henry Hardy (London: Chatto and Windus, 1996), 169–93 (192).
34. Ryan, *Manual*, 3.
35. Mary Midgley, *Science and Poetry* (2001; London and New York: Routledge, 2006), 67, 71.

religion or art, such aggressive assessments have ignored a vast number of works that have focused, through science, on the fraught relationship between the needs of humanity and the limitations of human perception. For instance, while it is true that in invoking the image of God, Ryan steers toward a view of medicine as an *appropriation* of God's alleged powers, he is careful to see himself as a pretender to the throne:

> The history of medicine, of all other sciences, comprises the most intimate acquaintance with the works of nature, and elevates the mind to the most sublime conceptions of the supreme Being, and expands the heart with the most pleasing ideas of Providence. It *nearly* extends through the whole range of the creation; and no other profession requires so extensive a knowledge of the works of Providence.[36]

Implicit in the voice of Ryan is recognition of a higher power, or a supreme standard of truth, which allows him to accept that *his* truth falls short of the absolute. Like Christison during the trial of Robert Reid, he is careful to indicate that his knowledge is indicative rather than certain.

A similar strategy occurs in a lecture delivered by one of Ryan's contemporaries, John Gordon Smith, in 1830. In his forensic career, Smith says, he "began to discover a sure and certain method of correcting every-thing, or at least, of making medicine as perfect as any-thing human (if it be not more than human, which for one, I consider that it is), any-thing confided to human management is capable of becoming; and this I saw to be done by MEDICAL JURISPRUDENCE."[37] Like Ryan, Smith saw the "whole truth" as beyond his powers. He did suggest that his discipline could be "more than human," yet the very word *human* falls like a hammer stroke to keep his ambitions pegged into the ground. What is also significant about Smith's statement is that it distills a vital point that is implied in both Oesterlen and Ryan: that the concept of an unattainable, absolute truth does not leave the savant in darkness but rather sets him on the right course. "Real detachment, full objectivity is," according to Anderson, "an 'aspiration' rather than a possible achievement."[38] Yet not only will steering toward its light keep the forensic examiner on the right path; it will also teach him the kind of methodological humility that is central to a good interpretation.

---

36. Ryan, *Manual*. Italics added.

37. John Gordon Smith, "Introductory Lecture on Medical Jurisprudence," *The Lancet* 15 (1830–31): 97–103 (98).

38. Paraphrased in Levine, *Dying to Know*, 14.

Indeed, the concept of an absolute, unattainable truth was central to forensic medicine's negotiation of both its limits and its potential. As the following quotation from Alexander Thomson's "Lectures on Medical Jurisprudence" (1837) indicates, the perceived challenge of a seemingly unattainable truth necessitated a continuous evaluation of *how* medicine knows what it knows:

> A witness must possess the *ability* to speak the truth,—a circumstance which must depend not only on the opportunities which he has of observing the facts, but on the accuracy of his powers of observing, and the faithfulness of his memory in retaining them, when they have been once observed and known. These qualifications are common to, and required from, all witnesses; but as medical witnesses are required to testify to opinions which are wholly or particularly the result of reasoning, exercised upon particular circumstances, it is obvious that the reasons of a witness for drawing his conclusions, are of most essential importance for the purpose of ascertaining whether his conclusions be correct.[39]

I noted above that the concept of "no reasonable doubt" was central to legal indictments; in medical jurisprudence a reasonable or *reasoned-upon* doubt was key to constructing trustworthy evidence. This view was suggested by Thomson, who makes it plain that his science did not seek to reject analysis in favor of "blind sight, seeing without inference, interpretation or intelligence"[40] but that a careful balancing of what *can* be known with *how* ought to be central to the approximate truth that all scientists seek.

With this strategic way of thinking, forensic experts of the nineteenth century appeared to have more in common with Enlightenment scientists than with their positivist cousins. The former, according to Lorraine Daston and Peter Galison, believed in science as a commitment to "truth-to-nature":

> For Enlightenment naturalists like Linnaeus, the reality did not entail a commitment to Platonic forms at the expense of the evidence of the sense. On the contrary, sharp and sustained observation was a necessary prerequisite for discerning the true genera of plants and other organisms. The eyes of both body and mind converged to discover a reality otherwise hidden to each alone.

---

39. Alexander Thomson, "Lectures on Medical Jurisprudence: Lecture 2," *The Lancet* 27: 113–18 (114). Italics in original.

40. Daston and Galison, *Objectivity*, 17.

To see like a naturalist required more than just sharp senses: a capacious memory, the ability to analyse and synthesize impressions, as well as the patience and talent to extract the typical from the storehouse of natural particulars, were all key qualifications.[41]

Writing about the same subject, though calling it *instrumentalism* instead of *truth-to-nature*, Lissa Roberts claims that figures like Etienne Bonnot de Condillac, the eighteenth-century empiricist philosopher, insisted on "the mind as a laboratory in which balancing acts are assembled and compounds disassembled in a search for the elements":

> Condillac repeatedly represented nature by analogy to a countryside vista in which everything, at first glance, exists simultaneously as an organic whole. An unstudied version of nature totality, however, teaches us nothing. Knowledge comes only through a mental process of analysis.[42]

Daston and Galison observe that "mechanical objectivity did not [. . .] extinguish truth-to-nature" but that the latter "continued to command the loyalty of some scientists and even whole disciplines throughout the nineteenth and twentieth centuries."[43] Medical jurisprudence was one of these disciplines. Its belief in its inability to work with anything but a hypothetical version of the truth encouraged a deep-rooted loyalty to the idea of expert interpretation.

JAMES HEYWOOD

We see this attachment to interpretation reflected in the way that opinions became one of medical jurisprudence's main weapons. Unlike nonspecialist witnesses (who were required to limit their evidence to what they had perceived), medical experts were encouraged to give their opinion in courts of law. Such was the case in the 1839 prosecution of James Heywood, a publican from Bury in the north of England. The defendant's wife Mary died suddenly after a scuffle with her husband. Margaret Walker, who was servant to the married couple, gave evidence as follows:

---

41. Ibid., 58.
42. Lissa Roberts, "Condillac, Lavoisier, and the Instrumentalization of Science," *The Eighteenth Century* 33:3 (1992): 252–71 (254, 258).
43. Ibid., 105.

On the 15th of April prisoner came home about half-past seven in the evening, in liquour. He went to bed about half-past twelve. [. . . Husband and wife] then began to count up the money they had taken that day, 24s. He said, "Is that all you have drawn, and yonder kegs were filled up last night?" She said "Yes." He said, "Is that all, thou nasty, drunken w—e!" She said she was not drunk (I saw her before she went to bed, perfectly sober.) Immediately after I heard a scuffle. She said "Oh, Jem, you will break my arm; don't punish me so bad." He said she was drunk. [. . .] I heard her groan for about four minutes. I then heard the prisoner say, "D—n thy soul, if I can find a stick I'll make thee to rise." He found a stick, and I heard him strike three times. All was then silent.[44]

The witness then described finding her mistress's corpse:

The rush-light was still burning. The deceased lay on her back, with her feet towards the head of the bed. She had her night-cap and chemise on. Prisoner asked me if she was dead, and I said, "Yes, quite dead." [. . .] In the morning the prisoner said, "Margaret, was you asleep? Did you hear your mistress fall off the bed?" I said, "No; mistress never was in." He said, "Yea, she was; and added that, if I was going to tell those tales I should do him at once; I should get him into a hobble." I said, "I shall tell the truth."[45]

Margaret's insistence on "the truth" is significant because the trial of James Heywood became key to discussions of the relationship between truth and the kind of basic empiricism reflected in Margaret's experiences. On the night of Mary's death, her body was examined by two specialists: John Parks, surgeon of Bury; and his apprentice Joseph Rothwell. The latter was the first on the scene, and he discovered "marks on the [deceased's] arm [that] were made by the fingers. The whites of the eyes were bloodless; the cheeks livid; the lips bloodless; [. . .] the right breast was almost black."[46] He believed that these signs indicated how Mary had been smothered. He quickly got his master out of bed and informed him that "Mrs. Heywood was either dead or dying."[47] When cross-examined in court, Rothwell admitted that he had never seen a case like Mary's before. The admission was italicized in the pages of the *The Lancet*: "*I have not witnessed any cases*

---

44. Unsigned, "Medical Jurisprudence: Trial for Murder," 896–900 (896).
45. Ibid.
46. Ibid., 897.
47. Ibid.

of apoplexy, nor attended cases of *suffocation* or *sudden death*."[48] Rothwell then made a rather naive statement: "I never witnessed a sudden death before; but I am prepared to swear the death had been caused by external violence."[49] John Parks, Rothwell's mentor, was a little more guarded. He found that "the deceased had undergone considerable violence" and agreed with his protégée that suffocation was the cause of death.[50] Cross-examined, however, he also admitted that he had "attended many cases of sudden death, but not of suffocation."[51]

The defending lawyer, Mr Wilkins, saw a good opportunity to strengthen his case. He made a great deal of both men's seeming lack of hands-on experience. Such naivety made their evidence unreliable, in his view, and he made the bold and unusual step of requesting further medical evidence from a couple of doctors who happened to be in the courtroom at that moment. Extraordinarily, "the application was conceded."[52] Mr William Rayner, one of the surgeons present, disagreed with the previous medical witnesses, testifying instead that "there are no decisive signs by which you can tell that suffocation has taken place." Another bystanding specialist, Mr Riordan, added, "It is not my opinion that the signs must necessarily have been produced by suffocation."[53] The judge reminded the jury that if they had any reasonable doubt that Heywood murdered his wife, they should acquit him. They spent about fifteen minutes agreeing on a verdict of "Not Guilty." In a summing up that matches any Dickensian satire for absurdity, the judge added that "he was perfectly satisfied with the verdict, but he would advise [the defendant] to be more careful in future."[54]

Like the Robert Reid case, the failure to condemn Heywood seemed, to some commentators, a failure of the medical evidence. In a certain light, of course, it was. But as part of the larger development of medical jurisprudence—a discipline comprising medical texts and criminal indictments—the case stressed the importance of considered interpretation and the value of reasonable doubt. Although there was a lack of consensus among the four medical witnesses, it is clear that the court favored the opinions of Rayner and Riordan as the more considered interpretations. While it was often said in criticism of medicine that its practitioners found it difficult to agree on just about everything, the complex discussions in the courtroom,

---

48. Ibid.
49. Ibid.
50. Ibid.
51. Ibid.
52. Ibid.
53. Ibid., 899, 900.
54. Ibid.

in medical journals, in newspapers, and in medical treatises paint a picture of a discipline that was careful exactly because it knew its interpretations were not "whole truths" but a set of opinions open to doubt and revision.

OLIVER TWIST

Oliver Twist was written in the same decade as the Reid and the Heywood trials, each of which had showcased the conflict between the law's need for certainty and medicine's need for doubt. As John Lucas has observed, *Oliver Twist* was "Dickens's first sustained effort at realism." Yet

> to call *Oliver Twist* a realist novel may seem merely perverse. There is after all some bad plotting to take account of, to say nothing of those excessive coincidences which give the novel a forced symmetry that is very unlike life. And in what sense can characters such as the Maylies, Losberne, Brownlow, Nancy, Monks, Oliver himself be thought of as realistic?[55]

Comments on the novel's failed realism have usually centered on its rather extravagant content. Thackeray's famous account in *Fraser's Magazine*, for instance, damned with faint praise—calling the novel's scenes and characters "pleasing, unnatural caricatures" rather than true-to-life representations:

> There are in some of these histories more fun—in all, more fancy and romance—than are ordinarily found in humble life; and we recommend the admirer of such scenes, if he would have an accurate notion of them, to obtain his knowledge at the fountain-head, and trust more to the people's description of themselves, than to [. . .] Dickens's startling, pleasing, unnatural caricatures.[56]

Dickens was annoyed by such interpretations. In his preface for the 1841 edition he defended the portraits of some of his "lowest" characters. On Nancy, he said:

> It is useless to discuss whether the conduct and character of the girl seems natural or unnatural, probable or improbable, right or wrong. IT IS TRUE. Every man who has watched these melancholy shades of life knows

---

55. John Lucas, *The Melancholy Man: A Study of Dickens's Novels* (London: Methuen, 1970), 24.
56. William Makepeace Thackeray, "Horæ Catnachianæ," *Fraser's Magazine* 19 (1839): 407–24 (407).

it to be so. Suggested to my mind long ago—long before I dealt in fiction—by what I often saw and read of, in actual life around me, I have, for years, tracked it through many profligate and noisome ways, and found it still the same. From the first introduction of that poor wretch, to her laying her bloody head upon the robber's breast, there is not one word exaggerated or overwrought. It is emphatically God's truth, for it is the truth.[57]

The reference to the "man *who has watched* these melancholy shades of life" raises the idea of a certain kind of expertise, and the image of Dickens "tracking" truth through "profligate and noisome ways" draws on a forensic, detective image of the professional in search of an answer. Such specialist searches, based on looking, knowing, and reading signs, provide a way of approaching a certain standard of truth.

Yet what is perhaps most interesting about the preface is the way it defends the *objectives*, more than the content, of *Oliver Twist*. Lucas is right to doubt whether it would be possible for Dickens to defend the realism of all of his characters (particularly the Maylies), yet it is difficult to find fault with the author's account of his narrative's aims in relation to "low-life" characters:

> But I had never met (except in HOGARTH) with the miserable reality. It appeared to me that to draw a knot of such associates of crime as really do exist, to paint them in all their deformity, in all their wretchedness, in all the squalid poverty of their lives; to shew them as they really are, for ever skulking uneasily through the dirtiest paths of life, with the great, black, ghastly gallows closing up their prospect, turn them where they may; it appeared to me that to do this, would be to attempt something which was greatly needed and which would be a service to society. And therefore I did it as best I could. (liv)

Hogarth, Dickens said, "compromise[d not] a hair's breadth" in his gritty portrayals of reality (lvi). Although such encomiums are based on accuracy of content ("as really do exist," "as they really are"), his reverence for the artist's methods suggests that the *attempt* to represent reality is as important to him as, if not more important than, the result. In the above passage, for instance, focus is laid on the objectives of Dickens's method: he will show, he says; he will attempt; he will do his best. What this suggests about his

---

57. Charles Dickens, *Oliver Twist*, ed. Stephen Gill (1837–38; Oxford: Oxford University Press, 1999), xvii. Subsequent references to this edition will be given in the main body of the text.

view of truthful representation is that, like forensic medicine's, it is based on an *attempt* to get at the "whole truth" rather than any particular success in doing so. In the words of Coleridge, "veracity does not consist in saying, but in the *intention* of communicating truth."[58]

Oliver Twist is a study of absolute goodness and, specifically, the ways in which that idea might be used as a guide and an ambition for the realist objectives of the novel form. The central character is frequently associated with truth, indicating how truth and goodness amount to the same thing. In Oliver's face, it is observed, "there was truth in every one of its thin and sharpened lineaments" (90), and Brownlow asserts that he will "answer for that boy's truth with [his] life" (108). Shortly before he is taken on the burglary expedition that almost kills him, he is described as

> lying, fast asleep, on a rude bed upon the floor; so pale with anxiety, and sadness, and the closeness of his prison, that he looked like death; not death as it shews in shroud and coffin, but in the guise it wears when life has just departed; when a young and gentle spirit has, but an instant, fled to Heaven: and the gross air of the world has not had time to breathe upon the changing dust it hallowed. (155)

Oliver's "hallowed" light is a rehearsal, perhaps, of the angelic characterization of Little Nell; lying here he represents, as she will, the light of absolute purity. His incorruptible goodness is what allows him to be the novel's principal source of illumination, and it is linked, as it is in texts on the duties of medical jurisprudence, to a sense of truthful representation. Take, for example, the scene in which Oliver first sees his sleeping quarters in the back of Sowerberry's shop:

> Oliver, being left to himself in the undertaker's shop, set the lamp down on a workman's bench, and gazed timidly about him with a feeling of awe and dread, which many people a good deal older than he will be at no loss to understand. An unfinished coffin on black tressels, which stood in the middle of the shop, looked so gloomy and deathlike that a cold tremble came over him, every time his eyes wandered in the direction of the dismal object: from which he almost expected to see some frightful form slowly rear its head, to drive him mad with terror. Against the wall were ranged, in regular array, a long row of elm boards cut into the same shape: looking,

---

58. Samuel Taylor Coleridge, *Biographia Literaria, or Biographical Sketches of My Literary Life and Opinions* (1817; London: Dent, 1967), 84. Italics added.

in the dim light, like high-shouldered ghosts with their hands in their breeches-pockets. Coffin-plates, elm-chips, bright-headed nails, and shreds of back cloth, lay scattered on the floor; and the wall behind the counter was ornamented with a lively representation of two mutes in very stiff neckcloths, on duty in a large private door: with a hearse drawn by four black steeds, approaching in the distance. The shop was close and hot; and the atmosphere seemed tainted with the smell of coffins. The recess beneath the counter in which his flock mattress was thrust, looked like a grave. (31–32)

The position of Oliver as observer, plus the representation of the undertaker's shop as a gothic dream, creates a number of interesting parallels with the ambitions of medical jurisprudence. What makes the passage an exercise in "truth-to-nature" is not the questionable accuracy with which the room's contents (clearly exaggerated by Oliver's terrified imagination) are observed, but the role given to the perspective of the observer. Narrative is channeled through the vision of the central character, which is not an uncommon strategy in the nineteenth century but one that is done self-referentially in *Oliver Twist*. Notice, for instance, how objects are described only after Oliver's eyes have "gazed timidly" at them or "wandered in [their] direction." Things are portrayed as they appear *to* Oliver who is the "pure" means through which the text achieves a level of detail. Dickens uses his central character as the light the story needs in order to see and to make sense of the dark areas of his interest. The lurid portraits that Thackeray complained of may sit awkwardly with any high standards of verisimilitude, but Dickens makes it absolutely clear in the 1841 preface, and in scenes like those quoted above, that his commitment to the "whole truth"—"God's Truth"—allows his exaggerations to say something very real.

Of course, the view that *Oliver Twist* "shone a startling light on the sins of the criminal and Pharisee alike"[59] is a common one in Dickens criticism, yet what is considered less frequently is how the author drew on medical ideas as a means of creating and making good use of a central light in the novel. In an essay titled "Dickens and Language" Patricia Ingham notes that the name "Oliver" had slang associations with moonlight in the nineteenth century. "The choice of name," she notes, "is illuminated by an item in the *Glossary* Dickens used: 'Oliver is in town: a phrase signifying that nights are moonlit, and consequently unfavourable to depredation.'"[60]

---

59. A. E. Dyson, "Introduction," in *Dickens: Modern Judgments*, ed. A. E. Dyson (London: Macmillan, 1968), 13.

60. Patricia Ingham, "Dickens and Language," in *A Companion to Charles Dickens*, ed. David Paroissien (Oxford: Blackwell Publishing, 2008), 126–41 (129).

The moon and moonlight are laden with vast amounts of symbolic meaning: femininity, lunacy, and so on; in the novel's context their primary function is one of illumination. Early in the novel the orphan visits a slum with Sowerberry. Their "professional mission" (37) as undertakers is to collect the body of a female pauper who has starved to death. In the following description of a slum, note how Oliver's perspective illuminates a space that has been a scene of neglect previous to his (and the narrative's) visit:

> They walked on, for some time, through the most crowded and densely inhabited part of the town: and then, striking down a narrow street more dirty and miserable than any they had yet passed through, paused to look for the house which was the object of their search. The houses on either side were high and large, but very old; and tenanted by people of the poorest class: as their neglected appearance would have sufficiently denoted, without the concurrent testimony afforded by the squalid looks of the few men and women who, with folded arms and bodies half doubled, occasionally skulked along. A great many of the tenements had shop-fronts; but these were fast closed, and mouldering away: only the upper rooms being inhabited. Some houses which had become insecure from age and decay, were prevented from falling into the street, by huge beams of wood reared against the walls, and firmly planted in the road; but even these crazy dens seemed to have been selected as the nightly haunts of some houseless wretches; for many of the high boards, which supplied the place of door and window, were wrenched from their positions, to afford an aperture wide enough for the passage of a human body. The kennel was stagnant and filthy. The very rats, which were here and there lay putrefying in its rottenness, were hideous with famine. (37–38)

Oliver's presence allows the novel to illuminate awful realities—specifically characters and places—that are *terra incognita* to many of the novel's original readers. John Bowen suggests:

> The novel itself contains a clear polemical edge turned against "philosophers," among whom Dickens includes Benthamite utilitarians, but which also cuts wider. There is a constant distrust of philosophical reasoning's complicity with social and familial exploitation; against this, the book sets the contradictory and anomalous truth of fiction.[61]

---

61. Bowen, *Other Dickens*, 83.

Set against the harsh reality of a world dominated by political economy is the "anomalous truth of fiction" or, as I choose to see it, absolute truth embodied by the spotless parish boy. I argue that Oliver represents the kind of objectivity that Stephen Williams saw as shedding "rays of knowledge and of light," and, as such, the orphan is fated to offer an untenable means of perceiving the subjects of the novel. Dickens wrote that he "wished to shew, in little Oliver, the principle of Good surviving through every adverse circumstance, and triumphing at last" (liii); and that the "principle of Good" is matched by a "principle of Truth" that runs through *Oliver Twist*, embodied by Oliver himself.

The idea of a central illuminating character would have had religious connotations for Dickens. The notion of an allegorical figure constantly striving toward the light recasts the progress of Bunyan's pilgrim, and the light imagery of *Oliver Twist* also borrows much from the Bible, particularly the book of Genesis, which establishes many of the cultural links that have been made between illumination, goodness, and knowledge. Before Oliver arrives in the slum accompanied by Sowerberry, for instance, it is "clear" that the area has been a space of primeval darkness. Without the light of Oliver's presence—a light that guides the narrative and determines its outline—all is obscured and hopeless:

> "Ah!" said the man [husband to the starved pauper]: bursting into tears, and sinking on his knees at the feet of the dead woman; "kneel down, kneel down—kneel round her, every one of you, and mark my words! I say she was starved to death. I never knew how bad she was, till the fever came upon her; and her bones were starting through the skin. There was neither fire nor candle; she died in the dark—in the dark. She couldn't even see her children's faces, though we heard her gasping out their names." (39)

This unfortunate pauper dies in the dark, yet her body is now exposed to the light of Oliver's view: "Oliver [. . .] cast his eyes towards the place. [. . .] Though it was covered up, the boy felt that it was a corpse" (38). With Oliver comes light; with light comes knowledge; with both comes truth. The man's injunction that everybody kneel before the emaciated remains of his wife, and his insistence that he will be heard now that those remains are enlightened by the presence of Oliver, invokes the awesomeness of God, who speaks, sheds light, and *knows* in the first lines of the Bible. In Genesis light is good: it is synonymous with knowledge, and it is responsible for the beginning (of everything, certainly, including understanding).

adventures with the novel's underclass, and it also marks the start of two other important trajectories: the narrative's exposé of London's criminal life and the not-unrelated downfall of Fagin.

Oliver may symbolize enlightenment and purity, yet there are several scenes where the boy is grossly ignorant, for example, when he imagines that pickpocket training is a game and he is taken on the burgling expedition with Sikes. These scenes are still illuminating, of course, because the narrator and the reader have a sagacity that Oliver's innocence precludes. The parish boy's purity, the source of many a critical grumble since first publication, remains uncontaminated despite Fagin's best attempts to render it otherwise:

> The Old Man would tell [the boys] stories of robberies he had committed in his younger days: mixed up with so much that was droll and curious, that Oliver could not help laughing heartily, and showing that he was amused in spite of all his better feelings.
>
> In short, the wily old Jew had the boy in his toils; and, having prepared his mind, by solitude and gloom, to prefer any society to the companionship of his own sad thoughts in such a dreary place, he was now slowly instilling into his soul the poison which he hoped would blacken it, and change its hue forever. (146–47)

Marlene Tromp has noted that Oliver's "angelic purity protects [him] from the criminals, whose efforts to corrupt him through mistreatment, bribery, and fear repeatedly fail."[64] Fagin underestimates the nature and power of Oliver's whiteness. It is not the whiteness of naivety, to be besmirched as the old villain sees fit, but the whiteness of a representative of absolute truth and goodness. Episodes in *Oliver Twist* that feature the boy's blissful ignorance usually lead to a moment of blinding biblical revelation. Lending the boy a copy of *The Newgate Calendar* (1774), or some other dismal "history of the lives and trials of great criminals" (157), Fagin hopes to infect Oliver's heart with admiration for its rascals:

> In a paroxysm of fear, the boy closed the book, and thrust it from him. Then, falling upon his knees, he prayed Heaven to spare him from such deeds; and rather to will that he should die at once, than be reserved for such crimes, so fearful and appalling. (157)

---

64. Marlene Tromp, *The Private Rod: Marital Violence, Sensation, and the Law in Britain* (Charlottesville, VA, and London: University of Virginia Press, 2000), 27.

When light finally dawns on Oliver's senses and he realizes he is being used in a robbery, he is duly mortified:

> And now, for the first time, Oliver, well nigh mad with grief and terror, saw that housebreaking and robbery, if not murder, were the objects of the expedition. He clasped his hands together, and involuntarily uttered a subdued exclamation of horror. A mist came before his eyes; the cold sweat stood upon his ashy face; his limbs failed him; and he sunk upon his knees. [. . .]
> "Oh! for God's sake let me go!" cried Oliver, "let me run away and die in the fields. I will never come near London; never, never! Oh! pray have mercy on me, and do not make me steal. For the love of all the bright Angels that rest in Heaven, have mercy upon me!" (172)

As truth flashes on the boy, his supplications to God and the invocation of heavenly goodness take center stage. Goodness, knowledge, and enlightenment go hand in hand, underscoring how the characterization of Oliver seemingly relies upon these absolutes to drive the momentum of the narrative's exposés. What Oliver comes across in the catalogue of crimes he is given to read are images of "bodies hidden from the eye of man in deep pits and wells; which would not keep them down, deep as they were, but had yielded them up at last, after many years, and so maddened the murderers with the sight" (157). Like *The Terrific Register*, these narratives are all about truth coming to light without human agency; they tally with the traditional view that truth comes to light because God's gaze is all-seeing and all-settling.

One other aspect of John Elliotson's "well-lit Pall Mall" image worth mentioning is how it brings the enlightening qualities of intelligence and morality to the streets of London. Light in the passage behaves like the typical flâneur: moving through and illuminating the streets, remaining untouched by the city's filthier qualities. Michael Ryan had a similar image for the forensic expert: he rarely participates in "the commotions which occupy societies and empires. He avoids politics and political assemblies, while engaged in the peaceful pursuits of his profession. He takes no interest in the quarrels of sovereigns. [. . .] In time of war medical men feel equally bound to aid friends and enemies, according to the law of nations."[65] With knowledge of Dickens's later work, we are also reminded, ironically enough, of the representation of disease in *Bleak House* (1852–53), which has the ability to infect people from all levels of society, regardless

---

65. Ryan, *Manual*, 69–70.

of whether they are good, bad, rich, poor, benevolent, or indifferent. One of the most striking motifs of that novel is the invisible network of channels that binds all members of society together—a motif made manifest at various points by smallpox and the infection of Chancery. In 1836 Michael Ryan suggested, more optimistically, that medical skill might employ a similar sort of indiscrimination: the good work of medicine was all about seeking to transcend the common interests of man by shedding light, ironically, on that most common and material of things: the body.

If, therefore, Oliver Twist represents the light of knowledge, a "light" that he appears to share with God and men of medicine, it becomes clear why he needs to be an orphan, a solitary traveler, a force of incorruptible goodness. When Oliver is taken from Miss Mann's establishment, we are told that "a sense of [Oliver's] loneliness in the great wide world, sank into the child's heart" (8), and traveling from Mudfog to London, he is "cold and hungry, and more alone than he had ever felt before" (55). The boy is isolated, unrelated (seemingly) to other characters in the novel—an apparent tabula rasa. Some characters question Oliver's origins: "Where does he come from?" Grimwig asks. "Who is he? What is he?" (107), whereas Noah Claypole boasts that he does not share the boy's "blank" history: "Noah was a charity-boy, not a workhouse orphan. No chance child was he, for he could trace his genealogy all the way back to his parents, who lived close by; his mother being a washerwoman, and his father a drunken soldier" (34). Oliver's apparent lack of mortal connections allows him to adopt the role of detached observer in the places he visits and of the people he meets. Like the portrait of scientific knowledge painted by Elliotson and Ryan, he is able to move nimbly across boundaries and dark spaces. "Truth," observes Bowen with reference to the novel, "is not a matter of probability or inference, but stands above them, 'God's truth,' the meeting of apparently irreconcilable forces of ideas in a knowledge beyond the claims or judgement of reason or nature."[66] As Oliver moves from the pauper class to the affluent middle class, he brings characters like Rose Maylie and Nancy together, and he is required on more than one occasion to creep into small holes and apertures. Mr Gamfield, the chimney sweep, "knowing what the dietary of the workhouse was, well knew [Oliver] would be a nice small pattern: just the very thing for register stoves" (17). Mrs Sowerberry and Charlotte drag "Oliver, struggling and shouting, but nothing daunted, into the dust-cellar" (47), and Sikes, of course, passes the boy through a small window after observing that "he is just the size I want" (153). Seemingly

---

66. Bowen, *Other Dickens*, 82.

unconnected to any group or geographical space throughout much of the novel, Oliver is perfectly suited to infiltrate the dark recesses he is required to visit and, importantly for the aims of the novel, he sheds his light within.

The characterization of Oliver as light-giver in fact lends a specific power to the method and purpose of Dickens's text. *Oliver Twist* is a novel, according to Lucas, in which "the crusading journalist [is] determined to make his readers confront the truth. This is important. For *Oliver Twist* confronts its readers with a society which is rapidly becoming incapable or unwilling to recognize itself and which in the process is becoming rapidly dehumanized."[67] But the novel would seem to have none of its crusading powers were it not for the illumination spread by the central character who remains untouched by London's grime. He is, according to Karín Lesnik-Oberstein, "neither the main topic of, nor in any unambiguous sense a 'self' in, the novel."[68] A character of undeniable whiteness, he is a stylistic device that apparently allows the story to access the tools associated with a "whole truth."

As I hinted above, however, Oliver's association with absolute truth and goodness is unsustainable in the nightmarish world of Dickens's London. The novel concedes, in accordance with the theories of forensic medicine, that the incorruptible version of truth and goodness, as embodied in the central character, is neither possible nor essential. The novel has a significant turn in focus in the scene where Oliver dreams he is being watched by Fagin and Monks at the Maylies' rural home. Lucas notes:

> In the notion of a "safe" rural world which is inexplicably terrorized by Fagin and Monks' appearance, it is perfectly possible to see a prolepsis of the dream of revolutionary horror that infects much of the literature of the 1840s. Rousseau's prescription for avoiding corruption was to withdraw from society; Dickens's realism has much to do with his recognition that such a withdrawal is impossible.[69]

Oliver's dream represents the questioning of absolute goodness linked with whole truth. Famous for having attracted the notice of G. H. Lewes, the scene begins as follows:

---

67. Lucas, *Melancholy Man*, 29.
68. Karín Lesnik-Oberstein, "*Oliver Twist*: The Narrator's Tale," in *Textual Practice* 15:1 (2001): 87–100 (98).
69. Lucas, *Melancholy Man*, 37.

There is a kind of sleep that steals upon us sometimes, which, while it holds the body prisoner, does not free the mind from a sense of things about it, and enables it to ramble at its pleasure. So far as an overpowering heaviness, a prostration of strength, and an utter inability to control our thoughts or power of motion, can be called sleep, this is it; and yet we have a consciousness of all that is going on about us; and if we dream at such a time, words which are really spoken, or sounds which really exist at the moment, accommodate themselves with surprising readiness to our visions, until reality and imagination become so strangely blended that it is afterwards almost a matter of impossibility to separate the two. (271)

In this borderland between sleep and wakefulness Oliver believes he sees Monks and Fagin peering at him through the window:

Good Heaven! what was that, which sent the blood tingling to his heart, and deprived him of his voice, and of power to move! There—there—at the window; close before him; so close, that he could have almost touched him before he started back: with his eyes peering into the room, and meeting his: there stood the Jew! And beside him, white with rage, or fear, or both, were the scowling features of the very man who had accosted him in the inn-yard. (272)

This moment of panic is a reversal of the earlier scene where Oliver half awakes to find himself watching Fagin. Once the watcher, the boy now finds himself being watched. When Harry Maylie and Mr Losberne search for the two rogues, their efforts turn out to be "all in vain. There were not even the traces of recent footsteps, to be seen" (275). It is verified later that Fagin and Monks did travel out to the country in search of Oliver; their appearance at the window is no illusion then, but this does not seem to be the most important revelation at this point in the text. What matters most is the seeming fact that we can no longer trust Oliver's observations. The long theoretical passage that leads up to the boy's "seeing" of Fagin and Monks is concerned with subjective thinking only: Oliver experiences an "inability to control [his] thoughts or power of motion"—a far cry from the way he has seemed to embody purity of thought and the power of incorruptibility. His inability to control his physical movements is also a marked change from his skills of moving in and out of inaccessible spaces. The actual world, we are told, blends into a dream, and "visions" cast a ghostly shadow over the "real." The change represents a poignant parallel with the kinds of discussions being had by experts in the field of medical jurisprudence: like them, the text deconstructs its "objective centre" and develops a form of realism that views key revelations through the interpretations and experiences of its flesh-and-blood characters.

In the second part of *Oliver Twist* there is no central symbol of enlightenment, yet we are left with neither chaos nor a primeval world of darkness. What we have instead are a number of subjective observations and coincidences—strategies that are intended to represent the human faculty of *interpretation* as a valuable alternative to a doomed objectivity. In Brian Cheadle's reading of *Oliver Twist*, the second half of the novel sees Nancy "replace [. . .] Oliver both as the novel's main victim and as the 'the principle of Good' surviving."[70] In several later scenes it certainly appears as though the knowing and worldly prostitute has appropriated the orphan's position of observer, as we see in the following passage where she spies on Fagin and Monks:

> The girl drew closer to the table, and glancing at Monks with an air of careless levity, withdrew her eyes: but as he turned his towards the Jew, she stole another look: so keen and searching, and full of purpose, that if there had been any bystander to observe the change, he could hardly have believed the two looks to have proceeded from the same person. (316)

Whereas Oliver represents the brilliant light of truth and clarity, Nancy conducts her observations in the dark:

> Before the sounds of their footsteps had ceased to echo through the house, the girl had slipped off her shoes; and drawing her gown loosely over her head, and muffling her arms in it, stood at the door, listening with breathless interest. The moment the noise ceased, she glided from the room; ascended the stairs with incredible softness and silence; and was lost in the gloom above. (Ibid.)

Nancy also appears to replace Oliver's role as the novel's symbolic corpse. In the first stages of the book, the parish orphan, "more dead than alive" (173), looking "like death" and bearing a "hallowed" glow (155), prefigures Little Nell's saintly body, yet in the closing installments, Nancy becomes the text's principal cadaver: "You look like a corpse come to life

---

70. Brian Cheadle, "*Oliver Twist*," in *A Companion to Charles Dickens*, ed. David Paroissien (Oxford: Blackwell Publishing, 2008), 308–17 (314).

again," observes Sikes (318). She is a very different spectacle, however, from the hallowed body of Oliver:

> It is a common thing for the countenance of the dead, even in that fixed and rigid state, to subside into the long-forgotten expression of sleeping infancy, and settle into the very look of early life; so calm, so peaceful do they grow again, that those who knew them in their happy childhood, kneel by the coffin's side in awe, and see the Angel even upon earth. (185–86)

Compare with Nancy's foresight of her own death:

> "I don't know why it is," said the girl, shuddering, "but I have such a fear and dread upon me to-night that I can hardly stand. [...] Horrible thoughts of death, and shrouds with blood upon them, and a fear that has made me burn as if I was on fire, have been upon me all day. I was reading a book to-night, to wile the time away, and the same things came into the print. (371)

Previously, it was Oliver who was haunted by such visions: in Sowerberry's shop, remember, he was disturbed by "gloomy and death-like" fancies (32), and the pages of *The Newgate Calendar* that Fagin hands him "seemed to turn red with gore" (157). Yet there are key differences between Oliver's and Nancy's embodiments of death. The prostitute's visions of dying are horrible, sanguinary, and corporeal, while the orphan's resemblances to death are angelic and sentimental; whereas he embodies the light of a heavenly view, she represents the grimy and sullied nature of human reality.

The foulest crime in the book and the one that cries out more than any other for retribution is the savage murder of Nancy herself. The beginning of this well-rehearsed sequence begins "two hours before daybreak" (377), a time when rigor mortis seems to hang over the city:

> [It is a] time which, in the autumn of the year, may be truly called the dead of night; when the streets are silent and deserted; when even sounds appear to slumber, and profligacy and riot have staggered home to dream: it was at this still and silent hour, that the Jew sat watching in his old lair, with face so distorted and pale, and eyes so red and bloodshot, that he looked less like a man, than like some hideous phantom moist from the grave, and worried by an evil spirit.
>
> He sat crouching over a cold hearth, wrapped in an old torn coverlet, with his face turned towards a wasting candle that stood upon a table by

his side. His right hand was raised to his lips, and, as absorbed in thought, he bit his long black nails, he disclosed among his toothless gums a few such fangs as should have been a dog's or a rat's. (377–78)

Dickens describes a candle "with a long-burnt wick drooping almost double, and hot grease falling down in clots upon the table" (378). Fagin becomes "a hideous phantom moist from the grave"—an incubus conjured from the pages of a gothic romance with all the added corporeality of a forensic subject. As in death, all movements and processes associated with life are stilled; grave and cadaver imagery run throughout, and the only things that move or develop are the grisly reminders of decomposition: a livorish blackening of Fagin's fingernails, the receding of his rotten gums, and the greasy candle dripping on the table like deliquescing anatomical matter. More importantly, and ironically, the lack of light during the murder (and shortly afterwards) becomes enlightening:

> There was a candle burning, but the man hastily drew it from the candlestick, and hurled it under the grate. Seeing the faint light of early day, without, the girl rose to undraw the curtain.
> "Let it be," said Sikes, thrusting his hand before her. "There's light enough for wot I've got to do." (382)

After Sikes has beaten Nancy to death, there is a break in chapters. Then:

> Of all the bad deeds that, under cover of the darkness, had been committed within wide London's bounds since night hung over it, that was the worst. Of all the horrors that rose with an ill scent upon the morning air, that was the foulest and most cruel.
> The sun,—the bright sun, that brings back, not light alone, but new life, and hope, and freshness to man—burst upon the crowded city in clear and radiant glory. Through costly-coloured glass and paper-mended window, through cathedral dome and rotten crevice, it shed its equal ray. It lighted up the room where the murdered woman lay. It did. He tried to shut it out, but it would stream in. If the sight had been a ghastly one in the dull morning, what was it, now, in all that brilliant light! (384)

Whereas the murder is committed in the obscurity of darkness, the results and the evidence are exposed to a "clear and radiant" light. The image of the sun shedding its glow through a wide and varied range of windows reminds us of the heliocentric characterization of Oliver and the moral-epistemological ideals he embodied. As we have been led to expect in scenarios featuring brilliant light, illumination amounts to some form of restitution through truth, yet this light is linked to two forms of subjectivity: the narrator's self-conscious interpretation of the scene and Sikes's guilt. The glorious sunlight becomes, for Sikes, the source of guilty torment:

> He had not moved; he had been afraid to stir. There had been a moan and motion of the hand; and, with terror added to hate, he had struck and struck again. Once he threw a rug over it; but it was worse to fancy the eyes, and imagine them moving towards him, than to see them glaring upward, as if watching the reflection of the pool of gore that quivered and danced in the sunlight on the ceiling. He had plucked it off again. And there was the body—mere flesh and blood, no more—but such flesh and so much blood! (384)

We might wonder why Dickens adds so much detail about the appearance of Nancy's corpse when the trajectory of the story does not demand it. He could have, for instance, described how "the murderer stagger[ered] backward to the wall, and shutting out the sight [of Nancy] with his hand, seized a heavy club and struck her down" (383) and then moved silently to Sikes's flight. Instead, the novel pauses to provide a vivid and weirdly beautiful portrait of the crime scene. The red blood reflects the sunlight, which then dances on the ceiling in graceful forms. This unexpected moment of "visual" poetry, in an otherwise graphic scene, marks the crime out as a source of "reflection" and interpretation. Dickens links the minutiae of the place to the burgeoning guilt of the murderer, suggesting that it is his (Sikes's) *interpretation* of the sight, not any self-evident truth, which brings the fruits of his violence to harvest.

Sikes becomes plagued by the vision of Nancy's eyes, which, according to Cheadle, are invested with "panoptical power" and "given the full force of retributive justice."[71] I am not sure that *panoptical* is quite the correct term here; like *omniscient* it is a term based on the idea of seeing *all*, whereas Nancy's ghostly eyes see only the guilt of one man. This is an important distinction because it portrays Sikes's punishment as having been brought about by a subjective interpretation. Although much of the novel figures the parish boy as a transcendent embodiment of light, knowledge, and goodness, the darker denouement depicts a man hanged largely by his own thoughts. The ending does not portray a rejection of the idea of

---

71. Cheadle, "*Oliver Twist*," 314–15.

omniscience but offers a picture of how human approximations of moral truth might do the same job.

Although the "great, black, ghastly gallows" cast a shadow over much of *Oliver Twist*, the figures of the legal system are either absent or inadequate. In the chasing of Oliver that follows the pickpocketing of Mr Brownlow, it is the blow of a "lubbering" civilian, not a policeman, that stops the boy (75); in the burglary sequence it is the shot of Mr Giles that immobilizes Oliver; and Mr Fang, the appalling magistrate, shows *his* inadequacy by being prepared to send the orphan to three months of hard labor on the basis of scanty evidence. Yet the most revealing absence of legal intervention occurs after Nancy's murder. Sikes flees the scene and afterwards reads the hue and cry raised in the newspapers. The crowd that eventually pursues him to his death has none of the objective calm and deliberation that, one would hope, the law might use in bringing a murderer to justice:

> There were lights gleaming below, voices in loud and earnest conversation, the tramp of hurried footsteps—endless they seemed in number—crossing the nearest wooden bridge. One man on horseback seemed to be among the crowd; for there was the noise of hoofs rattling on the uneven pavement. The gleam of lights increased; the footsteps came more thickly and noisily on. Then, came a loud knocking at the door, and then a hoarse murmur from such a multitude of angry voices as would have made the boldest quail. [. . .] On pressed the people from the front—on, on, on, in a strong struggling current of angry faces, with here and there a glaring torch to light them up, and shew them out in all their wrath and passion. (411)

The mob carries light with it, which indicates, in accordance with the symbolic use of illumination throughout the novel, that it brings moral truth and restitution. But the torches shed more light on the people themselves than they do upon the object of pursuit. What we see is a chaos of writhing subjectivities: animal rage, passionate feeling, and blind prejudice. It forms a link to the earlier chase scene where Oliver is hunted by a seeming pack of wolves:

> The tradesman leaves his counter, and the carman his wagon; the butcher throws down his tray; the baker his basket; the milk-man his pail; the errand-boy his parcels; the schoolboy his marbles; the paviour his pick-axe; the child his battledore. Away they run, pell-mell, helter-skelter, slap-dash: tearing, yelling, and screaming: knocking down the passengers as they turn

the corners: rousing up the dogs, and astonishing the fowls; and streets, squares, and courts, re-echo with the sound. (74)

Both crowd scenes are examples of Dickens's extraordinary ability to combine style with subject. Describing crazy mobs, the text becomes frenetic: synonym is piled on synonym, and verb follows verb, in hectic velocity. The novel's earlier dream of an absolute truth has disappeared, it seems, along with the dream of a dispassionate method of dealing with crime.

What follows is the account of Sikes's "execution":

> The murderer, looking behind him on the roof, threw his arms above his head, and uttered a yell of terror.
> "The eyes again!" he cried in an unearthly screech.
> Staggering as if struck by lightning, he lost his balance and tumbled over the parapet. The noose was on his neck. It ran up with his weight, tight as a bow-string, and swift as the arrow it speeds. He fell for five-and-thirty feet. There was a sudden jerk, a terrific convulsion of the limbs; and there he hung, with the open knife clenched in his stiffening hand. (412)

The image that gets implanted on the very morning that Sikes sits and contemplates the horrors of his violence plays a central role in bringing the murderer to justice. Nancy's eyes determine how the criminal's subjectivity, like the chaos of the crowd, fulfills the work of the "whole truth." In the text, then, there is a strategy similar to what we perceive in medical jurisprudence where certain truth, an epistemological and moral absolute, is established in order for it to be put beyond the reach of the narrative. What replaces it is not the pessimistic idea that, in the words of Dodger, "This ain't the shop for justice" (356), but rather that "justice" (a concept that both forensic science and *Oliver Twist* tie to "truth") might be furnished by human, rather than godly, perceptions.

OUR MUTUAL FRIEND

If parts of the second half of *Oliver Twist* present us at times with a range of interlinking subjectivities, then *Our Mutual Friend,* a novel "concerned with questions of epistemology,"[72] tests whether it is possible to make sense,

---

72. Hutter, "Dismemberment and Articulation," 135–75 (137).

or get any use, of such subjectivities. Dickens's last completed novel shares medical jurisprudence's tendency to rationalize a form of interpretation that falls short of the "whole truth." In *Charles Dickens: The World of his Novels* (1958), Hillis Miller studies the novel's epistemological aims, noting that "there is no realm of pure spirit or pure freedom":

> *Our Mutual Friend* presents a fully elaborated definition of what it means to be interlaced with the world. [. . .] Character after character is presented living imprisoned in his own nature and in his own milieu. [. . . The novel] apparently differs from its predecessors only that it presents a greater number of characters in terms of the intermingling of their inner natures and outer surroundings. There is no central protagonist in *Our Mutual Friend*.[73]

As there is no "realm of pure spirit or pure freedom" in the novel and "no central protagonist," there can be no fantasy of truth/goodness like what we get in the characterization of the Parish Boy in the first half of *Oliver Twist*. *Our Mutual Friend* presents a world where, if truth-to-nature exists, it is out of the reach of the characters and the narrator; there is no spotless orphan to guide the narrative, no hallowed light, no position of totality. In the words of Nicholas Royle, "*Our Mutual Friend* invites us into the dark, into other scenes of reading, leading us along strange waterways, into the desiccation of headstones and crypts, the silence of the tomb."[74]

Faced with a similar challenge in their (re)presentations of the modern world, writers on medical jurisprudence, as noted above, chose to stress the importance of expert judgment: they suggested that forensic subjectivity—tried and tested knowledge and reflection—was the thing that determined the strength of a forensic view. *Our Mutual Friend* does something very similar. It presents what Hillis Miller calls "a large number of interlocking perspectives on the world, each what [Alfred North] Whitehead would call a special *prehension* of the same totality. But Dickens can never present the totality as it is in itself":

> In the "memorandum book" which Dickens kept between 1855 and 1865, while he was writing, among other novels, *Our Mutual Friend* [. . .], [he] imagines a story "representing London—or Paris, or any other great place—in the new light of being actually unknown to all the people in the story

---

73. Hillis Miller, *Charles Dickens*, 280–81.
74. Nicholas Royle, "Our Mutual Friend," in *Dickens Refigured: Bodies, Desires and other Histories*, ed. John Schad (Manchester: Manchester University Press, 1996), 39–54 (40).

and only taking the colour of their fears and fancies and opinions. So getting a new aspect, and being unlike itself. An *odd* unlikeness of itself."[75]

This passage from Dickens's memorandum book is revealing because of its contradictions. The idea of a place being formed from characters' fears, fancies, and opinions is all about the nature of subjective imposition, but how do we make sense of the oxymoronic "*actually* unknown"? The word *odd* in the final sentence, emphasized by Dickens himself, is surely out of place: how could an "unlikeness" be anything *but* odd in this context? Indeed, words like *unlikeness, unlike,* and *unknown,* similar to that loaded term *unheimliche,* carry a world of meaning because they negate something familiar and certain. In Dickens's memorandum book, these *un*-terms suggest that there *is* a likeness—an accurate form of truth—but the author will concern himself only with modes of knowing that fall short of it. Where my interpretation differs from Hillis Miller's is that I suggest that these "interlocking perspectives" are an idea appropriated from the kinds of sophisticated critical strategies discussed in medical jurisprudence. This is most clear in the fact that when a character's perspective turns out to be accurate or useful in *Our Mutual Friend,* it is analytical; it is concerned with the particular details and telltale signs associated usually with bodies and other "matter." It does not suit the story to have any character build a "high tower in his mind," as Inspector Bucket does in *Bleak House* (1852–53). Instead, truth, signs, and documents have all to be pulled out of the river, read upon the bodies of the dead, or extracted from the middens of modern London.

The character whose work comes closest to that of a forensic examiner in *Our Mutual Friend* is Mr Venus, taxidermist and dealer in "human warious."[76] By his own account, his interpretive skills are "perfect":

> Mr Wegg, not to name myself as a workman without an equal, I've gone on improving myself in my knowledge of Anatomy, till both by sight and by name I'm perfect. Mr Wegg, if you was brought here loose in a bag to be articulated, I'd name your smallest bones blindfold equally with your largest, as fast as I could pick 'em out, and I'd sort 'em all, and sort your wertebrae, in a manner that would equally surprise and charm you. (89)

After he has assisted in the foiling of Wegg, Mr Venus says that "it was his fixed intention to betake himself to the paths of science, and to walk in the

---

75. Hillis Miller, *Charles Dickens,* 291–93.
76. Charles Dickens, *Our Mutual Friend,* ed. Stephen Poole (1864–65; London: Penguin, 1997), 88. Subsequent references to this edition will be given in the body of the text.

same all the days of his life; not dropping down upon his fellow-creatures until they were deceased, and then only to articulate them to the best of his humble ability" (572). The verb *articulate* has two meanings: one being to express oneself, the other to connect (skeletal remains) through artificial joints. Both definitions are appropriate in the context of Venus's science, as he goes about assembling bones with wire and, through that process, is able to speak on the behalf of bodies: he names their bones, small and large.

Reading bodies textually in this way, and articulating the meaning of their clues, is a preoccupation similar to that which occupied forensic experts. Mr Wegg, in attempting to persuade Venus to join him in his search of the dust heaps at Boffin's Bower, makes the connection between his companion's anatomical skills and the search for "justice":

> Mr Wegg then goes on to enlarge upon what throughout has been uppermost in his crafty mind:—the qualifications of Mr Venus for such a search. He expatiates on Mr Venus's patient habits and delicate manipulation; on his skill in piecing little things together; on his knowledge of various tissues and textures; on the likelihood of small indications leading him on to the discovery of great concealments. "While as to myself," says Wegg, "I am not good at it. Whether I gave myself up to prodding, or whether I gave myself up to scooping, I couldn't do it with that delicate touch so as not to show that I was disturbing the mounds. Quite different with YOU, going to work (as YOU would) in the light of a fellow-man, holily pledged in a friendly move to his brother man." [. . .] Lastly, he returns to the cause of the right, gloomily foreshadowing the possibility of something being unearthed to criminate Mr Boffin (of whom he once more candidly admits it cannot be denied that he profits by a murder), and anticipating his denunciation by the friendly movers to avenging justice. (300–301)

These words echo what is written in textbooks like Michael Ryan's, where the skills of the medical man are similarly glorified as a search for moral justice in the signs and stories inscribed on bodies. In "Chambers" (1860), an article Dickens wrote for *All the Year Round*, he made an even more overt link between dust heaps and bodies. Speaking of Gray's Inn, he asks, "Can anything be more dreary than its arid Square, Sahara Desert of the law, [. . .] the dry, hard, *atomy-like* appearance of the whole dust heap?"[77]

---

77. Charles Dickens, "Chambers," *All the Year Round* (18 August 1860), *Journalism* 4: 157–69 (160). Italics added.

The mention of "tissues and textures" in *Our Mutual Friend* is almost certainly a reference to Xavier Bichat, the French anatomist whose theory that in the human body there are a finite number of "tissues" resisting death, stressed "a simplicity of causes reconciled with a multiplicity of effects."[78] In an 1849 letter to Forster, Dickens had complained that medical practitioners have a "miserable folly of looking at one bit of a subject" and "settl[ing] solemnly" on a diagnosis;[79] it was a "folly" that Bichat's insistence on sympathies and shared tissue structures sought to correct by highlighting the interlinking nature of "animal" matter. Venus's "patient habits and delicate manipulation" belong to a follower of Bichat rather than to the "miserable folly of looking at one bit of a subject." Instead of offering an objective view of the whole organism, Bichat's model is all about noticing, in painstaking detail, the *connections* between anatomical components.

Like the wire he uses to articulate his collections of bones, Mr Venus can be found at several of the novel's key joints, overseeing, like medico-legal investigation, the evidentiary signals of human action. Wegg's suggestion that he assist him in rummaging through Old Harmon's dust heaps, for instance, will not be the first time the anatomist has examined the bits and pieces to be found there. He says to Wegg, "The old gentleman wanted to know the nature and worth of everything that was found in the dust; and many's the bone, and feather, and what not, that he's brought to me" (90). It later emerges that Venus was by the riverside on the day the body of Radfoot (mistaken for young John Harmon) was fished out of the Thames. He had been, he says, "looking for parrots" and "a nice pair of rattlesnakes, to articulate for a Museum" (492). Yet it is the greasily lit shop in Clerkenwell that best symbolizes how Venus is in the crux of everything. The setting for a number of key revelations, the shop is described as follows:

> From these, in a narrow and a dirty street devoted to such callings, Mr Wegg selects one dark shop-window with a tallow candle dimly burning in it, surrounded by a muddle of objects vaguely resembling pieces of leather and dry stick, but among which nothing is resolvable into anything distinct, save the candle itself in its old tin candlestick, and two preserved frogs fighting a small-sword duel. Stumping with fresh vigour, he goes in

---

78. Xavier Bichat, *Anatomie Générale: Appliquée à la Physiologie et à la Médecine* (1801), trans. George Hayward as *General Anatomy: Applied to Physiology and Medicine* (Boston: Richardson and Lord, 1822), 11. See Pamela K. Gilbert, *Cholera and Nation: Doctoring the Social Body in Victorian England* (New York: State University of New York Press, 2008), 92.

79. Charles Dickens, letter to John Forster, late August 1849, *Letters* 5, 604–6 (605).

at the dark greasy entry, pushes a little greasy dark reluctant side-door, and follows the door into the little dark greasy shop. It is so dark that nothing can be made out in it, over a little counter, but another tallow candle in another old tin candlestick, close to the face of a man stooping low in a chair. [. . .] But, the little shop is so excessively dark, is stuck so full of black shelves and brackets and nooks and corners, that he sees Mr Venus's cup and saucer only because it is close under the candle, and does not see from what mysterious recess Mr Venus produces another for himself until it is under his nose. (83–84)

The shop has much in common with some of the descriptions we have encountered in the second part of *Oliver Twist*. The idea of everything being obscured, or half peeping out of the darkness, recalls both the central preoccupation of the narrative's exposé and Nancy's spying. However, whereas the earlier text represents epistemological challenges as either obstacles to be overcome or a riddle to be solved, an air of inventive ignorance settles around Venus's shop. "Nothing is resolvable into anything distinct": the light being thrown by a dim candle occasionally illuminates something, but that "something" is barely as enlightening as it is ridiculous or incredible: dueling frogs, a dead bird "drooping on the one side against the rim of Mr Venus's saucer" like a soggy biscuit (84), babies in jars, a half-built Frenchman, and a smiling crocodile. Everything appears to be here, and yet despite the anatomist's confidence in his perceptive abilities, there are indications that Venus's knowledge is no more "perfect" than the next man's:

> Mr Wegg, looking back over his shoulder as he pulls the door open by the strap, notices that the movement so shakes the crazy shop, and so shakes a momentary flare out of the candle, as that the babies—Hindoo, African, and British—the "human warious," the French gentleman, the green glass-eyed cats, the dogs, the ducks, and all the rest of the collection, show for an instant as if paralytically animated; while even poor little Cock Robin at Mr Venus's elbow turns over on his innocent side. (91)

> As the fire cast its flickering gleams here and there upon the dark greasy walls; the Hindoo baby, the African baby, the articulated English baby, the assortment of skulls, and the rest of the collection, came starting to their various stations as if they had all been out, like their master and were punctual in a general *rendezvous* to assist at the secret. (488)

As Nicola Bown has commented, "Mr Venus's shop [. . .] is full of dead things that come back to life";[80] the notion of the objects in the shop being "paralytically animated" is one of those Dickensian oxymorons which indicates that something *is* and *is not* all in the same moment. The glare of the candle and the fire make the objects come alive; it articulates them, renders them objects of knowledge, while simultaneously drawing attention to the darkness—and to the fact that the animation is an illusion. According to Royle, "The singularity of Mr Venus's shop consists in the fact that it does not figure anything: with all its crammed figures and forms of suspended animation and taxidermic productions, it makes the very space of figuration tremble and crack."[81] Indeed, the two key scenes in which Mr Venus's shop is described feature Silas Wegg, a character whose unsettled gaze fits these carnival objects to the illusory action. These descriptions anticipate the famous, hypothetical account in *Middlemarch* (1871–72) of a candle placed in front of a scratched mirror giving an illusion of ordered arrangement and providing a parable of perception as a form of "egoism."[82] The objects in Venus's queer emporium take on life and meaning only when the light of a character's egoism falls upon them. Here "things" conceal as much as they reveal, and they speak in a way that highlights the subjectivity of interpretation. This is not the "whole truth" fantasized about in the law courts, but rather the forensic model of *interpreted* truth. On the characterization of Mr Venus, Albert D. Hutter has said, "He is more than a taxidermist and less than a god; but as a parody of a godlike creator, he fulfils within the novel the function of the artist, of the novelist himself."[83] I agree in the sense that Venus allows the novel to personify one of the major epistemological questions asked at the border between law and medicine and the theme running through the novel: namely, the issue of converting the limits and the reaches of human perception into a reconstructive account. Within Venus's shop we have an entire world: a chaos of moving, speaking, gesturing, and preserved and decaying "warious." Like the dust heaps, the river, and the slum in *Oliver Twist*, it is a repository for society's waste: a place of *both* darkness and potential enlightenment. The light that falls

---

80. Nicola Bown, "What the Alligator Didn't Know: Natural Selection and Love in *Our Mutual Friend*," in *19: Interdisciplinary Studies in the Long Nineteenth-Century* 10 (2010), www.19.bbk.ac.uk [accessed October 2015].
81. Royle, "*Our Mutual Friend*," 51.
82. George Eliot, *Middlemarch*, ed. Rosemary Ashton (1871–72; London: Penguin, 1994), 267.
83. Hutter, "Dismemberment and Articulation," 152.

on Venus's strange objects allows them to come alive, but only in a way that underscores the egoism of the gaze.

Dickens's sense of the challenges of interpretation became less optimistic in the novels that followed his great middle period. Following and including *Bleak House*, the later works show less confidence in the powers of narrative perception and appear to relish the playfulness that a fundamentally flawed subjectivity gives to a story. Take, for example, his representations of the Thames. Always in a "nightmare condition" while it flows through urban areas, the river of *David Copperfield* (1849–50) is a place of both answers and grim suggestion. In the scene where the fallen Martha stands by the riverbank it is written:

> A sluggish ditch deposited its mud at the prison walls. Coarse grass and rank weeds straggled over all the marshy land in the vicinity. In one part, carcases of houses, inauspiciously begun and never finished, rotted away. In another, the ground was cumbered with rusty iron monsters of steam-boilers, wheels, cranks, pipes, furnaces, paddles, anchors, diving-bells, windmill-sails, and I know not what strange objects, accumulated by some speculator, and grovelling in the dust, underneath which—having sunk into the soil of their own weight in wet weather—they had the appearance of vainly trying to hide themselves. [. . .] Slimy gaps and causeways, winding among old wooden piles, with a sickly substance clinging to the latter, like green hair, and the rags of last year's handbills offering rewards for drowned men fluttering above high-water mark, led down through the ooze and slush to the ebb-tide. There was a story that one of the pits dug for the dead in the time of the Great Plague was hereabout; and a blighting influence seemed to have proceeded from it over the whole place. Or else it looked as if it had gradually decomposed into that nightmare condition, out of the overflowings of the polluted stream.[84]

The way in which Dickens lists the objects around the river—"rusty iron monsters of steam-boilers, wheels, cranks, pipes, furnaces, paddles, anchors, diving-bells, windmill-sails"—suggests that a realistic picture is being built up using detail. It is the sort of detailism to be found in the work of Hogarth, or in Théodore Géricault perhaps, where a subject might be grim and nightmarish, but where the stylistic proliferation of "things" adds to an overall sense of verisimilitude. The objects in the *David Copperfield* passage

---

84. Charles Dickens, *David Copperfield*, ed. Malcolm Andrews (1849–50; London: J. M. Dent, 1993), 643.

are noted as having "the appearance of vainly trying to hide themselves," underscoring the perceptive powers of the flâneuristic narrator: nothing escapes him.

When Dickens was about halfway through serializing *Bleak House*, however, he had the idea to write an article about Waterloo Bridge as a popular suicide spot. "Down with the Tide" (1853) has descriptions of the river that are notably different from those that appear in *David Copperfield*:

> Every colour but black seemed to have departed from the world. The air was black, the water was black, the barges and hulks were black, the piles were black, the buildings were black, the shadows were only a deeper shade of black upon a black ground. Here and there, a coal fire in an iron cresset blazed upon a wharf; but one knew that it too had been black a while ago, and would be black again soon. Unfortunate rushes of water suggestive of gurgling and drowning, ghostly rattlings of iron chains, dismal clankings of discordant engines, formed the music that accompanied the dip of our oars and their rattling in the rullocks. Even the noises had a black sound to me—as the trumpet sounded red to the blind man.[85]

Ending with an example of synesthesia from John Locke's *Essay Concerning Human Understanding* (1690), an 1824 edition of which Dickens owned,[86] the passage anticipates the depiction of Venus's shop, whose contents get illuminated, in part, by the flickering of a fire or a candle. It also anticipates "Night Walks" (1860), one of Dickens's papers for *All the Year Round*:

> The river had an awful look, the buildings on the banks were muffled in black shrouds, and the reflected lights seemed to originate deep in the water, as if the spectres of suicides were holding them to show where they went down. The wild moon and clouds were as restless as an evil conscience in a tumbled bed, and the very shadow of the immensity of London seemed to lie oppressively on the river.[87]

---

85. Charles Dickens, "Down with the Tide," *Household Words* (5 February 1853), *Journalism* 3: 113–21 (115).

86. Stonehouse, *Catalogue*, 73. Locke writes: "A studious blind man, who had mightily beat his head about visible objects, and made use of the explication of his books and friends, to understand those names of light and colours which often came in his way, bragged one day, That he now understood what scarlet signified. Upon which, his friend demanding what scarlet was? The blind man answered, It was like the sound of a trumpet." John Locke, *An Essay Concerning Human Understanding*, ed. Roger Woolhouse (1690; London: Penguin, 1997), 127.

87. Charles Dickens, "Night Walks," *All the Year Round* (21 July 1860), *Journalism* 4: 148–57 (151).

There are a number of key similarities between these depictions and the portrait we get of the river in *Our Mutual Friend*. In all there is a link between the water and dead bodies; in the novel no fewer than six carcasses are dredged out of the water—some more dead than others: George Radfoot, Gaffer Hexam, Rogue Riderhood, Eugene Wrayburn, Bradstone Headstone, and, for a second time, Rogue Riderhood. In *Our Mutual Friend*, as well, Dickens describes the Thames as a place "where accumulated scum of humanities seemed to be washed from higher grounds, like so much moral sewage, and be pausing until its own weight forced it over the bank and sunk it into the river" (30). Things appear partially in order to signify the epistemological challenge that the narrator faces in trying to represent a world that furnishes nothing but questions, echoing—as we shall see in the next chapter—the hermeneutic challenges that faced experts in medical jurisprudence during their interpretations of bodies. The references to suicides in the journalistic piece nod toward the forensic activity of recovering and reading bodies. The idea of color having departed from the world, however, implies a lack of specificity—a dark inability to focus, to interpret, and to make realistic representations. Forensic strategies are in place, yet they are to have no easy time of it.

Considering how her father is suspected of the murder of John Harmon, Lizzie Hexam notices that

> as the great black river with its dreary shores was soon lost to her view in the gloom, so, she stood on the river's brink unable to see into the vast blank misery of a life suspected, and fallen away from the good and bad, but knowing that it lay there dim before her, stretching away to the great ocean, Death. (77)

This is one of the moments in the novel where the river comes to symbolize a thwarted wish to know something. The Thames becomes a metonym, not of ignorance, but of the desire to understand things, and the difficulties involved in the same. While the water blackens things, obscures them, keeps their secret, it also yields up clues (like bodies). The opening scene, where Radfoot's cadaver is fished out of the river by Gaffer and his daughter (and is then mistaken for the corpse of John Harmon), creates an atmosphere that "hangs over the whole novel."[88] It features

> a slant of light from the setting sun glanc[ing] into the bottom of the boat, and touching a rotten stain there which bore some resemblance to the

---

88. Hillis Miller, *Charles Dickens*, 316.

outline of a muffled human form, coloured it as though with diluted blood. This caught [Lizzie's] eye, and she shivered. (14)

John R. Reed has suggested that "the narrator gives us a lesson in reading signs and establishes the basis for some of the central themes of the narrative—preying and scavenging, the transformative powers of water, and the contrast of fancy with pragmatic thought." And "while the Gaffer's gaze is utilitarian, Lizzie's is affected by emotion and fancy."[89] Here we perceive the danger of assuming that because something elicits an emotional response, it is the product of emotional thinking. Lizzie's horror at the stain in the bottom of the boat is a rational reaction to a perceived fact. She may not share her father's ruthless entrepreneurship, but she has inherited his ways of looking, interpreting, and gathering meanings. The fact that father and daughter find different meanings and motivations in the river serves to highlight the subjective nature of the knowledge to be obtained from the Thames.

The river, then, offers epistemological challenges, like the dust heaps and Mr Venus's shop.[90] It is there (in the river) that all manner of clues get washed, and the novel frequently establishes encounters between this grand sewer and characters who need to search it. When Gaffer's body is pulled out of the river, the question of how he came to be drowned becomes a forensic one. A police inspector based, in all probability upon a member of the Thames Police whom Dickens had met while writing "Down with the Tide," examines the body: "It was an awful sort of fishing, but it no more disconcerted Mr Inspector than if he had been fishing in a punt on a summer evening by some soothing weir high up the peaceful river" (174). The novel becomes preoccupied with Gaffer's body as a thing to be perceived and interpreted. Notice in the following extract how often the words *see* and *observe(d)* are used:

> "Now see," said Mr Inspector, after mature deliberation: kneeling on one knee beside the body, when they had stood looking down on the drowned man, as he had many a time looked down on many another man: "the way of it was this. Of course you gentlemen hardly failed to observe that he was towing by the neck and arms. [...] And you will have observed before, and you will observe now, that this knot, which was drawn chock-tight round his neck by the strain of his own arms, is a slip-knot": holding it up for demonstration.

---

89. Reed, *Dickens's Hyperrealism*, 87, 86.
90. Karl Ashley Smith notes, "The Thames now becomes a force as powerful as the fog in *Bleak House* to blur all proper categories of things." Smith, *Dickens and the Unreal City*, 169.

> "Plain enough.
>
> "Likewise you will have observed how he had run the other end of this rope to his boat. [. . .] Now see," said Mr Inspector, "see how it works round upon him. It's a wild tempestuous evening when this man that was," stooping to wipe some hailstones out of his hair with an end of his own drowned jacket, "—there! Now he's more like himself; though he's badly bruised,—when this man that was, rows out upon the river on his usual lay." (175)

We have a number of indications that Mr Inspector's interpretation is, after all, just an interpretation. The notion of Gaffer appearing as himself but badly bruised reminds us of the remains of Elizabeth Reid, whose bruises were mistaken for livor mortis (or livor mistaken for bruises; we can never know which). The inspector concludes that Gaffer, reaching for a dead body in the water, must have fallen in the river and gotten tangled in his own rope (a fate similar to Sikes's). The inspector also points to that classic forensic clue, the clenched fist, as an indication that the man died for the sake of a few pieces of silver in a drowned man's pocket: "'How do I make that out?' he asks triumphantly. 'Simple and satisfactory. Because he's got it here.' The lecturer held up the tightly clenched right hand" (177).

In spite of such evidence, the text situates the inspector's interpretations within a world where certainty is unlikely: this is a world of a thousand possible meanings, where no single standard of truth might be trusted. We are reminded of this fact when John Harmon describes the discovery of Radfoot's corpse, also taken out of the river:

> I examined the newspapers every day for tidings that I was missing, but saw none. Going out that night to walk (for I kept retired while it was light), I found a crowd assembled round a placard posted at Whitehall. It described myself, John Harmon, as found dead and mutilated in the river under circumstances of strong suspicion, described my dress, described the papers in my pockets, and stated where I was lying for recognition. [. . .] I perceived that Radfoot had been murdered by some unknown hands for the money for which he would have murdered me, and that probably we had both been shot into the river from the same dark place into the same dark tide, when the stream ran deep and strong. (365–66)

The mistaken interpretation of Radfoot's remains is an indication, put simply, that things are not always what they seem. The use of the word *dark* reminds us of the water as observed by the Hexams plus the black river of

"Down with the Tide." The free indirect discourse, which blends Harmon's internal monologue with the text's main revelation, highlights how there is nothing outside interpretation: no method of knowing, apparently, that may be termed the "whole truth." This key chapter, often discussed as the novel's best success or its worst failure, is a moment where the lessons of the river, the dust heaps, and Venus's shop blend with the style of the novel. Hutter observes that

> when Dickens reveals to his readers, less than halfway through the novel, that Handford, Harmon and Rokesmith are one and the same, he does so in a passage remarkable not for revelation but for revelation undercut by a simultaneous vision of chaos, of the failure of memory, of nightmare, of entrapment in an urban maze.[91]

Hutter is correct to indicate that revelation, though undercut, is still possible in this chapter; yet I would invert his "vision of chaos" to "chaos of vision" to suggest that revelation is not *threatened* by chaos in these scenes but is assisted in the sense that subjectivity—or the nightmares, visions, and bad memories of the mind—build *some* form of knowledge and representation.

Before Harmon thinks out the inward soliloquy that reveals the mystery of his disappearance, he takes a stroll by Limehouse Church, trying to remember the events of the night he was robbed:

> The wind was blowing so hard when the visitor came out at the shop-door into the darkness and dirt of Limehouse Hole, that it almost blew him in again. Doors were slamming violently, lamps were flickering or blown out, signs were rocking in their frames, the water of the kennels, wind-dispersed, flew about in drops like rain. (359)

We note, once again, the flickering illumination that Dickens uses to symbolize partial knowledge elsewhere in the text. The "signs" rocking in their frames also give an impression of an unsteady relationship between interpretation and interpreted and lead to a narrative sense of disorientation:

> Indifferent to the weather, and even preferring it to better weather for its clearance of the streets, the man looked about him with a scrutinizing glance. "Thus much I know," he murmured. "I have never been here since

---

91. Hutter, "Dismemberment and Articulation," 158.

that night, and never was here before that night, but thus much I recognize. I wonder which way did we take when we came out of that shop. We turned to the right as I have turned, but I can recall no more. Did we go by this alley? Or down that little lane?" (ibid.)

The context for Harmon's revelation is as much about remembering as it is about forgetting. Rather than providing a scene in which complete ignorance frustrates, the novel focuses on what Harmon *does* know and what he *can* recognize:

He tried both [directions], but both confused him equally, and he came straying back to the same spot. "I remember there were poles pushed out of upper windows on which clothes were drying, and I remember a low public-house, and the sound flowing down a narrow passage belonging to it of the scraping of a fiddle and the shuffling of feet. But here are all these things in the lane, and here are all these things in the alley. And I have nothing else in my mind but a wall, a dark doorway, a flight of stairs, and a room." (Ibid.)

What Harmon does or does not know depends on his ability to make sense of the details around him: drying clothes, a low public house, the shuffling of feet, and so on. He calls his memories "sick and deranged impressions [. . . with] spaces between them" and "not pervaded by any idea of time" (362). He knows that his perception cannot be trusted entirely; memories sometimes mislead, and interpretations are flawed. Yet the novel continues to orchestrate an extraordinary picture of London through Harmon's mind: "the great iron gate of the churchyard" leads to "a high tower spectrally resisting the wind," "white tombstones, like [. . .] the dead in their winding-sheets," and "nine tolls [from] the clock-bell" (360). This London is, as Harmon himself points out, "the fanciful side of the situation." It has "a real side," he thinks; however, "Don't evade it, John Harmon; think it out!" (360).

Harmon's subjectivity is creative in the sense that it makes details, geographies, and histories subjects that may be thought out, worked through, and interpreted rather than simply known. This crystallizes a strategy the novel has for presenting the London streets, as well as its river, as an enigma: "such a black shrill city, combining the qualities of a smoky house and a scolding wife; such a gritty city; such a hopeless city, with no rent in the leaden canopy of its sky; such a beleaguered city" (147). There is, once again, a synesthetic combination of sights and sounds; obscurity seems to be the "hopeless" keynote. Compare with the churchyards described in "The City of the Absent" (1863), a sketch that Dickens published in *All the Year Round*:

> Such strange churchyards hide in the City of London; churchyards sometimes so entirely detached from churches, always so pressed upon by houses; so small, so rank, so silent, so forgotten, except by the few people who ever look down into them from their smoky windows. As I stand peeping in though the iron gates and rails, I can peel the rusty metal off, like bark from an old tree. [. . .] I look in at the rails and meditate [. . .].[92]

The scene is designed for interpretation: Dickens peeps and he meditates, but what he sees has lost any wholly "true" meaning: a churchyard without a church, man-made rails that peel like tree bark. Analogy, often used by Dickens as a means of explaining himself further, now seems to move the object of interpretation away from its "real" purpose. In *Oliver Twist*, London's darkness gets illuminated by the Parish Boy, the character who is compared to light and all that is good. In later writings the narrator seems to revel in the city's obscurity. In the following extract from *Our Mutual Friend* a corporeal metaphor is used to construct a London that is both "visible and invisible," managing to be "wholly neither":

> It was a foggy day in London, and the fog was heavy and dark. Animate London, with smarting eyes and irritated lungs, was blinking, wheezing, and choking; inanimate London was a sooty spectre, divided in purpose between being visible and invisible, and so being wholly neither. Gaslights flared in the shops with a haggard and unblest air, as knowing themselves to be night-creatures that had no business abroad under the sun; while the sun itself when it was for a few moments dimly indicated through circling eddies of fog, showed as if it had gone out and were collapsing flat and cold. [. . .] From any point of the high ridge of land northward, it might have been discerned that the loftiest buildings made an occasional struggle to get their heads above the foggy sea, and especially that the great dome of Saint Paul's seemed to die hard; but this was not perceivable in the streets at their feet, where the whole metropolis was a heap of vapour charged with muffled sound of wheels, and enfolding a gigantic catarrh. (417)

Whereas the fog in *Bleak House* is used to open possibilities for differing interpretive methodologies, as we shall see, there is a sense in *Our Mutual Friend* that any strategies to know are strangled by their limitations. In Elliotson's description of Pall Mall, gas lamps are symbols of brilliant

---

92. Charles Dickens, "The City of the Absent," *All the Year Round* (18 July 1863), *Journalism* 4: 260–69 (262).

illumination, but in this passage they "have no business" in the novel's dark world. The gigantic catarrh, an image of sick corporeality, keeps everything weighed down to human level; nothing rises to a standard of wholeness, though the dome of St. Paul's makes a valiant attempt at transcendence. *Catarrh*, an inflammation of the mucus membrane, reminds us of the anatomical materiality of *Our Mutual Friend*'s London. In the context of a foggy day, where signs mislead and meaning cannot be pinned down, the word also sounds like *cataract*—opacity of vision. In her fine essay "Omniscience in *Our Mutual Friend*" (1987), Audrey Jaffe notes that "this novel is [. . .] wonderful for the relativity of its truths—the absence of a fixed center or omniscient overseer."[93] Yet, she continues, "the novel traces a pattern of epistemological one-upmanship [. . .]. The easily identifiable omniscient voice may have disappeared, but concern with omniscience has not."[94] It is a point supported by a thought of Reverend Frank Milvey's in *Our Mutual Friend*: "He only learned that the more he knew, in his little limited human way, the better he could distantly imagine what Omniscience might know" (327), which is itself an echo of Oesterlen's view that omniscience is a useful *aspiration* rather than something that might be achieved. The only way to be responsive to "real life" (as either a perception or a representation) is to accept one's inevitable limitations and make the best of one's powers of interpretation.

Hence descriptions of London as "hopeless," choking, blind, and lost give some impression that any project based on the "whole truth" is a doomed one; yet, as Jaffe points out, the quest for omniscience, or—as I choose to see it—the impulse to interpret, is never abandoned by *Our Mutual Friend*. Instead, the novel reminds us of "the potential depth of our insecurity—the possible existence, always, of knowledge we haven't got."[95] It also reminds us of the knowledge that we *can* get: of the power of interpretation. And this corresponds with the idea we see, explored in medical jurisprudence and in *Oliver Twist*, that while one can never hope to capture absolute truth, limited, self-aware, and self-distrusting truth is a powerful compromise.

The sacrifice that *Our Mutual Friend* has to make in its representation of a bleak world of catarrh is the sense of a fundamental link between the far-off light of truth and goodness. In the novel several characters appropriate the skills of specialist interpretation (Bradley Headstone, Jenny Wren, Fascination Fledgeby, the Lammles), and not all of them are

---

93. Jaffe, "Omniscience," 91–101 (94).
94. Ibid.
95. Ibid., 97.

working toward the sense of right. Rogue Riderhood, for instance, is perhaps the best example of a man whose subjectivity is not out of synchronicity with his ability to adopt analytical strategies. While working at Plashwater Weir Mill Lock, he works out that Bradley Headstone is intent on killing Eugene Wrayburn and on framing him (Riderhood) for the offense. The deductions he makes remind us of the analytical work of the forensic expert and that which is undertaken by the inspector when Gaffer Hexam is pulled out of the water:

> [Riderhood] rose and looked at [Headstone] close, in the bright daylight, on every side, with great minuteness. He went out to his Lock to sum up what he had seen.
> "One of his sleeves is tore right away below the elber, and the t'other's had a good rip at the shoulder. He's been hung on to, pretty tight, for his shirt's all tore out of the neck-gathers. He's been in the glass and he's been in the water. And he's spotted, and I know with what, and with whose. Hooroar!" (686)

> Rogue Riderhood had been busy with the river that day. He had fished with assiduity on the previous evening, but the light was short, and he had fished unsuccessfully. He had fished again that day with better luck, and had carried his fish home to Plashwater Weir Mill Lock-house, in a bundle. (696)

That bundle is the clothing that Headstone wore on the night he attacked Wrayburn. It is the evidence that will incriminate him, but—unlike forensic examiners whose work, ideally, aided the law in bringing the guilty to justice and in exonerating the innocent—Riderhood's examinations are performed only to exhort money from the murderer. It highlights how truth garnered from the world of humans will always risk being tainted by human motivations. All the more need, then, for a forensic scrutiny of the investigative process.

CHAPTER 3

BODIES
Early Journalism and *Bleak House*

COMBUSTING MR KROOK

The famous disagreement that Dickens had with G. H. Lewes over the combustion of Mr Krook indicates that the author not only shared forensic medicine's distrust of the "absolute truth" but also believed that the kind of positivism preached by Lewes and his circle was in danger of reproducing the pernicious effects of taking evidence at face value. Despite appealing to the research of a number of medical authorities in his discussions of spontaneous combustion and his representation of Krook's demise,[1] Dickens himself leaned most heavily on Robert MacNish's *The Anatomy of Drunkenness* (1827), an 1840 edition of which he owned at the time of his death.[2]

---

1. Altogether, Dickens referenced the works of François-Emmanuel Fodéré, Theodric Romeyn Beck, Charles Marc, John Paris, and Anthony Fonblanque.

2. Stonehouse, *Catalogue*, 77. MacNish's textbook harvested most of its examples from an article by Pierre-Aime Lair titled "On the Combustion of the Human Body, produced by the long and immoderate Use of Spiritual Liquors," in *The Philosophical Magazine* 5 (1800): 133–46. That Dickens took his examples from MacNish is clear from the way he reproduces the latter's errors. In referring to "Mere" in *Bleak House* (425), Dickens means Charles Marc, the forensic analyst who first attributed spontaneous combustion to the build-up of inflammable gases in the gut. In *The Anatomy of Drunkenness*, MacNish made the same error. In a response to G. H. Lewes's criticism of the credibility of combustion, Dickens urged him to read the 1773 edition of *The Annual Register*, which, he thought, contained the account of Mary Clues's death by spontaneous combustion. That account actually appears in the 1775 edition of *The Annual Register*. This inaccuracy can also be traced to MacNish. See Robert MacNish, *The Anatomy of Drunkenness* (1827; Philadelphia: Carey, Lea and Carey, 1828), 141, 143.

MacNish avoided committing to any overt belief in the reality of spontaneous combustion, noting that "all [...] cases rest on vague report, and are unsupported by such evidence as would warrant us in placing much reliance upon them"; the same cases "wear, unquestionably, the aspect of fiction; and are, notwithstanding, repeated from so many quarters, that it is nearly as difficult to doubt them altogether as to give them our entire belief."[3] MacNish's opinions encapsulate the kind of conflict that fueled mid-century debates over spontaneous combustion: on the one hand, there was a lack of hard evidence (any "facts" that did exist were purely circumstantial or anecdotal), yet the numbers of learned people willing to testify to the existence of the phenomenon carried obvious weight—even among men of science. There was a disparity between proofs that might be used for a reliable, positivist deduction and the clues that might be used for interpretation. Indeed, MacNish's *Anatomy*'s main source of information, an article by the French agronomist Pierre-Aime Lair, adopts a position of skepticism-made-fuzzy by the many case histories that make it difficult to discredit the phenomenon entirely:

> I confess that at first they appeared to me worthy of very little credit, but they are presented to the public as true by men whose veracity seems unquestionable. Bianchini, Massei, Rolli, Le Cat, Vicq-d'Azyr, and several men distinguished by their learning, have given certain testimony of the facts. [...] This collection of instances is supported [...] by all those authentic proofs which can be required to form human testimony; for, while we admit the prudent doubt of Descartes, we ought to reject the universal doubt of the Pyrrhonists. The multiplicity and uniformity even of these facts, which occurred in different places, and were attested by so many enlightened men, carry with them conviction.[4]

It was not just the *amount* of "human testimony" that favored the existence of spontaneous combustion but also the "enlightened" nature of those who swore by it. Such was the tenor of Dickens's defense of Krook's conflagration in *Bleak House* (1852–53), which he makes strongly in the thirty-third chapter of the novel:

> Out of the court, and a long way out of it, there is considerable excitement too; for men of science and philosophy come to look, and carriages set

---

3. MacNish, *Anatomy*, 146–47.
4. Lair, "Combustion," 132.

down doctors at the corner who arrive with the same intent, and there is more learned talk about inflammable gases and phosphuretted hydrogen than the court has ever imagined. Some of these authorities (of course the wisest) hold with indignation that the deceased had no business to die in the alleged manner; and being reminded by other authorities of a certain inquiry into the evidence of such deaths, reprinted in the sixth volume of the Philosophical Transactions [Lair]; and also of a book not quite unknown, on English Medical Jurisprudence [Paris and Fonblanque]; and likely the Italian case of the Countess Cornelia Baudi [sic Bandi], as set forth in detail by one Bianchini, prebendary of Verona, who wrote a scholarly work or so, and was occasionally heard of in his time as having gleams of reason in him; and also of the testimony of Messrs Foderé and Mere [sic Foderé and Marc], two pestilent Frenchmen who *would* investigate the subject; and further, of the corroborative testimony of Monsieur Le Cat, a rather celebrated French surgeon once upon a time, who had the unpoliteness to live in a house where such a case occurred, and even to write an account of it;—still they regard the late Mr Krook's obstinacy, in going out of the world by such any such by-way, as wholly unjustifiable and personally offensive.[5]

At the point of writing this defense, Dickens had received criticism from Lewes who had suggested in *The Leader* that the author had no business dispatching one of his characters in such an incredible way. Writing about what could be scientifically refuted was, according to Lewes, a mark of bad fiction. At the time, he was in the throes of his passion for Auguste Comte's positivism, and he was encouraging Marian Evans to write her masterpiece *Adam Bede* in the realist mode. In "Realism in Art: Recent German Fiction" (1858), an article penned for the *Westminster Review*, he observed:

> Realism is thus the basis of all Art, and its antithesis is not Idealism, but *Falsism*. When our painters represent peasants with regular features and irreproachable linen; when their milkmaids have the air of Keepsake beauties, whose costume is picturesque, and never old or dirty; when Hodge is made to speak fine sentiments in unexceptional English, and children utter long speeches of religious and poetic enthusiasm; when the conversation of the parlour and drawing-room is a succession of philosophical remarks, expressed with great clearness and logic, an attempt is made to idealize,

---

5. Charles Dickens, *Bleak House*, ed. Andrew Sanders (1852–53; London: J. M. Dent, 1994), 424–45. Subsequent references to this edition will be given in the body of the text.

but the result is simply falsification and bad art. [. . .] Either give us true peasants, or leave them untouched; either paint no drapery at all, or paint it with the utmost fidelity; either keep your people silent, or make them speak the idiom of their class.[6]

Unwittingly similar to Gradgrind's "one thing needful" sermon, "Realism in Art" is one of a number of pieces in which Lewes argued for "utmost fidelity" in literary representation. It should come as no surprise, then, that he disliked the way Mr Krook was dispatched. "As a novelist," he conceded, Dickens "is not to be called to the bar of science," yet his representation of spontaneous combustion "is a fault in Art, and a fault in Literature, overstepping the limits of Fiction, and giving currency to vulgar error."[7] The phenomenon is a spurious one, he complains, because it is decidedly "unscientific." In a book published the same year that the volume edition of *Bleak House* appeared, Lewes stated, "Science is a knowledge of the laws of nature. This knowledge is the only rational basis of man's action on nature."[8] Hence,

> even supposing [. . .] clairvoyance and Spontaneous Combustion to be scientific truths, and not the errors of imperfect science, still the simple fact that they belong to the extremely questionable opinions held by a very small minority, is enough to render their introduction into Fiction a mistake. They are questions to be argued, not to be treated as ascertained truths.[9]

The problem with Krook's combustion, apart from its alleged impossibility in chemico-physiological terms, is that its evidence is composed entirely of "questionable opinions" rather than "observations and classifications."

Dickens took advantage of the nature of serial publication to respond to Lewes's *Leader* piece in the subsequent number of *Bleak House* by parodying the "men of science and philosophy" who have "come to look" at Krook's remains. "Humorous," Lewes responded soon after in *The Leader*, "but not convincing!"[10] Lewes took this new opportunity to go through the

---

6. Quoted in Rosemary Ashton, *G. H. Lewes: A Life* (Oxford: Oxford University Press, 1991), 191–92.

7. George Henry Lewes, "Literature," *The Leader* (11 December 1852): 1189.

8. George Henry Lewes, *Comte's Philosophy of the Sciences: Being an Exposition of the Principles of the* Cours de Philosophie Positive *of Auguste Comte* (London: Henry G. Bohn, 1853), 41.

9. Lewes, "Literature," 1189.

10. George Henry Lewes, "Spontaneous Combustion: Two Letters to Charles Dickens," *The Leader* (5 and 12 February 1853): 137–38; 161–63 (137).

problems with Dickens's sources, focusing mainly on the fact that his key references were anecdotal. Addressing Dickens openly, he said:

> I have [. . .] become aware of a serious fact,—viz., that the belief is very current among medical men, and has grace authorities to support it. [. . .] It is due to you that I should declare a large majority on your side. Works on medical jurisprudence, Dictionaries, and Encyclopædias, lend the theory their authority. Medical men frequently adopt it. So that you, not specially engaged in any subjects of this nature, may well be excused for having adopted it.[11]

Lewes's patronizing tone is likely to have offended Dickens, who in *Bleak House* had made a point of showing that his research had been thorough. What is more, Lewes set about teaching Dickens the principles of "proper science" (an area in which he himself would be taken to task by T. H. Huxley in 1854[12]):

> What are medical dictionaries and works on jurisprudence compared with the authorities of such commanding eminence as LIEBIG, BISCHOFF, REGNAULT, GRAHAM, HOFMANN, and OWEN? [. . .] When I mentioned the subject to Professor GRAHAM, the other evening, he replied, "*There is no more completely exploded error in chemistry*. It has been carefully examined, and found to have no vestige of probability." [. . .] In the last edition of his *Letters on Chemistry* [1843], Liebig devotes a chapter to this subject.

Justus von Liebig, pioneer of laboratory chemistry, is then quoted as follows:

> The distinct and unhesitating way in which, in many works on medical jurisprudence, the known cases are related and the different theories of spontaneous combustion are explained, has had the bad effect of inducing many well-formed practical physicians, contrary to their better conviction, to allow spontaneous combustion to pass for established truth, and not to contradict the statements and opinions of the supporters of that theory, in order to avoid being regarded as heretics of medicine.[13]

---

11. Ibid., 137.
12. Huxley noted in the *Westminster Review* that the mistakes in Lewes's scientific writings were due to the fact that the latter was "without the discipline and knowledge which result from being a worker" as opposed to someone with "mere book-knowledge." Quoted in Ashton, *G. H. Lewes*, 146.
13. Lewes, "Spontaneous Combustion," 137. Italics in original.

The circulation of combustion stories had allowed an error to preponderate, according to Liebig, a view upheld by Lewes with positivist enthusiasm: "I have attentively read about forty cases [. . . and] there is not one which carries with it the evidence necessary to shake a skeptic. It is miserable stuff for the most part, to be thrown into the lumber room with witchcraft evidence."[14] He concludes:

> Let us not deceive ourselves respecting the value of reported cases. You, Dickens, would not believe a whole neighbourhood of respectable witnesses who should declare that the lamp-post had been converted, by a flash of lightning, into an elm tree. No, not if they swore to having *seen* it. Why? Simply because you would rather believe these witnesses in error than disbelieve the millions of testimonies *implied* in the establishment of those scientific truths which contradict such a transmutation.[15]

Anecdotal testimony is imperfect, according to Lewes, even when it comes from respectable sources. Scientific truths like those developed in the laboratories of men like Liebig are worth a million such stories.[16]

Part of Dickens's response, as we have seen, was to underscore the amount of research he had done on spontaneous combustion which, all things considered, was likely to have been exaggerated.[17] Possibly feeling that the bonds of their friendship were under some strain, Dickens replied in a private letter to Lewes, insisting that he had "looked into a number of books, with great care, expressly to learn what the truth was. I examined the subject as a judge might have done. And without laying down any law upon the case, I placed the evidence impartially before myself, the Jury, as I will place it before you."[18] His reference to what a judge might have done is incredibly revealing. Aware that in *Bleak House* and in *Household Words* he had attacked the "barbarous custom" of legal precedent, Dickens avoids the idea of his judgment having binding potential, yet he believes in a legal model that, by 1853, had learned to value the testimonies and opinions of specialists. No less obsessed with "the whole truth" than science, the

---

14. Ibid.

15. Ibid., 138.

16. Liebig himself was once called to testify in a case following the death of the Countess of Gorlitz. According to an early biographer, Liebig "demonstrated the complete absence of any real evidence in support of its truth." See William Ashwell Shenstone, *Justus von Liebig, His Life and Work (1803–1873)* (London, Paris, New York, Melbourne: Cassell, 1901), 189–91.

17. See Peter Denman, "Krook's Death and Dickens's Authorities, *The Dickensian* 82 (1986): 131–41.

18. Charles Dickens, letter to G. H. Lewes, 25 February 1853, *Letters* 7, 28–31 (29).

legal system, as it had been shaped by the rise of medical jurisprudence, suggested that it was possible to get to an approximate version of the truth through the interpretive talents of the expert witness. What may seem surprising about Dickens's responses to Lewes, given what we know of his love of the "romantic side of familiar things," is how he does not insist on the need for portraying "lumber-room" fairytales in fiction, nor, as Daniel Hack suggests, does he sidestep Lewes's challenge "by emphasizing the episode's allegorical function."[19] Instead, he chooses to underscore the reliability of his sources by insisting on the importance of specialist interpretation. In his private letter to Lewes, he holds steadfastly to the belief in spontaneous combustion as a "fact" suggested by "scientific evidence":

> Liebig is a great man, deserving of all possible respect, and receiving no greater deference from any one than from me. But I cannot set his opinion—his mere opinion and argument—against full scientific evidence of a fact. That evidence appears to me to exist, on the subject of what is called (rightly or wrongly) spontaneous combustion. If I take anything on evidence, I must take that. I have the greatest regard for, and admiration of, Owen. But if I had such evidence of the existence of a Sea Serpent as I have of cases similar to Krook's, I could not for a moment set even his ingenious argument against such human experience.[20]

For all the powers of his laboratory, Liebig is, after all, a man with "mere opinion and argument" like any other. Lewes appears to have forgotten that scientific knowledge, gained through "human experience," is necessarily restricted by human limitations, and, more importantly, testimony has as much value, certainly in a legal setting, as hard evidence. In the preface to the volume edition of *Bleak House* Dickens stipulates, more publicly, that "before I wrote that description" of Krook's death, "I took pains to investigate the subject." By his own account he encountered

> about thirty cases on record, of which the most famous, that of the Countess Cornelia de Bandi Cesanate, was minutely investigated and described by Giuseppe Bianchini. [. . .] The next most famous instance happened at

---

19. Hack, "Sublimation Strange," 129–56 (135). James Mussell has pointed out quite recently that "for both Dickens and Lewes science was an important instrument in establishing the probability of phenomena, fictional or non-fictional, but their conceptions of what constituted science were different. See "Science," in *Charles Dickens in Context*, ed. Sally Ledger and Holly Furneaux (Cambridge: Cambridge University Press, 2011), 326–33 (331).

20. Dickens, letter to Lewes, 25 February 1853, 28.

Rheims, six years earlier; and the historian in that case is LE CAT, one of the most renowned surgeons produced by France. (xlii)

He goes on to underscore the reliability of Bianchini and Le Cat: "I shall not," he notes, "abandon the facts until there shall have been a considerable Spontaneous Combustion of the testimony on which human occurrences are usually received" (xlii), a sentiment that backs up something he wrote in his letter to Lewes:

> The question is a question of evidence. Have people been found almost consumed when there were no external agencies by which they could have been reduced to that state? If so, have there usually (not without exception, but usually) been pervading circumstances of age, sex, or previous habits, or all three, suggesting the presence of pretty uniform conditions, essential to the extraordinary law (extraordinary that is to say, within our small experience) governing such cases?[21]

At first glance, it appears as though Dickens relies upon a popular idea of "common sense" here: the truth of spontaneous combustion appears self-evident. Yet he is careful to enumerate his sources, all of which, he urges, are credible and lead to one pregnant "fact": that spontaneous combustion is a "truth" supported by authoritative testimony: "I champion no hypothetical explanation of the fact," he says, "but I take the fact upon the testimony, which I considered quite impartially and with no preconceived opinion."[22] In measuring his forms of evidence against those of Lewes, he made the claim that informed testimony is as viable, if not more so, than chemical and physiological proofs. As we shall see, he had the weight of forensic theory and court decree to back him up on this broader point.

Dickens's sources, Bianchini and Le Cat especially, are given credence by the author, not because they offer material suitable for "an author of emotion, sentimental throughout,"[23] nor because the "romantic" appeal' of spontaneous combustion spoke to Dickens more than "trifling doubts as to scientific veracity,"[24] but rather because they reveal how expert nar-

---

21. Dickens, letter to Lewes, 25 February 1853, 29.
22. Ibid., 31.
23. Gordon Haight explained the differences between the two men by suggesting "Dickens was a man of emotion, sentimental throughout; Lewes was a man of intellect, philosophical and scientific." See Gordon S. Haight, "Dickens and Lewes," *PMLA* 71:1 (March 1956): 166–79 (166–67)
24. Winyard and Furneaux, "Dickens, Science and the Victorian Literary Imagination," www.19.bbk.ac.uk [accessed October 2015].

ration furnishes a valuable, alternative interpretative system to Lewes's positivism. In *The Annual Register*'s account of the death of the Countess Cornelia Bandi, the discovery of the woman's remains had been outlined by Bianchini with a clear attention to detail:

> At the distance of four feet from the bed was a heap of ashes, in which could be distinguished the legs and arms untouched. Between the legs lay the head, the brain on which, together with half the posterior part of the cranium, and the whole chin, had been consumed: three fingers were found in the state of a coal; the rest of the body was reduced to ashes, which, when touched, left on the fingers a fat, fœtid moisture. A small lamp which stood on the floor was covered with ashes, and contained no oil; the tallow of two candles was melted on a table, but the wicks still remained, and the feet of the candlesticks were covered with a certain moisture. The bed was not damaged; the bed-clothes and coverlid were raised up and thrown on one side, as is the case when a person gets up. The furniture and tapestry were covered with a moist kind of soot of the colour of ashes, which had penetrated into the drawers and dirtied the linen.[25]

It is worth noticing how an opportunity for a sermon on the deleterious effects of alcohol is not taken up by Bianchini or by *The Annual Register*. Avoiding any mention of the alleged links between drinking and combusting, the account describes the Countess's remains using the unobtrusive testimony of an expert.

Similarly, in Le Cat's account of the case he witnessed, details are presented in such a way that the reader must do his or her own sermonizing, should he or she feel that way inclined:

> Having spent several months at Rheims in the years 1724 and 1725, I lodged at the house of Sieur Millet, whose wife got intoxicated every day. [. . .] This woman was found consumed on the 20th of February 1725, at the distance of a foot and a half from the hearth in her kitchen. A part of the head only, with a portion of the lower extremities and a few of the vertebræ, had escaped combustion. A foot and a half of the flooring under the body had been consumed, but a kneading-through and a powdering-tub, which were very near the body, had sustained no injury. M. Chretien, a surgeon, examined the remains of the body with every juridical formality.[26]

---

25. Quoted in Lair, "Combustion," 133–34.
26. Quoted in ibid., 136–37.

In his preface, Dickens appropriates legal language to say that "the appearances beyond all rational doubt observed in [these cases] are the appearances observed in Mr Krook's case" (xlii). And, indeed, they have much in common with the demise of the rag and bottle merchant. Offering no "moral" commentary beyond that supplied by the trajectory of Krook's story, *Bleak House*'s appropriation of the details of Bianchini and Le Cat highlights how the particulars of those cases are open, like all details, to a process of interpretation:

> Mr Guppy takes the light. They go down, more dead than alive, and holding one another, push open the door of the back shop. The cat has retreated close to it, and stands snarling—not at them; at something on the ground, before the fire. There is a very little fire left in the grate, but there is a smouldering suffocating vapour in the room, and a dark greasy coating on the walls and ceiling. The chairs and table, and the bottle so rarely absent from the table, all stand as usual. [. . .] Here is a small burnt patch of flooring; here is the tinder from a little bundle of burnt paper, but not so light as usual, seeming to be steeped in something; and here is—is the cinder of a small charred and broken log of wood sprinkled with white ashes, or is it coal? O Horror, he IS here! and this from which we run away, striking out the light and overturning one another into the street, is all that represents him. (414)

As in Bianchini and Le Cat, unsparing detail is considered crucial to the outline of a "true" account, but so too is the perspective of the witnesses. For example, the present tense of *Bleak House*'s narrative encourages the reader to take the journey of discovery with Guppy and Weevle: observations are made, one by one, until the grim detection of Krook's remains completes the process. In a letter responding to Lewes's criticism in *The Leader*, one correspondent named George Redford defended Dickens on the basis that a phenomenological interpretation of detail, though he does not call it such, is a more powerful mode of investigation than the sort of analyses undertaken by scientists. Addressing Lewes, he observes:

> The universal affection of our race for the supernatural, the love of a miracle, the determination to hunt up mysteries and try to solve them, is not a bad tendency. When not counterpoised by the "positive" temperament, by a wholesome resolve to apply the two and two make four principle to everything, we get all the metaphysical vagaries about "vital force," "mental principle," and the "vis medicatrix naturæ"; yet it is the same disposition

that leads the most positive of the scientific to be always treading upon the confines of knowledge, hovering between the known and the unknown, led captive by the charm of mystery. It is when the qualities of the hodman are combined with the forecast of the speculator that any territory is reclaimed.[27]

Redford has an idea of science in which speculation and uncertainty are crucial to the process of knowing; he believes that the positivist qualities of "two and two make four" must be supplemented with curiosity in order for any "territory to be reclaimed." In Dickens's outline of spontaneous combustion, the relationship between certainty and speculation is a much tighter analysis of the same question. The episode is not, as Jude V. Nixon has suggested, "one of the few poor lights in which Dickens is seen in relation to science"[28] but an indication of how, in line with forensic ideas, Dickens believed in a sort of realism that laid out its evidence so that it might be examined like it would be in a court of law. His interpretations seem to be unwilling to abandon themselves to what they find: they turn ideas and images over and over in order to inspect their details and contradictions.

THE STREETS OF LONDON

It is no coincidence that Dickens is most overt in his discussions of truth and testimony when he is talking about a body (in this case Mr Krook's combusted body). Garnered in large part from medical jurisprudence, ideas of bodies as unruly, unstable, and misleading are a vital part of Dickens's sense of realism. We can see as much when we look at what is traditionally seen to be his greatest series of successes in the realist mode: namely, his representation of the city streets.[29] On the earliest of his works John Forster noted:

---

27. George Redford, letter to *The Leader*, 26 March 1853, 303–5.
28. Jude V. Nixon, ""Lost in the Vast Worlds of Wonder": Dickens and Science," *Dickens Studies Annual* 35 (2005): 267–333 (277).
29. Forster, *Life*, vol. 1, 17. Texts that have insisted on Dickens's realism have been matched in number by those insisting on the lack of realism in the same works. George Eliot famously complained in *The Westminster Review* that the melodrama of his characters got in the way of his texts' verisimilitude. C. P. Snow hesitated over whether to include Dickens in *The Realists* (1978) because "he is only realistic occasionally" (9). Although Peter Brooks's treatment of Dickens's realism is a good deal more thoughtful than Snow's, he admits, "I am of course not sure that it is right to talk about Dickens in the context of realism at all, since so much of Dickens appears as the avoidance or suppression of realism" (40). See George Eliot, "The Natural History of German Life," *Westminster Review* 66 (1856): (51–79); C. P. Snow, *The Realists: Portraits of Eight Novelists*

The observation shown throughout is nothing short of wonderful. Things are painted literally as they are. [. . .] It was a picture of everyday London at its best and worse, in its humours and enjoyments as well as its suffering and sins, pervaded everywhere not only with the absolute reality of the things depicted, but also with that subtle sense of mastery of feeling which gives to the reader's sympathies invariably right direction, and awakens consideration, tenderness and kindness precisely for those who most need such help.[30]

Sir Arthur Helps, speaking of Dickens just after his death, said, "His powers of observation were almost unrivalled [. . .]. Indeed, I have said to myself when I have been with him, he sees and observes nine facts for any two that I see and observe";[31] Helps's friend G. H. Lewes overlooked his usual ambivalences toward Dickens's work to note in his journal of 1861 that "no one has ever combined the niceties of observation, [. . .] the perception of character, and accuracy of description, with the same force that he has done."[32] George Levine, more recently, has observed in *Darwin and the Novelists* (1988) that "Dickens begins his career as a reporter whose skills are based on his powers of observation, with an uncanny eye for the ordinary. In his eyes the ordinary is transformed, not by miraculous or catastrophic intrusions, but by intense and minute perception."[33] And Robert Douglas-Fairhurst adds that "there is very little Boz does not know by sight. He can retrieve whole biographies at a glance. [. . .] No object is free from the force of [his] curiosity [. . .]. Boz's eyes waste nothing."[34]

Yet while it is widely acknowledged that Dickens aimed to present an accurate picture of city life in his works, he is known also to have been

---

(London: Macmillan, 1978); and Peter Brooks, *Realist Vision* (New Haven: Yale University Press, 2005).

30. Forster, *Life*, vol. 1, 70.

31. Quoted in Frank T. Marzials, *Life of Charles Dickens* (London: Walter Scott, 1887), 32.

32. Quoted in Ashton, *G. H. Lewes*, 24–25. In "Dickens in Relation to Criticism," published two years after the death of Dickens, Lewes famously noted that "Dickens sees and feels, but the logic of feeling seems the only logic he can manage. Thought is strangely absent from his works" and "keenly as he observes the objects before him, he never connects his observations into a general expression, never seems interested in general relations of things" (quoted in ibid., 257). Ashton is correct, in my view, in that Dickens suffered in Lewes's account because his style was compared to that of George Eliot. Despite their disagreements over spontaneous combustion in the 1850s, and despite Lewes's unchanging impression that Dickens was not a man of sophisticated intellect, the men remained on good terms, the former admitting, later in life, that he had learned a great deal from the accounts of dreams he had heard in person from Dickens.

33. George Levine, *Darwin and the Novelists*, 131–32.

34. Robert Douglas-Fairhurst, *Becoming Dickens: The Invention of a Novelist* (Cambridge, MA: Belknap Press of Harvard University Press, 2011), 154–55.

attracted to the idea of demystifying scenes that had become too familiar to his readers. As I discussed in the previous chapter, he had a unique skill of making his narratives go astray; the world of certain and absolute knowledge was not his world. His works became preoccupied with chaos, ugliness, and uncertainty. Writing on the art of Lucien Freud, Peter Brooks notes that "the ugly is often used [. . .] as a call to attention: look, see. [. . .] The discovery of the ugly is part of the process of disillusioning in which realism deals."[35] If we substitute the word *ugly* for *grotesque* and call up the work of Michael Hollington, we note that the same applies to the realness of Dickens's London. Grotesquery involves the "'making strange' of the familiar world that may serve to renew and radicalize automatic or stereotyped perception of reality."[36] Yet, developed early in the author's career, the obsession with London as a thing of real and ugly details is about much more than a drive to confront readers with the squalors they had chosen to ignore. In addition to what some critics have identified as Dickens's use of figurative, metaphoric, and spiritual language to describe the city,[37] he was preoccupied with the tangible, corporealized details of the same. Dickens medicalized London so that he could lead his narratives astray and underscore, in the same process, how looking at the real city involved an exploration of what it means to interpret. Dickens's realism knew, through its links with medical jurisprudence, how a human view is only ever a partial one. The author did have an extraordinary eye for the realities of London, but this was due, in no small part, to his appropriations of the technique of forensic science. The crucial evidence in support of this point is Dickens's corporealization of the city and his determination to undercut the realist possibilities of his own interpretations by imposing overt elements of fiction.

This is an investigation that ought to begin with early journalism. In a sketch that first appeared in the *Evening Chronicle* in 1835, for instance, the following comparison is made between Greenwich Fair and the sick body:

> If the parks be "the lungs of London," we wonder that Greenwich Fair is—a periodical breaking out, we suppose, a sort of spring-rash: a three days' fever, which cools the blood for six months afterwards, and at the

---

35. Brooks, *Realist Vision*, 8.
36. Michael Hollington, *Dickens and the Grotesque* (London: Croom Helm, 1984), 11.
37. See Efraim Sicher, *Rereading the City, Rereading Dickens: Representation, the Novel, and Urban Realism* (New York: AMS, 2003); Robert Alter, *Imagined Cities: Urban Experience and the Language of the Novel* (New Haven, CT: Yale University Press, 2005); and Smith, *Dickens and the Unreal City*.

expiration of which London is restored to its old habits of plodding industry, as suddenly and completely as if nothing had ever happened to disturb them.[38]

What Dickens portrays here is an "ordinary" London disturbed and thrown into a state of unease by the breaking out of the springtime rash called Greenwich Fair. His physiological metaphors capture a sense of disrupted regularity: the "old habits of plodding industry" pulsate like a beating heart or a pair of lungs, yet these usual movements are interrupted by the springtime event.

In another sketch the contents of a pawnbroker's shop are itemized minutely: "a flute, complete with the exception of the middle joint; a pair of curling-irons; and a tinder-box. In front of the shop window are ranged some half-dozen high-backed chairs, with spinal complaints and wasted legs."[39] Edgar Allan Poe noticed this sketch as one of Boz's finest and drew attention to the way in which it "engages and enchains our attention." Using bodily imagery we can all relate to, it has us "enveloped," according to Poe, "in its atmosphere of wretchedness and extortion."[40] The objects described by Dickens, "rags and bones," "labelled separately, like the insects in the British Museum,"[41] are to be found in a "squalid neighbourhood," where there are also "adjoining houses, straggling, sunken, and rotten, with one or two filthy, unwholesome-looking heads, thrust out of every window, and old red pans and stunted plants exposed on the tottering parapets."[42] None of the objects described may be termed *healthy*: flutes have missing joints like broken fingers; buildings totter, sag, and sink like bodies racked by disease; and high-backed chairs have fractured spines. In such images of sickness and disfigurement the young journalist develops a method of describing the city that he would continue using throughout his career: the imposition of corporeal metaphors befuddles as much as it immerses us in the real world. Little wonder, then, that London is associated with the dead—not with ghosts or other spiritual figures necessarily—but with cold and rigid bodies similar to the one he encounters in the Paris Morgue.

---

38. Charles Dickens, "Greenwich Fair," *Evening Chronicle* (16 April 1835), *Journalism* 1: 112–19 (112).

39. Charles Dickens, "Brokers' and Marine-store Shops," *Morning Chronicle* (15 December 1834), *Journalism* 1: 176–79 (177).

40. Edgar Allan Poe, "Watkins Tottle," in *The Fall of the House of Usher and Other Writings*, ed. David Galloway (London: Penguin, 1984), 361–63 (363).

41. Dickens, "Brokers' and Marine-store Shops," 178; and Dickens, "The Pawnbroker's Shop," *Evening Chronicle* (30 June 1835), *Journalism* 1: 186–93 (188).

42. Ibid.

As has been noted by Pamela K. Gilbert, Dickens responded to professional attempts to explain the metropolis by "using medical knowledge to create a poetics of the city which allowed for a particular kind of bildungsroman to be mapped onto London's 'body.'"[43] What I add is that this corporealization of London allowed Dickens to adopt analytical methods similar to those developed through autopsies; like his medical counterparts, his aim was to transform his subject into a system of clues and symbols, yet, like the dead body, the city was as misleading as it was edifying.

In 1761 the Italian anatomist Giovanni Battista Morgagni published *The Seats and Causes of Disease Investigated by Anatomy*. Translated into English eight years later, the text contained "seven hundred case reports with a detailed clinical history followed by a report of the pathology found at autopsy." According to Hector O. Ventura, "One can first witness [in Morgagni] the meticulous clinical description of a disease process [in] correlation with anatomo-pathological findings."[44] Following John Hunter's popularization of Morgagni's methods through the practice of autopsy,[45] the perception of the corpse as a thing that might hold a number of details about life, death, and everything in between became a fairly established idea. In 1832, for instance, the *London Medical Gazette* noted that

> in the darkness of the grave we are taught to behold the brightness of futurity; and in the passive structure of the corpse, we are led to discover the active mechanism of life in all its functions. [. . .] In exploring the dead body, the anatomist is in pursuit of truth, and is perpetually endeavouring to ascend from death to life, from the mere organism of matter to the laws which govern matter itself when alive. [. . .] From the filthiness of death, he learns the excellence of life; he unfolds the nice inter-dependence of different organs; he traces throughout every part the slender rudiments of minute anatomy.[46]

This author would find himself contradicted by a growing number of physiologists who held the opposing view that *life* provided more enlightenment

---

43. Gilbert, *Mapping*, xviii.
44. Hector O. Ventura, "Giovanni Battista Morgagni and the Foundation of Modern Medicine," *Clinical Cardiology* 23 (2000): 792–94.
45. Hunter's "expertise in post-mortems was in regular demand, and he became the central figure in the gradual acceptance of autopsy investigations." Moore, *The Knife Man*, 232.
46. "Mediculus," "Dissection Viewed with reference to the Resurrection," letter to the editor, *London Medical Gazette* (25 February 1832): 789–91 (790).

(through vivisection mainly) than analyses of the dead.[47] Yet he expects, in accordance with the ideas of Morgagni, that cadavers will yield truths to an explorative gaze. "Death is more interesting than life," he insists.

Thus, at the time Dickens started writing in the 1830s dead bodies had developed new identities as objects to be interpreted; the young author established a technique for comparing the city's features with the characteristics of a dead body. In "The Streets—Morning," for example, a sketch that originally appeared in *The Evening Chronicle* of 1835, he writes:

> The appearance presented by the streets of London an hour before sunrise, on a summer's morning, is most striking [. . .]. There is an air of cold, solitary desolation about the noiseless streets which we are accustomed to see thronged at other times by a busy, eager crowd [. . .]. The drunken, the dissipated, and the wretched have disappeared; the more soberly and orderly part of the population have not yet awakened to the labours of the day, and the stillness of death is over the streets; its very hue seems to be imparted to them, cold and lifeless as they look in the grey, sombre light of daybreak.[48]

In setting up his portrait of London through the figure of the observer, Dickens presents the deathly hues of the city as something that requires experienced observation. The illustration that George Cruikshank supplied for the 1836 volume edition of *Sketches by Boz* (figure 3.1), which Dickens would have overseen and commented on, portrays the streets and their inhabitants as objects to be examined: a policeman in the background watches three figures who occupy the foreground, presaging the function that would be served by Dickens's urban inspector Mr Bucket. Taking up, according to Jeremy Tambling, "a position of surveillance,"[49] the sketch's policeman reminds us that the streets are a visual phenomenon: a place where a guide might be needed for the impulse to know. Also prominent are the street lamps that cast an unforgiving light over the streets—providing enlightenment and performing the work that the rising sun (referred to in a pub sign) has yet to do. Indeed, the lights and the spectator illustrate how observing the streets, the *dead* streets, is an activity for which Dickens has some empirical interest. In his journalism, he is trying detailed methods

---

47. In 1865, for instance, Claude Bernard noted that "vivisection is only an autopsy on the living. [. . .] To know something about the functions of life, you must study them in the living." Bernard, *Introduction*, 104, 108.

48. Charles Dickens, "The Streets—Morning," *Evening Chronicle* (21 July 1835), *Journalism* 1: 49–54 (49).

49. Jeremy Tambling, *Going Astray: Dickens and London* (Harlow: Pearson, 2009), 40.

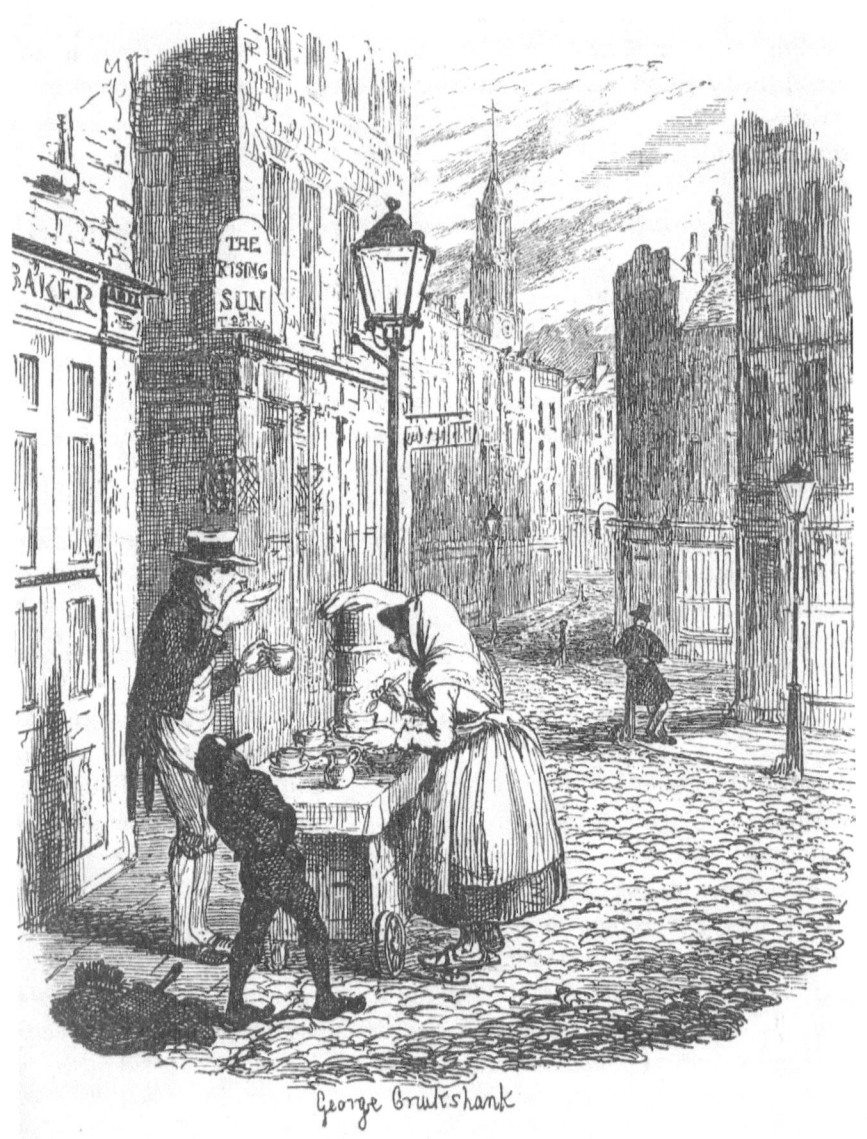

FIGURE 3.1. "The Streets—Morning," *Sketches by Boz* (1836)

of reconstruction similar to those that characterized morbid anatomy. Boz notices signs and objects and sets himself the task of interpreting them using a range of analogies and techniques that the new culture of medical jurisprudence has opened up for him.

The streets of London, then, become medico-textual: like bodies, they bear some of the marks that medical examiners were urged to interpret. The first step, according to John Gordon Smith, was determining whether a body was alive or dead. His *Principles of Forensic Medicine, Systematically Arranged and Applied to British Practice* (1821) said of death:

> This state of the *human* body, for we speak of that only, is characterized (where no mechanical impediment exists) by the prostrate posture; absence of pulsation in the arteries, and stoppage of circulation in the veins; cessation of respiration; paleness or lividity of the surface and of the countenance, the latter ghastly; insensibility of all the parts; and coldness, accompanied by rigidity of the muscles.[50]

These characteristics are mirrored by the stillness with which Dickens portrays the London streets in "The Streets—Morning." In that sketch's description of the urban environment, the circulations and movements of everyday life are suspended, and, though his report is made during summer, the city is said to feel cold. When this coldness occurs alongside an apparent "arrest" of activity in the body's vital functions, it is one of the key signals that death has taken place, and, according to forensic experts, the cadaver soon enters into a state of rigor mortis.

RIGOR MORTIS

Cadaveric rigidity, as the process was more frequently understood in the age of Dickens, was, according to medical textbooks, a transformation that virtually froze the body in the position it held at the time of death. As Smith commented:

> Cessation of circulation and respiration, coldness combined with rigidity of the limbs, though not of themselves absolute proofs of death, amount when combined to very strong evidence. The stiffness of the limbs has been

---

50. John Gordon Smith, *The Principles of Forensic Medicine, Systematically Arranged and Applied to British Practice* (London: Thomas and George Underwood, 1821), 17. Italics in original.

observed to commence at a very early period, even before warmth has been diminished. [... This] stiffness is of greater importance. As long as the limbs retain their flexibility, the fact of death may in general be doubted, although in some particular cases they may continue to do so, even until putrefaction comes on, to place everything beyond a doubt.[51]

The process of rigor mortis was believed to benefit legal investigation because it preserved the bodies of murder victims in the active moment of dying. In the words of Robert L. Grimes, used in a different context, "to die is not to become powerless but to become powerful in a fixed mode."[52] In rigidifying, the cadaver became a "thing" that might be scrutinized, read, and evaluated. The process became, in the words of Suzy Anger, "interpretative[,] and [it] involve[ed] sign systems in ways that [...] closely replicate[d] nineteenth-century debates over textual interpretation."[53] It was even claimed that some corpses retained the facial expressions they wore at the time of death or, through the rigidification of their muscles, held tightly to the objects they grasped at the fatal moment. Smith noted:

> Where dirt, sand, &c. are found under the nails, or any substance likely to have been grasped in the water is discovered in the hand, it will be a strong inducement to believe that the person died in the water. [...] Not so certain are the means of discriminating between the event of a person having been forced into the water by others, and that of having thrown himself in. [...] Incidental circumstances may clear up the subject—as the marks of footsteps, &c. about the margin of the water; substances being found grasped in the hands of the deceased, that have been evidently laid hold of which making resistance.[54]

At the 1835 trial of Robert Reid physiologist John Fletcher testified that "we know that the features of the face often retain, till putrefaction supervenes, the expression of the last mental emotion; that in cases of death from cholera, the contractions of the extremities are often equally permanent."[55] If a body is found with an expression of terror on its countenance, specialists claimed that it was likely that the individual died by foul means.

---

51. Ibid., 26–27.
52. Richard L. Grimes, "Masking: Towards a Phenomenology of Exteriorization" (1975), quoted in Timothy Clark, "Dickens through Blanchot: The Nightmare Fascination of a World without Interiority," in *Dickens Refigured*, ed. Schad, 22–38 (29).
53. Anger, *Victorian Interpretation*, 87.
54. Smith, *Principles of Forensic Medicine*, 213, 215.
55. Quoted in Ryan, *Manual*, 495.

Similarly, if a corpse is dredged from the bottom of a river and is found to be holding a clump of grass from the riverbank, it may be deduced that the victim had made an attempt to avoid entering the water. It may be, also, that the corpse holds part of the murderer's clothing or hair. Before the days of photography the dead body seemed to become, in itself, a snapshot of the violence enacted upon it.

Forensic medicine and photography have always had much in common, and Ronald R. Thomas draws parallels between Dickens's work and the development of the latter.[56] On the broader question of Dickens's urban descriptions, Deborah Epstein Nord suggests that the author was faced with the ambitious task of seeing, and effectively recording, "everyday life and everyday people," and he planned to fix scenes that were ever-changing and bewildering:

> He focuses on one place and represents it as it changes, indeed, in the very process of change. Dickens turns the camera on and keeps it running, hoping to capture movement, above all, and to show how a variety of types occupy the same urban space. [. . .] Boz transforms the sketch, then, by mining the past, catching the city in the process of change.[57]

Hillis Miller expresses a similar idea when he says that "there appears the motif of the 'progress' frozen into a series of juxtaposed vignettes,"[58] and Murray Baumgarten adds that "Dickens's illustrations resemble the moving image of the diorama and Panorama shows that were the buzz of London in the 1840s and 50s."[59] These visual analogies might be supplemented with a medical one: Dickens appears to reproduce, through style and content, ideas of petrification, change, and decay—ideas that, at this time, were expressed through a predominantly medical vocabulary. Dickens's urban descriptions work like motion pictures, certainly, because they arrange a series of "stills" in order to give the overall illusion of action; yet attempts

---

56. Thomas, for instance, links *Bleak House* with the rise of forensic photography in *Detective Fiction*, 131–49.

57. Epstein Nord, *Walking*, 61.

58. J. Hillis Miller, "The Fiction of Realism: *Sketches by Boz, Oliver Twist*, and Cruikshank's Illustrations" (1971), repr. as "J. Hillis Miller on the Fiction of Realism," in *Realism*, ed. Lillian R. Furst (London and New York: Longman, 1992), 287–318 (301). Amanpal Garcha's work on sketch literature in the nineteenth century adds that "Dickens's long descriptions capture a scene at a particular moment; they tend to freeze time and stop objects' spatial movement in order to represent surroundings in great detail." See Amanpal Garcha, *From Sketch to Novel: The Development of Victorian Fiction* (Cambridge: Cambridge University Press, 2009), 123.

59. Murray Baumgarten, "Reading Dickens Writing London," *Partial Answers* 9:2 (2011): 219–31 (220).

to record and reorder stillness as a means of understanding movement and change is a scheme that also preoccupied medico-legal experts. As we perceive in the comments of Smith, on the subject of determining whether a person is dead or not, one of the principal objectives of medical jurisprudence was to understand the "living" act of crime by studying a frozen moment captured in the stillness of death.

Although to all appearances a corpse is an object of immobility and rigidity, death to the medical establishment was a process of transition. On a physical level, the body decays: "Putrefaction undergoes a train of varieties in its progress," wrote one forensic expert;[60] yet on a more figurative level, the body represents no moment of repose. "These attitudes," wrote Alfred Swaine Taylor in his *Principles and Practice of Medical Jurisprudence* (1865), are "not those of the relaxation of death, but rather of a seemingly active character, the muscles remaining rigid and inflexible as the result of spasmodic muscular action in the last moment of life."[61] Such references to movement and change indicate how medical writings shared with Dickens's urban descriptions an acknowledgment of the way ordinary sense perception may go astray when it comes to reading the signs of death. Medical authors suggested that the dead, like Dickens's London, could not be evaluated using the assumption that "the physical objects which we commonly perceive are, in a sense to be explained, directly 'given to us.'"[62] Although men of science had a sense of rigor mortis as a thing that might be looked to as an indicator of various things, they also knew that, in some cases, the body bore little resemblance to the way it looked in life. For the moment we shall discount all of the physical changes that may be brought about by *mode* of death (such as bloating after drowning and blackening after burning) and focus instead on the ways in which the "ordinary" effects of death change a body's appearance even before the disfigurements of putrefaction set in. In a book owned by Dickens, James Harrison wrote, with some ostentation:

> There is nothing more appalling and humiliating than the decomposition of the dead [. . .]; when changes manifest themselves, and we can no longer

---

60. Ryan, *Manual*, 500.
61. Taylor, *Medical Jurisprudence*, vol. 1, 59.
62. A. J. Ayer, *The Problem of Knowledge: An Enquiry into the Main Philosophical Problems that enter into the Theory of Knowledge* (London: Penguin Books, 1956), 79. Tambling has noted in *Going Astray* that "writing about [the city], or about the self formed by it, is like describing death, the unknowable. Writing the city becomes a form of 'going astray,' taking the writer from his knowledge" (35).

recognise the familiar features we have so often looked upon, we see the greatness of that alteration, and feel what it is to die.

Shall we "look upon those lips that we have kissed we know not how oft," pale, cold, and repulsive, and not experience the immensity of the change![63]

Alfred Swaine Taylor noted, with a little more gravity:

> As rigidity manifests itself, there is sometimes a remarkable change of expression. The face is pale or sallow, the jaws are fixed, the corners of the mouth are drawn downwards, the temples sunk, and the brow contracted. Even those who have known a person well during life, would scarcely recognise him at this time, were they to see the body in a strange locality.[64]

In an article that appeared in *All the Year Round* in 1861, it was reported:

> A resurrection-man was found guilty of raising the body of a young woman buried at Stirling. The body was identified by her relations, not only by the features, but by the fact of one leg being shorter than the other. But it was afterwards shown that, although the man really had lifted the body at Stirling, the body identified by the relations was that of another young woman taken out of the churchyard at Falkirk, and she also, besides the general resemblance, had one leg shorter than the other.[65]

There is a complex point behind this ironic notion of a body and its features being no necessary indication of identity. In the words of Ellen Samuels and Samira Kawash, there is a "simultaneous reliance upon and undermining of the visual knowability of bodily identity, the haunting 'possibility that the body, which is meant to reflect transparently its inner truth, may in fact be misrepresentation.'"[66] In her discussion of Dickens's trip to the Paris Morgue, Bianca Tredennick calls the "enigmatic smirking corpse" seen by Dickens there "a completely opaque image, resisting and mocking any effort to make it meaningful." Bodies, she adds, "invite and resist comprehension, as Dickens soon finds."[67]

---

63. Harrison, *Medical Aspects of Death* (Longman et al., 1853), 19–20.
64. Taylor, *Medical Jurisprudence*, vol. 1, 57.
65. Unsigned, "Medical Nuts to Crack," *All the Year Round* (6 July 1861): 358–60 (359).
66. Ellen Samuels, *Fantasies of Identification: Disability, Gender, Race* (New York: New York University Press, 2014), 17. Samuels quotes from p. 132 of Samira Kawash, *Dislocating the Color Line: Identity, Hybridity, and Singularity in African-American Narrative* (Stanford, CA: Stanford University Press, 1997).
67. Tredennick, "Some Collections," 72–88 (79, 74).

In forensic texts, observing things "literally as they are" is never a straightforward process when it comes to the dead, but this is not, in itself, reason to give up on the analytical powers of the medical approach. Rather, the dead body, like the obscurity of Mr Venus's shop, is a reminder that human prehension is a partial one. The thing needed, according to forensic experts, was a willingness to think critically about the evidence of one's senses—especially when those senses get challenged by the ambiguities of death. The "morbid appearances" of bodies, noted Alexander Thomson in his forensic lectures, "are not more to be relied upon than [. . .] general symptoms during life" which should lead the expert "to be more than usually cautious in conducting his inspections; not to be hurried away in forming his conclusions; to be particularly guarded in drawing inferences from striking appearances."[68]

SIGNS: CORPOREAL AND SARTORIAL

The body belonging to the eponymous character in "The Drunkard's Death" (1836), a short story Dickens wrote to flesh out the collection *Sketches by Boz*, shows a relatively straightforward relationship between signifier and signified:

> His dress was slovenly and disordered, his face inflamed, his eyes bloodshot and heavy. He had been summoned from some wild debauch to the bed of sorrow and death [his wife's demise]. He rushed from the house, and walked swiftly through the streets. Remorse, fear, shame, all crowded on his mind. Stupefied with drink, and bewildered with the scene he had just witnessed, he re-entered the tavern he had quitted shortly before. Glass succeeded glass. His blood mounted, and his brain whirled round.[69]

In spite of its melodrama, the passage, as Kostas Makras has noted, is "remarkably similar to several case studies recorded by the early nineteenth-century medical profession."[70] The Drunk's dissolutions are written indelibly upon his anatomy: the inflammation of the face, the

---

68. Thomson, "Lectures on Medical Jurisprudence: Lecture 1," 65–70 (70).

69. Charles Dickens, "The Drunkard's Death," *Sketches by Boz* (1836), *Journalism* 1: 463–72 (464).

70. Kostas Makras, "Dickensian Intemperance: The Representation of the Drunkard in 'The Drunkard's Death' and '*The Pickwick Papers*,'" in *19: Interdisciplinary Studies of the Long Nineteenth Century*, 10 (2010), www.19.bbk.ac.uk [accessed October 2015].

bloodshot eyes, and the whirling blood are all marks of the man's weaknesses. This is also a story that anticipates a key sequence in *Oliver Twist* (1837–38). As when Sikes is haunted by the image of Nancy's eyes, the Drunkard has to endure "the eyes so soon to be closed in death rested on his face," which cause him to shake "beneath their gaze."[71] These eyes, like Nancy's, have the determination of forensic analysis: they place the guilty at the point of an intense and inescapable surveillance, and they concentrate on his face—the part of his anatomy that best registers his history of sin.

In a scene that rehearses the death of Quilp in *The Old Curiosity Shop* (1840–41), the Drunkard eventually drowns in the Thames. Dickens outlines the drowning with relentless detail:

> Bright flames of fire shot up from earth to heaven, and reeled before his eyes, while the water thundered in his ears, and stunned him with its furious roar.
>
> A week afterwards the body was washed ashore, some miles down the river, a swollen and disfigured mass. Unrecognized and unpitied, it was borne to the grave; and there it has long since mouldered away![72]

This episode forms the conclusion of a rather unsettling story that is remarkably accurate in terms of what the period understood about drowning. Alfred Swaine Taylor outlined the case of a woman who was found drowned in 1845:

> A woman, in full health, was observed to be intoxicated on the banks of a river, about one hour before her body was discovered in shallow water [. . .]. The face was swollen, and of a mottled purple colour. [. . .] The arms and thighs presented patches of discoloration, and small quantity of whitish froth issued from the mouth [. . .]. All parts of the lungs were gorged with blood, and were much heavier and of a darker red colour than in the normal state.[73]

In the postmortem appearances of people found drowned, Taylor observes, blood is often congested in the brain, which explains why Dickens's Drunkard senses flashing lights and rushing sounds. Furthermore, in the "normal" process of putrefaction, the body fills with gas and, if submerged, will resurface. John Gordon Smith wrote:

---

71. Ibid.
72. Ibid., 472.
73. Taylor, *Medical Jurisprudence*, vol. 2, 15.

The truth is that a person, whether dead or alive, when first thrown into the water, will sink, unless buoyed up by external aid; but after the process of putrefaction has occasioned the evolution of a sufficient portion of gaseous matter, to render the body specifically lighter than the water, it will rise to the surface; which is a phenomenon familiar enough to vulgar observation.[74]

The face, he adds, will be unrecognizable because it will be purple, swollen, and livid; in the panic of drowning, the individual will swallow water, which the medical examiner should be able to discover when he dissects the stomach. It is fitting, however, that the Drunkard, like the intoxicated woman described by Taylor, should die as he does. Addicted to drink in life, he is forced to drink a less palatable liquid on the brink of death. Rendered swollen and purple by the pathological functioning of his alcoholic body, he eventually exhibits the same appearances when fished out of the river.

"The Drunkard's Death" has a relatively simple idea of what the relationship is between the body's signs and the truth. Like forensic scientists, Dickens had an interest in retelling histories from the evidence provided by marked bodies, and that process, in "The Drunkard's Death,'" seems as simple as translating one language into another. Yet in other early pieces Dickens explores the problems of linking the evidences of bodies with the imposed interpretations that experience might seem to demand. In "Meditations in Monmouth Street" (*The Morning Chronicle*, 1836), for instance, Dickens considers the human habits that threaten to deform any translations of anatomical markings. It was a sketch inspired by Thomas Carlyle's *Sartor Resartus* (1833–34), a book that featured similar "Meditations among the Clothes-shops"[75] and that exhibits the sort of interplay between "fact" and "fancy" that would characterize Dickens's works. Like Carlyle's Professor Teufelsdröckh, the narrator of the Dickens article finds himself obsessed with wonder in a world of details:

> We love to walk among these extensive groves of the illustrious dead, and to indulge in the speculations to which they give rise; now fitting a deceased coat, then a dead pair of trousers, and anon the mortal remains of a gaudy waistcoat, upon some being of our own conjuring up, and endeavouring, from the shape and fashion of the garment itself, to bring its former owner before our mind's eye. [. . .] There was the man's whole life written

---

74. Smith, *Principles of Forensic Medicine*, 211.
75. Thomas Carlyle, *Sartor Resartus: The Life and Opinions of Herr Teufelsdröckh* (1833–34; London: Routledge, n.d.), 252.

as legibly on these clothes, as if we had his autobiography engrossed on parchment before us.[76]

Like Carlyle, Dickens converts secondhand clothes into the "mortal remains" of their former owners. Teufelsdröckh admits:

> With awe-struck heart I walk through that Monmouth Street, with its empty Suits, as through a Sanhedrim of stainless Ghosts. Silent are they, but expressive in their silence: the past witnesses and instruments of Woe and Joy, of Passions, Virtues, Crimes and all the fathomless tumult of Good and Evil in "the Prison men call Life."[77]

Clothing and corpses amount to the same thing; a man's autobiography may be written on his garments, as it might also be written on his anatomy. Like the inebriate's countenance in "The Drunkard's Death," the description of a boy's set of clothing in Dickens's sketch uncovers a great deal about its former owner:

> This was the boy's dress. It had belonged to a town boy, we could see; there was a shortness about the legs and arms of the suit; and a bagging at the knees, peculiar to the rising youth of London streets. A small day-school he had been at, evidently. If it had been a regular boys' school they wouldn't have let him play on the floor so much, and rub his knees so white. He had an indulgent mother too, and plenty of halfpence, as the numerous smears of some sticky substance about the pockets, and just below the chin, which even the salesman's skill could not succeed in disguising, sufficiently betokened.[78]

With use of analytical tools that would match those of any scientist, the author combines a sensitive knowledge of London with a forensic capacity for noticing small clues. According to Levine, "All things imply histories but hide their pasts. [. . .] The mysteries of the ordinary are only there for those who, like the readers of Dickens's novels, have been taught to look for clues."[79] The sketch discovers how unnatural modes of living appear to stunt the growth of urban children—a theme that would be returned to

---

76. Charles Dickens, "Meditations in Monmouth Street," *The Morning Chronicle* (11 October 1836), *Journalism* 1: 76–82 (76–78).
77. Carlyle, *Sartor Resartus*, 250.
78. Dickens, "Meditations," 78.
79. Levine, *Darwin and the Novelists*, 135–36.

in the characterizations of Amy Dorrit, Fagin's boys, and Jenny Wren. The boy's suit with the baggy knees "grows" into several other articles of dress which tell tales of drunkenness, profligacy, and sin:

> We saw the bare and miserable room, destitute of furniture, crowded with his wife and children, pale, hungry, and emaciated; the man cursing their lamentations, staggering to the tap-room, from whence he had just returned, followed by his wife and a sickly infant, clamouring for bread; and heard the street wrangle and the noisy recrimination that his striking her occasioned. And then imagination led us to some metropolitan workhouse, situated in the midst of crowded streets and alleys, filled with noxious vapours, and ringing with boisterous cries, where an old and feeble woman, imploring pardon for her son, lay dying in a close dark room, with no child to clasp her hand, and no pure air from heaven to fan her brow. [...] We had no clue to the end of the tale; but it was easy to guess its termination.[80]

Like forensic specialists, the narrator believes in the analytical power of observing physical clues (the beginning of the above citation with "we saw" hints at some kind of relationship between perception and understanding), yet use of terms like "imagination led us" suggests that there is some visualization going on as well. The narrator admits that "we saw, or fancied we saw—it makes no difference which,"[81] a sentence that seems to indicate how seeing and imagining amount to the same thing. Such is certainly supported in the last sentence of the large extract above, where Dickens admits to guessing the end of the story. The boy's story is easy to predict, he implies, because it follows a familiar plot: this could be the Rake's Progress, or the story of Jack Sheppard. Hogarth's Rake is hanged and dissected, and Ainsworth's Jack Sheppard ends his days the same way. The boy with the baggy knees probably shares a similar fate, Dickens implies, which, as a kind of diagnosis, follows a particular medical method of making predictions based on expert experience.

"Experience," it was said, was what made a medic's opinion worth listening to. In his 1857 lectures on clinical observation and research, professor of medicine Thomas Laycock summed up the position as follows:

---

80. Dickens, "Meditations," 80.
81. Ibid., 79.

> The acquisition of a certain amount of medical knowledge, by instructed daily experience, is [...] illustrated by the proverbial saying, "A man is either a fool or a physician at forty."
>
> What, then, is the requisite conduct for the attainment of the wise experience of which I speak? Simply this; long-continued, sedulous, accurate observation of manifest external phenomena—observation independently of aids, and therefore prompt, because practicable under all circumstances, in which the eyes, the ears, and senses generally can co-operate with the instinctive exercise of the judgement, or common sense, as it is termed. [...] Experience will afford a power of intuition such as is sometimes really marvelous in its results.[82]

It is interesting how old terms associated with the common law creep into Laycock's summary: principles may become "practicable under all circumstances"; they may also become "common sense." A lifetime of observing an anatomical phenomenon will make a man expert, in other words, in that phenomenon. Thomas Sydenham once asserted that "for the same disease in different persons the symptoms are for the most part the same, and the selfsame phenomena that you would observe in the sickness of a Socrates you would observe in the sickness of a simpleton."[83] Another great authority, John Gregory, noted in 1772:

> A young physician who has drawn his knowledge only from books or lectures, although he may be ingenious and learned, and consequently able to talk plausibly, will yet be extremely embarrassed when he enters upon practice—Medicine is not merely a speculative science to be acquired by study alone; it is an active and practical art, the proper exercise of which can only be attained by long practice.[84]

Such principles also found their way into medical jurisprudence as we saw in the Reid and Heywood cases of the last chapter. As late as 1859 an article

---

82. Thomas Laycock, *Lectures on the Principles and Methods of Medical Observation and Research* (Philadelphia: Blanchard and Lea, 1857), 35.

83. Ibid., 36–37. In his history of medicine Douglas Guthrie observes that "Sydenham was essentially a clinician; [...] his method consisted in the careful observation and recording of the phenomena of disease [...]. The greatest service [...] which Sydenham rendered to medicine was to divert men's minds from speculation, and to lead them back to the bedside for there only could the art be studied." Douglas Guthrie, *A History of Medicine* (London: Thomas Nelson and Sons, 1945), 204.

84. Gregory, *Lectures*, 206–7.

titled "Pathological Contributions to Medical Jurisprudence" appeared in the *British Medical Journal* in which the physician William Boyd Mushet noted:

> The evidence derived from books may be accepted as a confirmation or corrective; but no authority should be unreservedly subscribed to if opposed to observation or experience, as a number of cases, arising from any given operation—whether accidence, violence, poison, or disease—necessarily exhibit diversities in the character and evolution of symptoms, and in the textual alterations revealed by the scalpel.[85]

In spite of his admiration for Sydenham, a man whom he saw as "stand[ing] out as one of the greatest men of the modern era,"[86] Laycock disagreed with his experiential theory and observed that "unlearned experience is not the best guide."[87] Hypothetically, a doctor may deal with six cases of a condition in which the patient died, but who is to say that the seventh case will not recover? Laycock warns that "no two cases are alike [. . .]. No diseased individual is exactly like another individual; nor, in the same, is the condition of one day like the condition of another. It is a mere assumption that they are."[88] One year later Thomas Inman, a surgeon based in Liverpool, wrote, also in the *British Medical Journal*:

> Experience [. . .] can only give wisdom when it is associated with a well stored mind, steady powers of observation, habits of continued thought, and a power of calm judgment. It demands memory, discrimination, elasticity of mind, and self-reliance. [. . .] It was my fortune once to know a surgeon whose boast it was that he never read any book on medicine, as he was determined to trust to experience alone for an increase of his knowledge.[89]

Each case needed to treated, according to the profession's more careful observers, as though its symptoms were entirely new to the practitioner. The gold standard for Inman was the work of John Hunter: "One of the characteristics of the man was, that his theories were constantly changing as new facts were developed. Eager to interrogate Nature, his interpretation

---

85. William Boyd Mushet, "Pathological Contributions to Medical Jurisprudence," *British Medical Journal* (15 January 1859): 42.
86. Laycock, *Medical Observation*, 36.
87. Ibid.
88. Ibid., 37, 44.
89. Thomas Inman, "Experience in Medicine," *British Medical Journal* (6 November 1858): 923–27, 942–45 (924–24).

of her teachings varied with every answer he received."⁹⁰ Assumption was bad, interpretation good: "The greater *experience* we have of *experience*," Inman concluded, "the less we can place implicit reliance upon it."⁹¹

Referring to "Monmouth Street," then, who is to say that the boy with the baggy knees did not take a difference course? The end of the sketch delights in a world of invention, yet the narrator finds himself brought to earth with a solid reminder that the world of speculation does not always sit comfortably with reality. According to Damian Grant, writing on French Naturalism, the nineteenth century was the age of "a crisis of confidence in the imagination—a crisis which entails a systematic repudiation of its function."⁹² Distrust of fancy forms the basis of Carlyle's complex dialogues between the transcendentalist Teufelsdröckh and his empiricist editor, and, according to Albert William Levi, "Pascal called imagination the 'mistress of the world.' But he did not say this in her praise. He meant that she is promiscuous, untrustworthy, deceptive, and disloyal, the dangerous and eternal enemy of reason."⁹³ In "Monmouth Street" the term *imagination* is used to denote a kind of unruly presence as well as a kind of happy visualization. What follows is from the piece's conclusion:

> We were in the full enjoyment of these festivities [an imaginary pantomime] when we heard a shrill, and by no means musical voice, exclaim, "Hope you'll know me agin, imperence!" [...] We were conscious that in the depth of our meditations we might have been rudely staring at [an] old lady for half an hour without knowing it.⁹⁴

The end of the sketch provides a sobering moment in which we are brought to realize that despite the article's journalistic claims to having been based on reality, the sketch is not, in the words of J. Hillis Miller, "a mirror of reality" but rather an "interpretation of interpretation."⁹⁵ Eschewing its own attention to reality, which has insisted on genuine acts of reportage and geographical identifications, "Monmouth Street" indulges in a fantastic pantomime that warns against our facility to assume too much. Like a number of experts in medical jurisprudence, the article deals with its

---

90. Ibid., 924.
91. Ibid., 945.
92. Damian Grant, *Realism* (London: Methuen, 1970), 29.
93. Albert William Levi, *Literature, Philosophy and the Imagination* (Bloomington: Indiana University Press, 1962), 44.
94. Dickens, "Meditations," 82.
95. Hillis Miller, "The Fiction of Realism," 309.

subject in a way that seems conscious of how perception is challenged as often as it is satisfied.

JOHN BODLE

That such interpretive challenges were seen as productive opportunities for forensic experts is apparent in a number of real forensic cases of the nineteenth century where failure necessitated invention; here the challenges of interpretation, far from being a disappointment or cause for frustration, led the way to some extraordinary new developments. One of the most significant of these cases was the 1833 trial of John Bodle.

The Bodles were a fairly prosperous family of farmers living in South East London. In November 1833, the head of the family, George, was murdered with poison. One of the family's servants, Mary Higgins, claims to have heard the victim's grandson, John, then aged twenty, say to his mother, "He [John] would not mind poisoning anyone he did not like" and "that he wished his grandfather dead, [because then] he should have a thousand [. . .] a-year."[96] Young Bodle was arrested, and when his belongings were searched by local police, two packets of arsenic were found among his possessions. The case against him seemed like a fairly straightforward one, but the actual, tangible evidence was weak. To begin with, no traces of poison could be found in the body of the victim. John Butler, a surgeon, was called to treat George before his death, and he performed the postmortem examination with two other doctors. He admitted that there were "no evident marks in the stomach that the deceased came to his death by taking arsenic" and that he "would not swear from the appearance of the stomach alone that he had taken arsenic."[97] Such lack of physical evidence was not unusual. As Robert Christison noted in his *Treatise on Poisons* (1829), "Many causes conspire to remove from the stomach during life poisons which have actually caused death," including vomiting, purging, and absorption.[98]

Notwithstanding, a couple of expert witnesses claimed that they could tell from the symptoms George Bodle had experienced that the dead man had been poisoned. Dr Bossey claimed, rather vaguely, that "he could not positively say from the *post-mortem* examination that death was caused by

---

96. *The Times*, 12 November 1833, 5.
97. *The Times*, 14 December 1833, 5.
98. Robert Christison, *A Treatise on Poisons in Relation to Medical Jurisprudence, Physiology, and the Practice of Physic* (1829; Edinburgh: Adam and Charles Black, 1845), 342.

arsenic; [but] there could be no doubt it was caused by some irritating substance," and his colleague Mr Solley maintained—still with no hard evidence—that "death was caused by arsenic administered in small quantities."[99] Such haphazard guesswork became a source of embarrassment for the prosecution: bold statements seemed to be made with an ill-formed confidence, and this served only to highlight the hole in the case against the young defendant.

The Crown Prosecution turned to chemical science, sending samples of the victim's stomach contents (and his coffeepot) to the chemist Michael Faraday for investigation. Faraday was busy at the time, so he handed the samples over to his assistant, James Marsh, who, despite the scientific methods at his disposal, could find no traces of arsenic in the stomach contents, though he did find some in the coffee. Cross-examined at the trial, he admitted that he found only tiny amounts of poison and had "very seldom made such experiments, and had never before made an experiment to detect arsenic."[100] Marsh, unlike Bossey and Solley, played down his experience. A product of laboratory science, he would have had little confidence in past events, choosing instead to rely on inductive reasoning and microscopic evidence.

Faced with the possibility of executing a man on the basis of a few traces of arsenic in a coffeepot, the jury decided to acquit Bodle. Rather than perceiving the case as a professional failure, however, Marsh looked upon it as a challenge. Seeming to baffle the powers of empirical observation, the poisoned body required a new form of analysis. Katherine Watson writes:

> Marsh set out to develop a test for arsenic that would detect even the tiniest amounts in organic samples, and by 1836 he had succeeded. Basing his method on the production of arsine, a gaseous compound of arsenic and hydrogen that, when burned, gives a deposit of metallic arsenic, what became known as the Marsh test was quickly established as the most delicate and reliable of all the tests of arsenic.[101]

What seems most important about the Marsh test was the precision it promised. According to Ian Burney, "It lowered the threshold for detection, enabling the toxicologist to detect significantly smaller amounts of

---

99. *The Times*, 13 November 1833, 3. Italics in original.
100. *The Times*, 14 December 1833, 5.
101. Katherine Watson, *Poisoned Lives: English Poisoners and Their Victims* (London: Hambledon and London, 2004), 17–18.

poison."[102] Yet from the comments he made about the similar case of Thomas Smethurst, it is clear that Dickens considered microscopic evidence inconsequential in cases where more circumstantial evidence was not wanting. In 1859 he wrote to Forster:

> I followed the case with so much interest, and have followed the miserable knaves and asses who have perverted it ever since, with so much indignation, that I have often had more than half a mind to write and thank the upright judge who tried him. I declare to God that I believe such a service one of the greatest that a man of intellect and courage can render to society. Of course I saw the beast of a prisoner (with my mind's eye) delivering his cut-and-dried speech, and read in every word of it that no one but the murderer could have delivered or conceived it. Of course I have been driving the girls out of their wits here, by incessantly proclaiming that there needed to be medical evidence either way, and that the case was plain without it. Lastly, of course (though a merciful man—because a merciful man I mean), I would hang any Home Secretary (Whig, Tory, Radical, or otherwise) who would step in between that black scoundrel and the gallows. I cannot believe—and my belief in all wrong as to public matters is enormous—that such a thing will be done.[103]

At a glance, it seems that Dickens rejected the medical evidence in favor of "plain truth"—a return, we might assume, to the old way of thinking of truth as self-evident. Yet, unlike many other commentators, he resisted dismissing the medical testimony on the basis that it is less reliable than "common sense." One comment made to the *Daily News* about the case, for instance, suggested that "common sense, after all, [. . .] is the most infallible means we possess of guiding us to the truth."[104] Dickens's view seems to have been better informed. He implied that good evidence had been provided through "broad facts" and "moral evidence"; like William Webber, a Fellow of the Royal College of Surgeons, he believed that "the heavy preponderance of the moral evidence of guilt has been fated to yield to the lamentable discrepancy in the meagre amount of medical information [. . .] adduced."[105] An editorial in *The Morning Chronicle*, published the same day Dickens wrote his letter to Forster, said:

---

102. Burney, *Poison*, 99.
103. Charles Dickens, letter to John Forster, 25 August 1859, in *Letters* 9: 111–13.
104. R. W., letter to the editor of the *Daily News*, 26 August 1859, 4.
105. William Webber, "Toxicotechnia, or the Scientific Poisoning Art," *The Bury and Norwich Post and Suffolk Herald*, 1 November 1859, 4.

It was his acts [. . .] that formed the case against him. [. . .] As Chief Baron Pollock wisely told the jury, if there had been no chemical evidence whatever, there would have been little difficulty in coming to a conclusion; and the reason for this observation is, that the law deals with a criminal on the broad facts of the case against him, and not on the defect, or apparent flaw in the metal of the link which helps to make up the chain of evidence.[106]

Like this writer, Dickens appeared to have disliked forms of science that perceived themselves to be providing definitive answers—especially when those answers contradicted, seemingly, a more careful interpretation of the circumstances. This view was particularly apparent in his response to G. H. Lewes on the subject of spontaneous combustion and suggests that Dickens saw positive proof as another potential sort of assumption, every bit as unruly as the undisciplined imagination in "Monmouth Street."

THOMAS SMETHURST

In 1858 Smethurst, a surgeon specializing in hydrotherapy, left his wife and bigamously married the wealthy Isabella Bankes. Soon afterwards Isabella "fell ill with diarrhœa, vomiting, and fever."[107] When her medical attendants became suspicious, they sent a sample of her evacuations to Alfred Swaine Taylor for analysis; he discovered metallic deposits which seemed to indicate the presence of either arsenic or antimony. Smethurst was arrested on 2 May 1859 and, on 3 May, Isabella died. As Dickens notes, the circumstances spoke against the defendant, yet Taylor undertook further analyses of Isabella's viscera and he found no evidence of poison. Next, Taylor and a colleague tested the liquids in Smethurst's medical cabinet, initially finding nothing until they came to "bottle number 21." As Burney explains:

[Taylor] submitted a portion of the liquid contained in this bottle to the Reinsch process for isolating arsenic. This process was developed in 1841 by the German chemist Hugo Reinsch, who proclaimed it a safer and simpler test than Marsh's. [. . .] Reinsch's [. . .] process involved the introduction of pure and highly polished copper gauze into the suspect liquid mixed with hydrochloric acid. If arsenic were present, it would combine with the acid to form a gas and leave a greyish film on the copper. [. . .] Taylor was

---

106. Unsigned, "Medical Testimony in the Smethurst and Palmer Cases," *The Morning Chronicle*, 25 August 1859, 4.
107. Burney, *Poison*, 164. My account of the Smethurst story is indebted to Burney's careful study.

much surprised [. . .] by his application of the Reinsch test to the contents of bottle 21. When the copper gauze was introduced, the liquid in the bottle rapidly dissolved it. In response, Taylor [. . .] took the unusual step of introducing more copper gauze into the liquid, until its capacity to dissolve the copper was finally exhausted. At this point, when they introduced a fresh copper gauze, it "at once received the arsenic." [. . .] The absence of arsenic in the body of [Isabella] was entirely explicable—[she] had been slowly, scientifically, poisoned with arsenic.[108]

Like the Marsh test, then, the Reinsch process indicated that science was able to chase evidence into the innermost hiding places of the human body. In a novel serialized in *Bentley's Miscellany* in 1845, physician-turned-novelist Albert Smith commented that

> toxicology is now more certain in its researches after hidden poison, and in this deadly drug [arsenic] especially. The merest trace of it, in whatever form it may be administered, even to the eye of the vulgar affording no more attributes than pure water for analysis, can be reduced to its mineral state [. . . so] as to place all matter of detecting its presence beyond the slightest doubt, even in the quantity of the most minute atom.[109]

Medical jurisprudence seemed to have developed the ability to detect traces of evidence with remarkable precision.

Yet along with such confidence there arose a critical suggestion that toxicology was creating the results it was most eager to find. As one correspondent to the *Daily News* argued:

> In this case it was first suspected and then assumed that a murder was committed, and from that assumption the prosecution traced the murder to Dr. Smethurst. Having assumed that he was the murderer, they interpreted all his acts in the light of that assumption. Now then, let me assume that he was innocent, and I will undertake to prove that all his acts were consistent with innocence.[110]

Matthieu Orfila conducted a series of experiments in 1838 and 1839 which revealed that "arsenical stains could be generated from the bones of bodies

---

108. Ibid., 164–65.
109. Albert Smith, *The Marchioness of Brinvilliers, or The Poisoner of the Seventeenth Century*, *Bentley's Miscellany* (1845): 17–18 17, 117–18.
110. J. Passmore Edwards, "A Plea for Dr. Smethurst," *Daily News*, 24 August 1859, 5.

that had not been exposed to arsenic in any obvious way. Arsenic, he concluded, might be a natural constituent of the human body."[111] Similarly, the chemist William Brande indicated that the arsenic detected by Taylor at the trial of Thomas Smethurst "had been deposited into the solution by impurities contained in the copper gauze. [. . .] By feeding tainted copper into the liquid to 'exhaust' its dissolving powers, Taylor had himself introduced the arsenic that he subsequently detected."[112] Smethurst was found guilty, but after protests about the incompleteness of the medical evidence, he was given a reprieve by the Home Secretary, much to Dickens's disappointment.[113]

Marsh's evidence in the Bodle case was vindicated eleven years after the trial when the erstwhile defendant confessed. In 1844 he was arrested for extortion; found guilty and transported; he then confessed to having killed his grandfather. The confession must have looked like a validation of the old maxim that "truth will out," a maxim that relied, as we saw in chapter 1, upon a notion of natural law which, sometimes consciously, sometimes otherwise, set itself against expert interpretation. The failure of the Reinsch test in the Smethurst investigation also appeared to raise questions about the reaches of forensic science. "The work of the poison hunter," notes Burney, "look[ed] quixotic at best, futile at worst."[114] Yet despite the failings identified with the Marsh and Reinsch tests, Burney is closer to the mark when he writes that "chemical evidence was not straightforward, but was the product instead of a complex and highly self-conscious work of analytical art."[115] As we also saw in chapter 1, the field of medical jurisprudence, speaking broadly, was not unaware of its limits. "Failures" like those connected to the trials of Bodle and Smethurst were converted into evidence of how the field needed to interpret its own methods carefully. An editorial in *The Era* noted:

> Through the bungling of Dr. Taylor, and the contempt he has thrown on medical jurisprudence, a benefit to the community will be affected, not only in rousing the profession to the importance of this branch of study, but by rendering it impossible for so lamentable a system to be again exposed to

---

111. Burney, *Poison*, 100.
112. Ibid., 165. At the time of his death Dickens owned a copy of Brande's *Dictionary of Science, Literature, and Art* (1852). See Stonehouse, *Catalogue*, 15.
113. "[Smethurst's] reprieve provoked [Dickens's] sarcastic 'Five New Points of Criminal Law,' (A[ll the] Y[ear] Round), 24 Sept[ember 18]59), suggesting reforms "grounded on the profound principle in such trials 'that the real offender is the Murdered Person,'" *Letters* 9: n8, 111–13.
114. Burney, *Poison*, 185.
115. Ibid., 103.

the pity and derision of the world. [. . .] A *higher* order of study, a *superior* class of special teachers are demanded.[116]

Although instances of professional "bungling" could be a source of personal embarrassment for experts like Taylor, the larger field of medical jurisprudence sought to gain from these reminders that the interpretive and analytical skills at its disposal were not infallible. Indeed, moments like the Smethurst trial confirmed a narrative that had been written into medical jurisprudence since the early parts of the nineteenth century: in the search for truth, nothing may be taken for granted; even tests that take precision and positive evidence as their strongest virtue can be as misleading.

BLEAK HOUSE

The "whole truth" is something that Dickens never seems to be aiming for, in any naive-empiricist sort of way, when writing the later works. In *Bleak House* there is a return to the Dickensian obsession with turning the city into a jumble of cadavers yet he is clearly more dissatisfied with the kinds of links, made in his own "Drunkard's Death," between bodies and "facts". At the burial ground of Nemo, for instance, the dead *become* the city as their bodies ooze into the earth. And death does ooze in *Bleak House*: the city of the novel is all about misleading signs and thwarted interpretation, and the novel exploits the image of death as a means of challenging the wish to know the "whole truth." As Lauren Goodlad has observed, the novel is infected with an "unnerving epistemological uncertainty."[117]

One man with an interest in truth, naturally, is the lawyer Tulkinghorn. On the night of his murder, the third-person narrator of *Bleak House* offers a panoramic view of London:

> A very quiet night. When the moon shines very brilliantly, a solitude and stillness seem to proceed from her that influence even crowded places full of life. Not only is it a still night on dusty high roads and on hill-summits, whence a wide expanse of country may be seen in repose, quieter and quieter as it spreads away into a fringe of trees against the sky with the grey ghost of a bloom upon them; not only is it a still night in gardens and in woods, and on the river where the water-meadows are fresh and green,

---

116. Unsigned, "Our Medical Jurisprudence in Relation to Dr. Smethurst," *The Era*, 11 September 1859, 9. Italics in original.
117. Goodlad, *Victorian Literature*, 88.

and the stream sparkles on among pleasant islands, murmuring weirs, and whispering rushes; not only does the stillness attend it as it flows where houses cluster thick, where many bridges are reflected in it, where wharves and shipping make it black and awful, where it winds from these disfigurements through marshes whose grim beacons stand like skeletons washed ashore, where it expands through the bolder region of rising grounds, rich in cornfield wind-mill and steeple, and where it mingles with the ever-heaving sea; not only is it a still night on the deep, and on the shore where the watcher stands to see the ship with her spread wings cross the path of light that appears to be presented to only him; but even on this stranger's wilderness of London there is some rest. Its steeples and towers and its one great dome grow more ethereal; its smoky house-tops lose their grossness in the pale effulgence; the noises that arise from the streets are fewer and are softened, and the footsteps on the pavements pass more tranquilly away. In these fields of Mr Tulkinghorn's inhabiting, where the shepherds play on Chancery pipes that have no stop, and keep their sheep in the fold by hook and by crook until they have shorn them exceeding close, every noise is merged, this moonlight night, into a distant ringing hum, as if the city were a vast glass, vibrating. (600–601)

The present-tense narration, concerned with the details of nocturnal London, reminds us of Boz the journalistic writer of up-to-date urban sketches. Tulkinghorn's meditations, in contrast, invoke old stories and inherited narratives: "Many [. . .] mysteries, difficulties, mortgages, delicate affairs of all kinds, are treasured up in his old black satin waistcoat" (599). The lawyer's downfall, in fact, is driven by his greed for knowledge—his obsession, specifically, with knowing *every* secret without ever being satisfied with the fact that there are some truths that he is not meant to find out. It is his wish to ferret out the secret of Lady Dedlock that leads him to get involved with the hot-headed woman who kills him.

The above description of London is as much concerned with obscuring details as it is with revealing them. It has an appreciation for abstractions and hidden stories that Tulkinghorn can never approximate. Having spent some time outlining a night scene, the passage intends the observer to lose his or her footing, though this is no panic or fall; instead it is a form of respite: "Even on this stranger's wilderness of London there is some rest." After the frenzied scramble for secrets and revelations that the novel has represented, the passage's celebration of indefinition seems restful. Everything becomes ghostly, "ethereal," and "softened." The harshness of Chancery is unstiffened into a pastoral image, and the noise of the city is converted into the unique and ghostly sound of a humming glass. This is not simply a demystification; it is a determination to find the power behind an interpretation that only half satisfies the impulse to know.

Hillis Miller observes:

> In the opening paragraphs the novel presents the corpse of a dead society, smothered in fog, immobilized in mud, paralyzed by the injustices of an outmoded social structure frozen in its stratifications, and enmeshed in the nets of inextricably tangled legal procedures. The rest of the novel initiates us into the nature and causes of this general paralysis.[118]

Writing on Dickens's perception of the urban more generally, F. S. Scharzbach compares the experience of Victorian London to Nazi concentration camps: "The immediate consequences of such an extreme dislocation, as one can well imagine, are profound and profoundly crippling. [. . .] The events surrounding the experience are perceived as arbitrary and meaningless. In addition, one's sense of identity is shattered, and the sense of self becomes uncertain."[119] This sense of disorientation is the ironic result of a "forensic" view that prioritizes "real" details and often finds them misleading. As we saw in chapter 2, medical authors stressed how the medicolegal understanding was a partial one—subservient always to an absolute truth that is unavailable to any human observer. That Dickens has a similar concept of truth is registered in the *Household Words* article "Gone Astray" (1853), where the boyish panic of the young subject, presumably Dickens himself, sets an obvious contrast to the preoccupations that the narrator of the same piece has with the shifting particulars of the city:

> So, I began to ask my way to Guildhall: which I thought meant, somehow, Gold or Golden Hall [. . .]. I remember how immensely broad the streets seemed now I was alone, how high the houses, how grand and mysterious everything. When I came to Temple Bar, it took me half-an-hour to stare at it, and I left it unfinished even then. I had read about heads being exposed on the top of Temple Bar, and it seemed a wicked old place, albeit a noble monument of architecture and a paragon of utility. When at last I got away from it, behold, I came, the next minute, on the figures at St. Dunstan's! Who could see those obliging monsters strike upon the bells and go? Between the quarters there was the toyshop to look at—still there,

---

118. Hillis Miller, *Charles Dickens*, 169
119. F. S. Schwarzbach, *Dickens and the City* (London: Athlone, 1979), 10.

at this present writing, in a new form—and even when that enchanted spot was escaped from, after an hour and more, then Saint Paul's arose, and how was I to get beyond its dome, or to take my eyes from its cross of gold?[120]

To scan, observe, and interpret the conflicting realities of the city involves going astray and experiencing, in turn, all the disorientation that comes with having a partial knowledge of the scene. In *Bleak House* a similar strategy is used in the narrative of Esther Summerson, which begins as follows:

> I have a great deal of difficulty in beginning to write my portion of these pages, for I know I am not clever. I always knew that. I can remember, when I was a very little girl indeed, I used to say to my doll, when we were alone together, "Now, Dolly, I'm not clever, you know very well, and you must be patient with me, like a dear!" And so she used to sit propped up in a great arm-chair, with her beautiful complexion and rosy lips, staring at me—or not so much at me, I think, as at nothing—while I busily stitched away, and told her every one of my secrets. [. . .] I had always rather a noticing way—not a quick way, O no!—a silent way of noticing what passed before me, and thinking I should like to understand it better. I have not by any means a quick understanding. (15)

According to some nineteenth-century scientists, Esther's reasons for her alleged inability to recall facts ought to qualify her as a good interpreter. Her "silent way of noticing" is, according to some, the best way to perform an analysis. Claude Bernard noted in his *Introduction to Experimental Medicine* (1865), for example, that the good scientist "puts questions to nature but [. . .] as soon as she speaks, [. . .] hold[s] his peace; he must note her answer, hear her out and in every case accept her decision."[121] An orphaned outsider brought into London for the first time, Esther is, in many ways, the best person to narrate half the story precisely because she has none of the preconceptions or precedents that cripple others. Indeed, the way in which her vinegary aunt orders her to "forget [her] mother" (17) creates a deliberate difference between Esther's orphaned identity and the way Lady Dedlock is made to carry the burden of the truths concerning her past. Of course, as Esther becomes entangled in the web that binds other characters to the law, so too does she become infected by the various diseases that plague the others. Yet her confession at the start of her narrative

---

120. Dickens, "Gone Astray," 157–58.
121. Bernard, *Introduction*, 22–23, 25.

prefaces the novel's larger sense that "bewilderment" is an inevitable part of interpreting the world. As in "Gone Astray," the novel combines the ambitions of one interpreter (the narration) with the self-doubts of another (the lost child/Esther) in order to evidence the kind of self-reflection that accompanies the giving of testimony.

I have already discussed in my first chapter Dickens's use of fog as a symbol of the infectious stalemate of Chancery. In the famous opening paragraphs of *Bleak House* the same element is used to represent a larger sense of crisis caused by the narrative preoccupation with knowing the city. There is an unequivocal full stop that follows the first word (*London*), making it clear that "this is no fiction, [. . . but] the modern city."[122] Yet for all its detailing of men, horses, dogs, and their respective bad tempers, the description goes astray: dogs become indistinguishable, horses lose their footing, snow is black, and primeval creatures might waddle through the picture at any moment. As equine and human pedestrians lose their footing, so does any hope of a clear interpretation. Like the corporeal evidence of forensic discourses, Dickens's city is an interpretation at best—a representation that bears all the fogginess and all the creativity of forensic analysis.

Dickens wrote to Forster about the idea he had had for *Household Words*: he imagined "a certain SHADOW, which may go into any place, by sunlight, moonlight, starlight, firelight, candlelight, and be in all homes, and all nooks and corners, and be supposed to be cognisant of everything, and go everywhere, without the least difficulty [. . .] a kind of semi-omniscience, omnipresent, intangible creature."[123] He contradicts himself here: an omnipresent "creature" (like the traditional idea of God) has no need to *investigate* at all because it/he is all-knowing; the vision of a "shadow" or a *semi-*omniscience, however, suggests a human level of perception, complete with the quirks and limitations of mortal observation. As in the earlier sketches by Boz, this "mortal observation" is what is used to describe the squalors of the city. On Tom-All-Alone's, Dickens writes:

> Much mighty speech-making there has been, both in and out of Parliament, concerning Tom, and much wrathful disputation how Tom shall be got right. Whether he shall be put into the main road by constables, or by beadles, or by bell-ringing, or by force of figures, or by correct principles

---

122. John Lucas, "Past and Present: *Bleak House* and *A Child's History of England*," in *Dickens Refigured: Bodies, Desires and Other Histories*, ed. John Schad (Manchester: Manchester University Press, 1996), 136–56 (149).

123. Forster, *Life*, vol. 2, 78–79.

of taste, or by high church, or by low church, or by no church; whether he shall be set to splitting trusses of polemical straws with the crooked knife of his mind or whether he shall be put to stone-breaking instead. In the midst of which dust and noise there is but one thing perfectly clear, to wit, that Tom only may and can, or shall and will, be reclaimed according to somebody's theory but nobody's practice. And in the hopeful meantime, Tom goes to perdition head foremost in his old determined spirit. (568)

We see a problem that cries out for a remedy—an issue that has been recognized and discussed "in and out of Parliament" by a range of professionals using a varying range of methodologies. Yet the one mode of analysis that comes to dominate Dickens's own attitude toward the slum is, according to Jonathan Arac, the scientific one: the author "conveys less a specific physical description of the slum [. . .] than an attitude of scientific precision about it."[124] That Tom-all-Alone's is imagined as a Dantean netherworld does nothing, I add, to moderate the sense of the place as a body that both challenges and benefits from forensic inspection:

> Darkness rests upon Tom-All-Alone's. Dilating and dilating since the sun went down last night, it has gradually swelled until it fills every void in the place. For a time there were some dungeon lights burning, as the lamp of life hums in Tom-all-Alone's, heavily, heavily, in the nauseous air, and winking—as that lamp, too, winks in Tom-all-Alone's—at many horrible things. But they are blotted out. The moon has eyed Tom with a dull cold stare, as admitting some puny emulation of herself in his desert region unfit for life and blasted by volcanic fires; but she has passed on and is gone. The blackest nightmare in the infernal stables grazes on Tom-all-Alone's, and Tom is fast asleep. [. . .]
>
> But he has his revenge. Even the winds are his messengers, and they serve him in these hours of darkness. There is not a drop of Tom's corrupted blood but propagates infection and contagion somewhere. It shall pollute, this very night, the choice stream (in which chemists on analysis would find the genuine nobility) of a Norman house, and his Grace shall not be able to say nay to the infamous alliance. There is not an atom of Tom's slime, not a cubic inch of any pestilential gas in which he lives, not one obscenity or degradation about him, not an ignorance, not a wickedness, not a brutality of his committing, but shall work its retribution through every order

---

124. Jonathan Arac, *Commissioned Spirits: The Shaping of Social Motion in Dickens, Carlyle, Melville, and Hawthorne* (1979), quoted in Levine, *Darwin and the Novelists*, 121.

of society up to the proudest of the proud and to the highest of the high. Verily, what with tainting, plundering, and spoiling, Tom has his revenge. (567)

The moon prefigures, in the first paragraph, the role it will take on in the landscape described immediately prior to the murder of Tulkinghorn. Light represents knowledge, and it is this very enlightenment that, like the few rays provided by the dungeon lamps, forsakes Tom—not only to express despair over the paralysis of slumming but also to offer the narrative a means of exercising the interpretive partial sightedness of its "omnipresent" narrator. The notion that the slum ought to be a source of common concern because of its ability to infect the full strata of society is a well-known attempt to make readers take common ownership of a real problem. However, references to chemists, and the minutest atoms of Tom's blood, gesture toward a specialist interpretation as well. As we saw in my account of the Bodle and Smethurst trials, forensic examiners prided themselves on their ability to find guilt in the innermost "nooks and corners" of the human body. Using the language of tainting, plundering, and spoliation, Dickens captures and appropriates some of this forensic confidence, yet in Tom-all-Alone's, as in the muddy and foggy London of the opening chapter, *dis-easing* is used to establish the city as a world that offers such analytical systems a fierce challenge.

Indeed, the act of observing London and its details is more rigorously self-reflective because it is explored through characters like Allan Woodcourt and Inspector Bucket—men whose visions of the city provide an analysis of the interpretive impulse with all the inventive freedom that fiction is able to provide and exemplify. Woodcourt and Bucket "share between them," according to Karl Ashley Smith, "the role of guide through Hell and both are equally conversant with Tom-all-Alone's."[125] Inspector Bucket, "attentive," "steady-looking," "sharp-eyed," and "in all manner of places, all at wanst" according to the crossing sweeper (281, 575), is the novel's most effective practitioner of the analytical method. "He has the power of God," Smith notes; he "personifies the narrative drive towards discovery inherent in the story, irresistibly dispending an even-handed justice operating by inscrutable methods."[126] His ubiquity and his "ghostly manner of appearing" (281) give him the silent, overseeing qualities that have led some scholars, such as Ronald R. Thomas, to interpret him as part of a complex new system

---

125. Smith, *Dickens and the Unreal City*, 112.
126. Ibid., 105.

of social discipline. He is, Thomas argues, a product of the age of forensic photography where new "mechanisms of observation exploit[ed] the double discourse around the personal image as a form of self-authentication and a tool of social discipline."[127] Peter Thoms is somewhat more pessimistic: "Some psychologically disfigure themselves," he claims, "by becoming detectives. [. . .] As a detective one separates oneself from one's own sense of criminality and powerlessness and assumes an authoritative and more comfortable position on the right side of the law." The "chilling reductiveness of [Bucket's] interpretations," it is added, "[. . .] implies an oppressive egotism that likewise threatens the self-expression of others."[128] The detective is indeed *Bleak House*'s most compelling account of the process and significance of interpretive observation, but whether this amounts to a force of social discipline or a "chilling reductiveness" is not so obvious to me. Bucket's role as the man who must solve the novel's murder mystery elevates him to a position of watchful authority, to be sure, but if we compare his machinations to those of his colleague-in-law Mr Tulkinghorn, we see how the detective's methods of surveillance are fairly open-ended.

Bucket's methods are both forensic and sharp as a tack; they lead to him outwitting the very woman who defeats Tulkinghorn. As the lawyer's remains wend their way toward their final resting place, the narrator says:

> Contrast enough between Mr Tulkinghorn shut up in his dark carriage and Mr Bucket shut up in HIS. Between the immeasurable track of space beyond the little wound that has thrown the one into the fixed sleep which jolts so heavily over the stones of the streets, and the narrow track of blood which keeps the other in the watchful state expressed in every hair of his head! (647)

The novel invites us to compare the two men and to marvel at the forensic acumen of the one and the ultimate failures of the other. Taken out of historical context, Bucket's defeat of Hortense can be read as a suppression of unruly (foreign, passionate, feminine) passions,[129] but—given what we have been exploring in relation to the interpretive narratives of the forensic

---

127. Thomas, *Detective Fiction*, 146. See also D. A. Miller, *The Novel and the Police* (Berkeley, CA, and London: University of California Press, 1988), 58–106.
128. Peter Thoms, "'The Narrow Track of Blood': Detection and Storytelling in *Bleak House*," *Nineteenth-Century Literature* 50:2 (1995): 147–67 (160, 162).
129. It is a well-known fact that Hortense is based on Maria Manning, the Swiss-born woman who murdered her lover, Patrick O'Connor, in 1849. For more on this case see Andrew Mangham, *Violent Women and Sensation Fiction: Crime, Medicine and Victorian Popular Culture* (Basingstoke: Palgrave Macmillan, 2007), 7–9.

process—it seems more accurate to say that the inspector's detective method embodies the kind of scientific quest that was believed to lead to a successful assertion of justice.

On the solving of the murder, Bucket says:

> The last point in the case which I am now going to mention shows the necessity of patience in our business, and never doing a thing in a hurry. I watched this young woman yesterday without her knowledge when she was looking at the funeral, in company with my wife, who planned to take her there; and I had so much to convict her, and I saw such an expression in her face, and my mind so rose against her malice towards her ladyship, and the time was altogether such a time for bringing down what you may call retribution upon her, that if I had been a younger hand with less experience, I should have taken her, certain. [. . .] What should I have lost? Sir Leicester Dedlock, Baronet, I should have lost the weapon. My prisoner here proposed to Mrs Bucket, after the departure of the funeral, that they should go per bus a little ways into the country and take tea at a very decent house of entertainment. Now, near that house of entertainment there's a piece of water. At tea, my prisoner got up to fetch her pocket handkercher from the bedroom where the bonnets was; she was rather a long time gone and came back a little out of wind. As soon as they came home this was reported to me by Mrs Bucket, along with her observations and suspicions. I had the piece of water dragged by moonlight, in presence of a couple of our men, and the pocket pistol was brought up before it had been there half-a-dozen hours. (672)

Interestingly, Bucket's "experience" plays an important role in the criminalization of Hortense, but not in a way that recalls how, in the system of legal precedent, the past was stiflingly in attendance upon the present. Rather, he has learned the art of patient observation and interpretation: he scrutinizes a series of signs and then makes an interpretative leap at the truth: "By the living Lord it flashed upon me, as I sat opposite to her [. . .] and saw her with a knife in her hand" (670).

Dickens outlines the detective process in one of the numerous articles he wrote for *Household Words* on the subject of modern policing. "A Detective Police Party" (1850) describes a visit paid by "the whole Detective force from Scotland Yard"[130] to the Wellington Street offices of the journal.

---

130. Charles Dickens, "A Detective Police Party (1)," *Household Words* (27 July 1850), *Journalism* 2: 265–75 (267).

Showing "keen observation, and quick perception when addressed,"[131] the detectives tell of a number of cases in which their patient skills of inspection succeed in solving intricate and complicated mysteries. The sketch concludes:

> For ever on the watch, with their wits stretched to the utmost, these officers have, from day to day and year to year, to set themselves against every novelty of trickery and dexterity that the combined imaginations of all the lawless rascals in England can devise, and to keep pace with every such invention that comes out. In the Courts of Justice, the materials of thousands of such stories as we have narrated—often elevated into the marvellous and romantic, by the circumstances of the case—are dryly compressed into the set phrase, "in consequence of information I received I did so and so." Suspicion was to be directed, by careful inference and deduction, upon the right person; the right person was to be taken, wherever he had gone, or whatever he was doing to avoid detection.[132]

In these articles Dickens links detection and science. Inspectors are guided by "careful inference" and "deduction," and later he writes that these men "are enough for justice. To compare great things with small, suppose LEVERRIER or ADAMS informing the public that from information he had received he had discovered a new planet."[133] In an earlier contribution to *Household Words* Dickens defined the "The Modern Science of Thief-Taking," thus modifying Thomas De Quincey's famous definition of murder as one of the fine arts. Yet "A Detective Police Party" also acknowledges how, like forensic science and the early journalism, truth must always do battle with "stories"—with the human impulse to elevate "circumstances" into the "marvellous and romantic." Such explains how Mr Bucket's mind works while attempting to locate Lady Dedlock. During his search, he "never relaxes in his vigilance a single moment" (701), and he switches between visualization and perception:

> He mounts a high tower in his mind and looks out far and wide. Many solitary figures he perceives creeping through the streets; many solitary figures out on heaths, and roads, and lying under haystacks. But the figure that he seeks is not among them. Other solitaries he perceives, in nooks of bridges,

---

131. Ibid., 268.
132. Charles Dickens, "A Detective Police Party (2)," *Household Words* (10 August 1850), *Journalism* 2: 276–82 (281).
133. Ibid., 282.

looking over; and in shadowed places down by the river's level; and a dark, dark, shapeless object drifting with the tide, more solitary than all, clings with a drowning hold on his attention.

Where is she? Living or dead, where is she? If, as he folds the handkerchief and carefully puts it up, it were able with an enchanted power to bring before him the place where she found it and the night-landscape near the cottage where it covered the little child, would he descry her there? On the waste where the brick-kilns are burning with a pale blue flare, where the straw-roofs of the wretched huts in which the bricks are made are being scattered by the wind, where the clay and water are hard frozen and the mill in which the gaunt blind horse goes round all day looks like an instrument of human torture—traversing this deserted, blighted spot there is a lonely figure with the sad world to itself, pelted by the snow and driven by the wind, and cast out, it would seem, from all companionship. It is the figure of a woman, too; but it is miserably dressed, and no such clothes ever came through the hall and out at the great door of the Dedlock mansion. (696)

As with the Scotland Yard detectives, the "enchanted power" of Bucket's mind intrudes on the detective process. Smith understandably notes that the inspector "has the power of God" because of the "high tower of his mind," which allows his gaze to stretch far and wide and appears to imitate omniscience. Yet, as in the imaginary pantomime in "Meditations in Monmouth Street," use of the word *enchanted* provides an unsteadying reminder of the human nature of interpretation. Bucket visualizes a "dark, dark, shapeless object" that clings to his attention, clogging his "observations" with the emotional conjectures that the object encourages. Also, as in the opening to the novel, physical properties of things make little sense: bricks get scattered in the wind like confetti, clay and water are hard, and a mill becomes an instrument of torture. Bucket does not have the "power of God," but, like forensic science, he has something that approximates it on a human level. He is an excellent examiner of the world he inhabits, but the weirdness of his semi-imagined interpretations reminds us of his human capacity to get driven off course. He is too late, after all, to save Lady Dedlock.

I do not mean to argue, however, that the imaginative intrusions on Bucket's mind are perceived by Dickens as a weakness. On the contrary, they are shown to be part of the valuable propensity to imagine stories while looking for facts. It falls short of the absolute truth, to be sure, but it is "enough for justice." It is Allan Woodcourt's compassion, in fact, that best highlights how the *human* aspects of forensic science's interpretation, as opposed to its chemical and animal precisions, were one of its best assets. Our first encounter with the young surgeon occurs when he examines the body of Captain Hawdon. He is accompanied by Mr Tulkinghorn, whose obvious disinterest in the dead man's story creates a marked contrast to Woodcourt's ability to read the emotional aspects of the same:

> "It is beyond a doubt that he is indeed as dead as Pharaoh; and to judge from his appearance and condition, I should think it a happy release. Yet he must have been a good figure when a youth, and I dare say, good-looking." He says this, not unfeelingly, while sitting on the bedstead's edge with his face towards that other face and his hand upon the region of the heart. [. . .] During this dialogue Mr Tulkinghorn has stood aloof by the old portmanteau, with his hands behind him, equally removed, to all appearance, from [. . .] the young surgeon's professional interest in death, noticeable as being quite apart from his remarks on the deceased as an individual. (129)

Woodcourt's act of resting his hand on the dead man's heart could be read in two ways: as an act of sentimentality that links the surgeon to the emotional facets of Nemo's history; or as an act of professionalism that allows him to ascertain whether the man still has a heartbeat. Tulkinghorn notices a disparity between the surgeon's professional interests in death and his (Woodcourt's) recognition of the deceased as an individual. The surgeon's comments on Nemo's death as a "happy release," combined with melancholy reflections on how he must have once been handsome, recalls the sad trajectory of Boz's boy with the baggy knees. There is a conflict, it seems, between professional interest in the body and a *human* interest in the emotional story behind it.

Indeed, Allan Woodcourt is a man for whom analysis and feeling cannot be made separate. This we see in his experiences of meeting Little Jo and Jenny the Brickmaker's wife:

> Attracted by curiosity, he often pauses and looks about him, up and down the miserable by-ways. Nor is he merely curious, for in his bright dark eye there is compassionate interest; and as he looks here and there, he seems to understand such wretchedness and to have studied it before.
>
> [. . .] As he retraces his way to the point from which he descried the woman at a distance sitting on the step, he sees a ragged figure coming very cautiously along, crouching close to the soiled walls—which the wretchedest figure might as well avoid—and furtively thrusting a hand before it.

> It is the figure of a youth whose face is hollow and whose eyes have an emaciated glare. He is so intent on getting along unseen that even the apparition of a stranger in whole garments does not tempt him to look back. He shades his face with his ragged elbow as he passes on the other side of the way, and goes shrinking and creeping on with his anxious hand before him and his shapeless clothes hanging in shreds. Clothes made for what purpose, or of what material, it would be impossible to say. They look, in colour and in substance, like a bundle of rank leaves of swampy growth that rotted long ago. (572)

What Woodcourt notices about Jo, particularly about the boy's sickly body, is detailed with clinical exactitude. As with his interpretation of the body of Nemo, however, it is difficult to see where his professional interests begin and where his human interests end: his "bright dark eye," for instance, has a "compassionate interest" as well as a scientific one. Such is clear when he meets Jenny:

> No waking creature save himself appears except in one direction, where he sees the solitary figure of a woman sitting on a door-step. He walks that way. Approaching, he observes that she has journeyed a long distance and is foot-sore and travel-stained. She sits on the door-step in the manner of one who is waiting, with her elbow on her knee and her head upon her hand. [. . .]
> "Let me look at your forehead," he says, bending down. "I am a doctor. Don't be afraid. I wouldn't hurt you for the world."
> He knows that by touching her with his skilful and accustomed hand he can soothe her yet more readily.
> [. . .] He cleanses the injured place and dries it, and having carefully examined it and gently pressed it with the palm of his hand, takes a small case from his pocket, dresses it, and binds it up. While he is thus employed, he says, after laughing at his establishing a surgery in the street, "And so your husband is a brickmaker?"
> "How do you know that, sir?" asks the woman, astonished.
> "Why, I suppose so from the colour of the clay upon your bag and on your dress. And I know brickmakers go about working at piecework in different places. And I am sorry to say I have known them cruel to their wives too." (570–72)

Again, the young surgeon exercises a forensic eye to detail, making deductions from the clues he reads on and around Jenny's body. Yet this is combined with a determination to reflect on her emotional story as well.

As in "The Drunkard's Death," where signs on bodies tell stories of misery and sin, so do the brick dust and Jenny's scars indicate that she has been mistreated by her husband. Yet Woodcourt's most compassionate interest comes from stories he has known in the past. Like the story of the boy with the baggy knees, Jenny's story may (or may not) fit a pattern that the observer has experienced, yet his ability to undertake in-depth analysis, combined with the inevitable, affective weight of a human observer, is what *Bleak House* seems to applaud. Indeed, in 1852, at the point of just beginning *Bleak House,* Dickens, according to Goodlad, was working with Angela Burdett Coutts in the clearing of a London slum. He "rejected the expert advice of Mr. Field—the real-life model for Inspector Bucket," preferring instead the advice of "Dr. Southwood Smith, a member of the General Board of Health." While the author was "disposed to doubt the efficacy" of the policeman's "peculiar sort of knowledge," he was certain that the physician knew "all about" the people and "how [they] live."[134] The key term here is "the people." Like Bucket, Field may know his subject very well, but knowing *the people* (as opposed to just their bodies) requires a medical view.

Janis McLarren Caldwell defines "romantic materialism" as "a form of double vision" developed by "leading doctors and writers" of the nineteenth century:

> Romantic because they were concerned with consciousness and self-expression, and materialist because they placed a particularly high value on what natural philosophy was telling them about the material world. [. . .] Romantic materialists accepted disjunctions between the two ways of knowing and called for an interpretive method which tacked back and forth between physical evidence and inner, imaginative understanding.[135]

What we see in Woodcourt, however, is how, to accept Caldwell's definitions for the moment, the "romantic" and the "material" are not separate forms of vision that encourage one to tack back and forth but are part of the same process of looking. The moral, inner life of Jenny is registered in the tangible, outer indications on her body, and for Woodcourt as well as for the forensic examiner, the moral meaning of a scar is to be understood through a clinical interpretation of its materiality. Moral and epistemological virtues are involved, and they have equal billing, in the forensic act of looking. But, as we have seen, it does not suit the forensic project to

---

134. Goodlad, *Victorian Literature,* 103.
135. Janis McLarren Caldwell, *Literature and Medicine in Nineteenth-Century Britain: From Mary Shelley to George Eliot* (Cambridge: Cambridge University Press, 2004), 1.

have these values exist in harmony; seeing the imagination as a potentially unruly and persistent "mistress," to redeploy Pascal's term, allowed professionals like Woodcourt the chance to weigh and balance these professional strategies carefully.

Hence, Dickens converts the forensic skill of interpretation into a style whereby the analytical realism of literature is made both uncertain and a great deal richer by an acknowledgment of the *human* faculties that shape and often mislead scientific interpretation. Little wonder, then, that Dickens should have disliked the kind of empirical approach he witnessed in the trial of Smethurst, and in Lewes's response to Krook's death, where the clamor for clinical fact appeared to silence the feats of opinion that had sought to make sense of the circumstantial clues.

THE MUDFOG PAPERS

The Mudfog Papers (1837–38), or the "stray chapters" by another name,[136] were written by Dickens for *Bentley's Magazine* at the time he was the periodical's editor. In them he made the point that positivism risked returning to a method of uncritically linking "signs" with "truth." The chapters imply, in particular, that forensic medicine had introduced the better practice of interpreting the world with a healthy degree of self-awareness. The papers concern themselves with the events of a conference held by the Mudfog Association for the Advancement of Everything, modeled on the British Association for the Advancement of Science, which had been established in 1831 to "elevate the status of the physical sciences."[137] In one meeting the aptly named Professor John Ketch produces the skull of a notorious murderer named James Greenacre.[138] After a "most animated discussion" of what the lumps and bumps of the skull indicate, it turns out that the object under consideration is a coconut.[139] It is a satire likely to have been

---

136. "Stray chapters" is how *The Mudfog Papers* were named in the index of *Bentley's Miscellany* (Bowen, *Other Dickens*, 87).

137. Richard Yeo, *Defining Science: William Whewell, Natural Knowledge and Public Debate in Early Victorian Britain* (Cambridge: Cambridge University Press, 1993), 222. See G. A. Chaudhry, *The Mudfog Papers*, *The Dickensian* 70 (1974): 104–12.

138. Jack Ketch was the famous executioner employed by Charles II. He died in 1686. Michael Slater notes in *Journalism* 1 that "a Dr Inglis had lectured on the skull of the famous scholar-murderer Eugene Aram (executed in 1759), seeking to prove by 'phrenological observations' that he had been innocent. Some members of the audience expressed considerable doubt as to whether the skull was, in fact, Aram's" (531).

139. Charles Dickens, "Full Report of the First Meeting of the Mudfog Association for the Advancement of Everything," *Bentley's Miscellany* 2 (October 1837), *Journalism* 1: 513–50 (549).

inspired by *Noctes Ambrosianæ*, a serial that ran in *Blackwood's Edinburgh Magazine* between 1822 and 1835. In this series a phrenologized skull turns out to be a turnip:

> You haven't heard of it, then?—I thought all the world had. You must know, however, that a certain ingenious person of this town lately met with a turnip of more than common foziness in his field; he made a cast of it, clapped it on the case of somebody's face, and sent the composition to the Phrenological [*The Phrenological Journal*], with his compliments, as a *fac-simile* of the head of a celebrated *Swede*, by the name Professor Tornhippson. They bit,—a committee was appointed,—a report was drawn up,—and the whole character of the professor was soon made out as completely *secundum artem*, as Haggart's had been under the same happy auspices a little before. In a word they found that the illustrious Dr Tornhippson had been distinguished for his inhabitiveness, constructiveness, philoprogenitiveness, &c.—nay, even for "tune," "ideality," and "veneration."[140]

In Dickens's *Mudfog Papers*, the like error is discovered not before "Mr. Blubb delivered a lecture upon the cranium before him, clearly showing that Mr. Greenacre possessed the organ of destructiveness to a most unusual extent, with a most remarkable development of the organ of carveativeness [*sic*]."[141] Such readings of the skulls of criminals were not uncommon in the early parts of the nineteenth century; Dickens's acquaintance John Elliotson gave a phrenological study of the heads of resurrection men Bishop and Williams in 1832: "The characters of the two criminals in question," he noted in *The Lancet*, "are well known. Their conduct originated not from morbid excitement, nor any diseased condition of the brain. It arose, not from any momentary impulse, but was deliberate and settled."[142] He adds:

> The head of WILLIAMS is by far the worse. The intellectual portion is very small—exceedingly low; the moral portion is equally wretched—exceedingly low; while that devoted to the animal propensities—the

---

140. Quoted in John Strachan, "'The Mapp'd out Skulls of Scotia': *Blackwood's* and the Scottish Phrenological Society," in *Print Culture and the Blackwood Tradition, 1805–1930*, ed. David Finkelstein (Toronto: University of Toronto Press, 2006), 49–69 (60).
141. Dickens, *Mudfog*, 549.
142. John Elliotson, "On the Phrenology of Williams, and Bishop, who were Lately Executed for Murder Committed to gain Money by the Sale of Dead Bodies to Anatomical Teachers," *The Lancet* 17 (1832): 533–39 (537).

lower-posterior and lower lateral parts, especially destructiveness, acquisitiveness, secretiveness—is immense. [...] There is no wonder that his whole life was low and villainous.[143]

On Bishop, he adds:

> The preponderance of the lower feelings over the superior, and over the intellect and ideality, are likewise in accordance with Bishop's character. [... He had a] a large development of the organ of acquisitiveness, with the small development of that of conscientiousness, and of the moral sentiments at large [...]. Popular tradition, as well as certain memoirs, accuse him of many murders, and these were committed without interest vengeance, or anger. He would shoot workmen engaged upon roofs, that he might have the barbarous pleasure of seeing them precipitated.[144]

The description of the *Phrenological Journal*'s examination of the turnip in *Noctes Ambrosianæ* and Blubb's examination of the coconut in *Mudfog* is clearly intended to satirize the sort of analysis given by phrenologists like Elliotson (who had founded the Phrenological Society in 1824). Although Dickens held "phrenology, within certain limits, to be true,"[145] he seemed to believe, at the time of writing *The Mudfog Papers*, that the "science" promised (or threatened) a system that would do away with expert opinion. "As a phrenologist, interested in cerebral psychology and physiology," Fred Kaplan notes, Elliotson "believed that criminal tendencies could be physiologically located in the brain and nervous system and scientifically analyzed."[146] In *The Mudfog Papers*, Dickens demonstrates how this view was based upon the kind of positivist ambition he would take G. H. Lewes to task on. When the coconut mistake is finally discovered, it is narrated:

---

143. Ibid.

144. Ibid., 534–35.

145. Charles Dickens, "A Little Dinner in an Hour," *All the Year Round* (2 January 1869), *Journalism* 4: 364–70 (367). Sally Shuttleworth's is the best discussion of phrenology in the context of the development of ideas of psychiatry in the nineteenth century; see Sally Shuttleworth, *Charlotte Brontë and Victorian Psychology* (Cambridge: Cambridge University Press, 1996). See also Jane Wood, *Passion and Pathology in Victorian Fiction* (Oxford: Oxford University Press, 2001); John Van Whyle, *Phrenology and the Origins of Victorian Scientific Naturalism* (Hampshire: Ashgate, 2004); Roger Cooter, *The Cultural Meaning of Popular Science: Phrenology and the Organization of Consent in Nineteenth-Century Britain* (Cambridge: Cambridge University Press, 2005); and David Stack, *Queen Victoria's Skull: George Combe and the Mid-Victorian Mind* (London: Hambledon Continuum, 2008).

146. Fred Kaplan, *Dickens and Mesmerism*, 62n.

Professor Ketch hastily repossessed himself of the cocoa-nut, and drew forth the skull, in mistake for which he had exhibited it. A most interesting conversation ensued; but as there appeared some doubt ultimately whether the skull was Mr. Greenacre's, or a hospital patient's, or a pauper's, or a man's, or a woman's, or a monkey's, no particular result was obtained.[147]

It would be easy to fall into the opinion that this is Dickens parodying the whole of science, but an understanding of the original context of Greenacre's crime suggests that Dickens conjured the ghost of the murderer in order to highlight the strengths of the alternative approach to the kind of materialism espoused by phrenology.

JAMES GREENACRE

It is unlikely that Dickens's readers could fail to remember the success that forensic science had made of the prosecution of James Greenacre, a real murderer whose beating and dismemberment of his fiancé in 1837 marked, according to David Newsome, the dawn of the Victorian age with the bloodshed it would become obsessed with.[148] When the *Penny Satirist* sought to parody Dickens's portrait of Sam Weller in the same year, it came up with the following Wellerism: "I can't stay longer—you know it's the natur of o'things that the best friends must part, as Mr. Greenacre said ven he sharpened his knife to cut Mrs. Brown's head off her shoulders."[149] In 1837 Matthias Ralph a lock-keeper working near Edgware Road, London, found that the canal gates he was trying to close obstructed by "an object." At the trial of Greenacre he recounted:

> I had occasion to abut the gates of the canal, and found something impede their shutting—I was called to by a bargeman, who told me there was something in the gate—I immediately went with a hitcher—I found the

---

147. Dickens, *Mudfog*, 549.
148. David Newsome, *The Victorian World Picture: Perceptions and Introspections in an Age of Change* (1997; London: Fontana, 1998), 14. Dickens maintained an unhealthy interest in dismembered corpses. In Harvard he visited the place where John Webster had dismembered and burned the remains of his friend, and in "Night Walks" (1860), an article he wrote for *All the Year Round*, he mentioned the "chopped-up murdered man," which refers to the mutilated remains found in a carpet bag on Waterloo Bridge in 1857. See Philip Collins, *Dickens and Crime* (1962; London: Macmillan, 1965), 253–54; and Willoughby Matchett, "The Chopped-up Murdered Man," *The Dickensian* 14 (1918): 117–19.
149. Unsigned, "Boz to the *Penny Satirist*," *Penny Satirist*, 13 May 1837, 2.

gates would not come to—I put the hitcher down, and pulled it along to the middle—I said, "It is a dead dog; close the gate"—they eased the gate—I pulled it up, and, to my surprise, I found the head of a human being.

Cross-examined, Ralph added:

Sometimes we pick bodies out of the canal—I have picked out several, and sometimes one that has been in the water three or four days will be a great deal worse than those which have been in ten days—picked them out when they have been in overnight—(*the hitcher was here produced*)—I put the hitcher down, and drew it along, and drew it up.[150]

Despite the injuries the head sustained, it was apparent that it had belonged to a woman and, soon after, her torso and limbs were found at different locations near Edgware Road.[151] Theodric Beck reported in an 1842 edition of his *Elements of Medical Jurisprudence*:

The head had been severed above the sternum, and the fifth cervical vertebra was sawn through, leaving only about the tenth of an inch of that bone. The legs were cut off immediately under the hip-joint. [. . .] There were no marks present of medical treatment—she had not been bled or blistered recently. [. . .] The head was found in the canal near *Mile End*, seven miles from the former place—it corresponded with the body. The face was very much bruised and wounded. [. . .] After an interval of some weeks, the legs were found in a parcel at Camberwell, also seven miles distant from each of the above places.[152]

Forensic examiners John Birtwistle and Gilbert Girdwood did an extraordinary job in putting the body back together and in identifying the deceased as Hannah Brown. She was a washerwoman who had gone missing some days before and she was identifiable from a scar she had had on her left

---

150. Central Criminal Court, 3 April 1837. Record: t18370403–917.

151. In a curious twist of circumstances, one suspect of the murder of Hannah Brown was named Dickens. According to *The Morning Post*, a workman with that name intended to steal a plank of wood that he had secreted beneath a sack containing some of Hannah's remains on Edgware Road. Not knowing what the sack contained, Dickens intended to return to the spot to reclaim the wood but forgot to do so. He was examined by the coroner's jury, but "his testimony showed him innocent of a participation in the dreadful affair." Unsigned, "The Mutilated Body," *The Morning Post*, 2 January 1837, 4.

152. Beck, *Elements*, 605–6.

ear. When police investigated her story, they discovered she had become engaged recently to Greenacre. Disappointed by the discovery that she was not a wealthy woman, Greenacre took up with another woman, Sarah Gale, and plotted to kill Hannah. Police also discovered that Greenacre sold a shawl belonging to the murdered woman after she had disappeared. Such facts were certainly damning, yet when Greenacre was arrested, he denied the murder. In a police interview he admitted arguing with Hannah, but said that her death was an accident:

> I must say that I put my foot to [her] chair—it was just after we had concluded tea, and she went back with great violence against a chump of wood that I had been using of, and that alarmed me very much—I went round the table, and took her by the hand, and kept shaking her, and she appeared entirely gone—as it regarded my own feelings, it is impossible for me to give any thing like a description, from the agitation I was in at the time—during this state of excitement I deliberated, and came to the determination of concealing her death in the manner it has been already laid before the world.[153]

Unfortunately for Greenacre, forensic examination told a completely different story. At the trial Bertwistle and Girdwood said that Hannah's body must have undergone considerable violence in addition to (and prior to) the blow that killed her. A. D. Hutter notes that the "evidence offers a remarkable example of sophisticated pathology early in the nineteenth century: [it] determined the nature of the victim's life and background and identity, and even something about the criminal himself."[154] Beck explains:

> What had been asserted from a review of all the facts noticed proved to be correct by his confession. She came to see him, and they quarrelled [sic]; he struck her with a rolling-pin and she fell down either dead or insensible; in about an hour afterwards, he dismembered the body, and removed its parts to the different place where they were found.
>
> The medical testimony of Mr. Girdwood and Mr. Bartwhistle [sic] in this case is highly creditable to them; and the opinions they advanced, particularly as to the wounds inflicted during life and after death, evince accurate discrimination. It is almost needless to say that the murderer met his deserved doom.[155]

---

153. Central Criminal Court, 3 April 1837. Record: t18370403–917.
154. Albert D. Hutter, "Dismemberment and Articulation," 135–75 (142, 144).
155. Beck, *Elements*, 606.

Hutter is correct to note that the evidence of Girdwood and Bertwistle was remarkable; the surgeons were able to reconstruct what happened on the night Hannah died from the clues left on her scattered body. Beck's language indicates just how thoughtful and careful their professional analysis was: in their evidence they expressed "opinions," not facts, and they had shown "accurate discrimination" rather than the materialist zeal which might lead to the phrenological reading of a coconut.

Greenacre was found guilty, hanged, and his body sent for dissection. Sarah Gale was transported for the offense of aiding and inciting. Popular opinion agreed with Beck's view that it was the measured methods of forensic science that had secured the convictions. *The Examiner* said:

> One of the best features of our age is the increasing application of the results of improved theory and scientific research to the common uses of society. In few directions could this disposition of the times extend itself with better effect than in the advancement of the knowledge of forensic medicine. Of the value of good medical evidence we have recently had a striking example in the case of atrocity expiated on Tuesday last.[156]

Before execution, Greenacre was given a phrenological reading by Elliotson. Sadly, the results of the examination appear not to have survived, yet the *Penny Satirist* reported on the visit Elliotson paid to the convicted man, interestingly taking a verbatim extract from the *London Medical and Surgical Journal*:

> Dr. Elliotson, whose phrenological tact far exceeds even his stethoscopical acumen, [examined] the head of Greenacre, which through the official channel of Mr. M'Murdo, the Newgate apothecary, he was enabled to accomplish. We understand the doctor's examination was highly satisfactory. Greenacre submitted to the application of *callipers* [sic] without a frown, and appeared intensely anxious that the measurement of his head should coincide with his confessions.[157]

---

156. Unsigned, "Forensic Medicine," 299.
157. Unsigned, "Phrenology," 4. In the following week's edition there was featured an epitaph for Greenacre which ran as follows:

> Here festering lies a ruthless scourge of earth,
>   To virtue and to honest shame unknown;
> Low cunning on a dunghill gave him birth,
>   And villainay [sic] confessed him for her own.

Even without Elliotson's report, we are in fairly safe territory when we suggest that the measurement of Greenacre's head probably corroborated the "evidence" of his confession. Such is what the *The Mudfog Papers* implies when the text's phrenologists find evidence of Greenacre's guilt on a coconut. In the actual case, however, bodily evidence proved to be a great deal more credible because Girdwood and Birtwistle did not lean on the kind of material fact that a "science" like phrenology relied upon. This is indicated by Beck's report of their "discrimination," which forms an obvious contrast to the theory that a bump in a certain place on the skull may indicate a propensity to violence, amorousness, cunning, and so on. *The Mudfog Papers* contrasts the success of the Greenacre trial with the aims of the Scientific Association, to support a view, made later by Dickens in his responses to G. H. Lewes, that a self-critical, forensic testimony is a more valuable "truth" than the principle of "two and two make four." Indeed, Dickens's vacillations between the imperatives of investigative journalism and the invented world of fiction find more common ground with methods of forensic analysis than one might expect.

    Dread was his purpose, and his soul was dark;
        In secret murder too was all his hope;
    No pains he spared, and seldom missed his mark,
        And gained from justice all he feared—a rope.

    If farther you his villainies would know,
        The many tales, all false, he did confess;
    Go read the story of his vice and woe,
        Printed at large by the rabble press.

Unsigned, "An Epitaph for Greenacre," *Penny Satirist*, 6 May 1837, 1.

CHAPTER 4

COLLATERAL EVIDENCE
The Pickwick Papers and *Great Expectations*

ROBERT SEYMOUR

In April 1836 the first illustrator of *The Pickwick Papers,* Robert Seymour, walked into his garden and shot himself. One newspaper, *John Bull,* reported the discovery of his body as follows:

> Mr. John Mason, of Aston-place, deposed that he did not know the deceased. Between seven and eight o'clock on Wednesday morning, witness was passing Park-place West, Liverpool-road, when he was called by a gentleman named Cave, who exclaimed, "For God's sake come in; here is a dreadful sight!" Witness accordingly went into the residence of the deceased, [. . .] and passing through the house into the back garden, discovered the deceased stretched on the ground, weltering in blood, which proceeded from a dreadful wound in the chest. The unfortunate gentleman was apparently quite dead. A fowling-piece was lying near his person, which had recently discharged. Mr. Burrows, a surgeon, attended in a very short time, and declared life extinct.[1]

In seemingly objective and precise detail, the exact positions of the body, the weapon, and the wound are noted here; the method through which the narrative follows Mason into the garden, shifting attention to certain

---

1. Anon., Untitled Report, *John Bull,* 25 April 1836, 131.

"things" and constructing a vision of the whole scene from constituent parts, seems to anticipate a forensic form of analysis. Such attention to detail is not unusual in newspaper reports of suicides, where there is an obvious need to determine how an individual died, yet the style of the article also mirrors the meticulousness of a crime scene investigation.

Most important in the investigation, there was found at the scene a suicide note in which Seymour seemed to be keen to absolve all others of any direct or indirect involvement in his decision to kill himself. *Bell's Life in London,* the first home of many of Dickens's sketches, printed the letter, which was addressed to Seymour's wife, as follows:

> Best and dearest of wives—for best of wives you have been to me—blame I charge you not any one, it is my own weakness and infirmity, I don't think anyone has been a malicious enemy to me; I have never done a crime my country's laws punish with death. Yet I die, my life it ends; I hope my Creator will grant me peace, which I have prayed so [*sic*] for in vain whilst living.[2]

In addition to its obvious emotional qualities, the note provides hard, tangible proof that Seymour had died by his own hand, and, accordingly, the coroner's jury returned a verdict of "temporary derangement."[3] The relatively uncomplicated nature of the investigation was determined by the fact that one crucial object/text had been discovered. All other forms of evidence—the wound, the position of the weapon, the state of the illustrator's affairs, his psychiatric instabilities—all became secondary to this one important "thing"—a readable object that said in no uncertain terms, "Blame I charge you not any one."

CRIME SCENE EVIDENCE

In a series of lectures delivered at the University of London the following year, forensics expert Alexander Thomson mentioned one of the thousands of cases in which a suicide note was *not* found. In the absence of this key item, he said, other objects, such as the weapon and the accessories surrounding the dead body, necessarily take on added importance. The investigators of one scene, in particular, exercised none of the thoroughness that

---

2. Anon., Untitled Article, *Bell's Life in London and Sporting Chronicle,* 24 April 1836, 1.
3. Ibid.

had come to be associated with medical jurisprudence. Taking appearances for granted, and assuming that the death was a case of suicide, they tidied the corpse and took the weapon away: "If the body and the gun had not been moved by those who found the body," Thomson concludes, "it might have been ascertained whether the death was accidental or not. [. . .] Doubts remain to this day, whether [the] death was accidental or an act of suicide."[4] Investigators lost key parts of the evidence in this case because they had overlooked their importance. On the topic of bodies "found dead," Thomson insisted:

> Every collateral circumstance must be taken into account: the situation and attitude of the body; the position of the instrument with which the wound is supposed to have been inflicted; the direction of the wound, and the part of the body in which it is situated. [. . .] If weapons be found near a dead body with certain wounds inflicted upon it, we must ascertain whether the wounds could have resulted from the use of those instruments. Thus in 1764, a citizen of Leige [sic] was found shot, and his own pistol lying near him; but on examining the ball, which was extracted from the wound, it was found too large ever to have entered that pistol; murder was therefore inferred; and the murderers were afterwards discovered.[5]

Thomson's lectures were an important milestone in the rise of forensic medicine. They were serialized in *The Lancet* throughout 1837, while the science was still in its vital stages of maturation—largely because, at that time, the periodical's founder and editor Thomas Wakley "embraced the cause of medical jurisprudence"; he saw it as providing "an exemplary demonstration of the importance of a progressive approach to medical education and accreditation."[6] A key part of medical jurisprudence's "progressive approach" was its sense that "things" could act as indications of human intentions, and Thomson was among the first to argue for the importance of what he called "collateral evidence"—evidence that, in relation to the body, must be concomitant, accompanying, and secondary. The forensic expert becomes involved, he insists, in an act of interpretation that goes beyond the obvious: "It is not enough," he said, that the medical examiner has "a general acquaintance with his profession; he ought to be able to apply

---

4. Alexander Thomson, "Lectures on Medical Jurisprudence: Lecture 33," *The Lancet* 28 (1837): 273–78 (273).

5. Thomson, "Lecture 33," 273–74.

6. Burney, *Poison*, 42. On the links between Dickens and Wakley, see Collins, *Dickens and Crime*, 179.

the information which he possesses, to the investigation of certain objects, with a degree of precision and accuracy which the ordinary duties of his practice do not demand."[7] In his Liege case, objects told unexpected stories; the ball removed from the body did not match the pistol, whose position signified that the dead man committed suicide. Medical jurisprudence steered toward a resolution, to be sure, but its business, as we have seen, was to distrust self-evident narratives; its ability to read all clues, including the unruly and untidy ones, seemed at first glance to be a substantiation of the accuracy of scientific induction, yet Thomson was one of the many nineteenth-century specialists to complicate the act of interpretation in order to foreground its importance; take nothing for granted, he advised his students; read everything with suspicion and distrust self-evident "truths":

> Every minute circumstance relative to the condition of the body when found should be noted down; the surrounding objects, and their state, both in relation to their usual appearance and to the body; the manner in which the rope is fixed, and, in fact, every circumstance, however minute, should be recorded.[8]

It is my view that what "thing theorist" Bill Brown writes about American Modernism can be said of the forensic culture of the nineteenth century: "At times it seems that the physical object world, once breathtakingly legible, has become opaque."[9] According to Thomson, the correct strategy for medical jurisprudence was to treat the crime scene as opaque; the expert needed to question his own methods of analysis and raise, by extension, larger, transferrable questions of what it means to link interpretation with tangible "things."

Dickens's fascination with objects, props, and background details is an obvious feature of his work—so much so that in Charles Kingsley's *Alton Locke* (1850), the narrator says, "By-the-by, I have as yet given no description of the old eccentric's abode—an unpardonable omission, I suppose, in these days of Dutch painting and Boz."[10] In *Dickens: The Dreamer's Stance* (1965), Taylor Stoehr explains that "Dickens's novels are rightly termed "crowded,"

---

7. Alexander Thomson, "Lectures on Medical Jurisprudence: Lecture 1," *The Lancet* 27 (1836–37): 65–70 (66).

8. Alexander Thomson, "Lectures on Medical Jurisprudence: Lecture 31," *The Lancet* 28 (1837): 209–214 (212).

9. Bill Brown, *A Sense of Things: The Object Matter of American Literature* (Chicago: University of Chicago Press, 2003), 14.

10. Charles Kingsley, *Alton Locke: Tailor and Poet: An Autobiography*, ed. Elizabeth A. Cripps (1850; Oxford: Oxford University Press, 1983), 62.

[. . .] because of the superabundance of "things" in his imaginative world, a superabundance that goes much further than the demands of verisimilitude, cluttered as the real world was."[11] Stoehr discusses the now-familiar view that the "things" in Dickens's novels carry a symbolic purpose or a metonymic meaning; the death masks in Jaggers's office, the bags of hair in Mr Krook's shop, Madame Defarge's knitting, Fagin's pitchfork, all tell stories that are bigger than their purely descriptive function.[12] The point has been updated by Elaine Freedgood in *The Ideas in Things* (2006). She notes of the Dickens novel, "It could be imagined as performing a massive cultural reclamation project, revivifying lost objects and lost persons without discrimination."[13] In his famous essay "The Fiction of Realism" (1971), J. Hillis Miller suggests that objects in Dickens are intended to constitute habits and crises of interpretation. Rather than providing a "straightforward" indication of any given story or character trait, "things" seem intended to mislead and prevaricate:

> These objects are the residue of the culture they have inherited and have coercive force not as physical energies but as signs, habits of interpretation, forms. Such inherited forms constitute a world in which nothing is what it is, but everything is the arrow pointing towards something else.[14]

Hillis Miller believed that the details of *Sketches by Boz*, in particular, "are not *mimesis* of an externally existing reality, but the interpretation of that reality according to highly artificial schemas inherited from the past [. . . and] from fictitious patterns." However, I argue that Dickens's understanding of the relationship between "things" and habits of interpretation

---

11. Taylor Stoehr, *Dickens: The Dreamer's Stance* (Ithaca, NY: Cornell University Press, 1965), 5.

12. John R. Reed notes in a discussion of *Dombey and Son* (1846–48) that "plain realism could describe the room and associate certain objects with malign intent, let us say, but Dickens goes beyond that to characterize the objects as metonymic of Carker's *inner* condition." John R. Reed, *Dickens's Hyperrealism* (Columbus: The Ohio State University Press, 2010), 58. In a way, this interpretation, in which objects take on an emotional or moral meaning, contrasts with the number of works that appeared in which the "commodification" of nineteenth-century culture is a primary concern. Andrew Miller, for instance, notices how Dickens's work signals the numbing "dangers of commodification." Andrew Miller, *Novels behind Glass: Commodity Culture and Victorian Narrative* (Cambridge: Cambridge University Press, 1995), 13. The forensic method involves an inversion of this construct—where rather than values becoming "things," things take on moral and emotional value. My reading learns much from the recent, critical leaning toward objects in the novel as emblems of larger historical, contextual, and symbolic systems. See Brown, *A Sense of Things*.

13. Elaine Freedgood, *The Ideas in Things: Fugitive Meaning in the Victorian Novel* (Chicago: University of Chicago Press, 2006), 99.

14. Hillis Miller, "The Fiction of Realism," 308.

(or misinterpretation, as it may be) comes from schemas he picks up from medical jurisprudence—a science that in the nineteenth century promoted a new culture of self-questioning interpretation based upon the evidences of bodies and objects. In contrast to the argument of Freedgood, I believe that the "things" in the Dickens novel are not "a kind of unsupervised metonymic archive" that has "remained largely unread."[15] (The implication of this argument is that Dickens and his readers did not see, or feel, the onus of interpretation as much as we do.) My view is that "things" littered the Dickens novel so that the author could create a world in which investigation was simultaneously encouraged and frustrated. These texts were an assault course for the interpreting mind, and they learned much of their representational trickery from medical jurisprudence.

As we have already glimpsed in the arguments of specialists like Thomson, attention to detail was a method that exploited "facts" as a way of serving the moral objectives of the legal process. In the investigation in Liege, minute observations of collateral evidence led to the capture of murderers while, in the other case cited, sudden death becomes mysterious only after faulty perceptions of the "crime" scene have taken place. Attention to detail is a method of getting at the truth but not in any reassuringly simple way: professionals like Thomson believed that the intellectual powers of observation and interpretation were required to guide the moral objectives of the law, but it is a central acknowledgment in medical texts that the crime scene is a world where "nothing is what it is."

THE PICKWICK PAPERS

After *Sketches by Boz* the first work to explore the ambitions of interpretation was *The Pickwick Papers*. In the serialized number that followed the death of Seymour, Mr Pickwick is to be found "contemplating nature" over the balustrades of Rochester Bridge. What he observes is worth citing at length in order to demonstrate its profound attention to detail:

> On the left of the spectator lay the ruined wall, broken in many places, and in some, overhanging the narrow beach below in rude and heavy masses. Huge knots of seaweed hung upon the jagged and pointed stones, trembling in every breath of wind; and the green ivy clung mournfully round the dark and ruined battlements. Behind it rose the ancient castle, its towers

---

15. Freedgood, *The Ideas in Things*, 84.

roofless, and its massive walls crumbling away, but telling us proudly of its old might and strength, as when, seven hundred years ago, it rang with the clash of arms, or resounded with the noise of feasting and revelry. On either side, the banks of the Medway, covered with cornfields and pastures, with here and there a windmill, or a distant church, stretched away as far as the eye could see, presenting a rich and varied landscape, rendered more beautiful by the changing shadows which passed swiftly across it as the thin and half-formed clouds skimmed away in the light of the morning sun. The river, reflecting the clear blue of the sky, glistened and sparkled as it flowed noiselessly on; and the oars of the fishermen dipped into the water with a clear and liquid sound, as their heavy but picturesque boats glided slowly down the stream.

Mr. Pickwick was roused from the agreeable reverie into which he had been led by the objects before him, by a deep sigh, and a touch on his shoulder. He turned round: and [a] dismal man was at his side.

"Contemplating the scene?" inquired the dismal man. "I was," said Mr. Pickwick.[16]

Many of the objects observed by Pickwick, the trembling seaweed, the mournful ivy, and the ruined castle underscore the Ozymandian transience of life, which could be, also, a moment of melancholy reflection on the death of *Pickwick*'s illustrator. Yet the style of the text also begins to coincide with the objectives of its main character; fascinated by details, Pickwick is the means through which the narrative becomes, in this scene, richly descriptive. His "reverie" is a Romantic one, to be sure, yet it also manages to comply with the alleged scientific proclivities of the hero. According to Hillis Miller:

> When Dickens "thought of Mr. Pickwick," he thought of someone who was to have the motivations of a *scientist*. [. . .] Pickwick, "his telescope in his great-coat pocket, and his notebook in his waistcoat, ready for the reception of any discoveries of being noted down" [. . . is] stimulated by his desire to investigate and report objectively on all the variety of the world.[17]

The humor of the novel is facilitated in no small part by Pickwick's taste for facts and his obsession with recording them. On stepping into a cab at the beginning of the novel, for instance, he asks the driver the age of his

---

16. Charles Dickens, *The Pickwick Papers*, ed. Mark Wormald (1836–37; London: Penguin, 2003), 70. Subsequent references to this edition will appear in the main body of the text.

17. J. Hillis Miller, *Charles Dickens*, 6. Italics in original.

horse and quickly writes down the answer when it transpires to be forty-two. Although he is only an amateur scientist, Mr Pickwick has achieved some celebrity through his paper "Speculations on the Source of Hampstead Ponds, with some Observations on the Theory of Tittlebats" (15). His best efforts are in theories on pond life, and Mr Pickwick duly fancies himself a great scholar of the empiricist tradition. His initial reaction to the medical students Sawyer and Allen shows how he considers them to be kindred spirits: "Fine fellows," he says to Weller, "very fine fellows, with judgments matured by observation and reflection; and tastes refined by reading and study" (391). Such ideals of medical "observation and reflection," against which Pickwick's bumbling lack of self-perception is starkly contrasted, were not uncommon in expert treatises of the early nineteenth century. In his celebrated *Medical Ethics* (1803), for example, Thomas Percival, physician at the Manchester Infirmary, noted that "no profession is more favourable, than that of physic, to the formation of a mental constitution, which unites in it very high degrees of intellectual and moral vigour."[18] Recast as Pickwick's vain admiration of his and the medical students' empirical skills, such visions become a source of satirical ambivalence as each character fails to embody their ideal.

Drawing upon popular prejudices against medical men as allegedly insensitive, profligate, and in love with a good fee, *Pickwick* demonstrates, in accordance with the teachings of Alexander Thomson, that objects do not always have the weight of truth or accuracy of interpretation to commend them. Sawyer and Allen are important in this context because they are men who ought to have an interest in scientific accuracy. Chapter 37 finds them, having passed their examinations, in their Bristol surgery: "something between a shop and a private-house, and which a red lamp, projecting over the fan-light of the street door" (507). Mr Winkle joins them for punch and pie, and the accompanying illustration (figure 4.1) portrays all three in the throes of their enjoyments. The image creates a scene that may be looked at and examined like the London of the early sketches, which is clear from the appearance of Sam Weller who has been sent by Mr Pickwick to collect Winkle and who may be seen peering through the back door. It is he who serves the function of observer while Sawyer and Allen evidence nothing of their profession's alleged penchant for perception and analysis. When Mr Winkle enters their surgery, objects are being used either for indifferent purposes or as props to misrepresent the two young doctors:

---

18. Thomas Percival, *Medical Ethics; or, a Code of Institutes and Precepts, adapted to the Professional Conduct of Physicians and Surgeons* (Manchester: S. Russell, 1803), 192.

> At the first knock, a sound, as of persons fencing with fire-irons, which had until now been very audible, suddenly ceased; at the second, a studious-looking young gentleman in green spectacles, with a very large book in his hand, glided quietly into the shop, and stepping behind the counter, requested to know the visitor's pleasure. (507)

Recognizing Winkle, he says,

> "Get out, you mouldy old villain, get out!" With this adjuration, which was addressed to the large book, the medical gentleman kicked the volume with remarkable agility to the farther end of the shop, and, pulling off his green spectacles, grinned the identical grin of Robert Sawyer, Esquire, formerly of Guy's Hospital in the Borough, with a private residence in Lant Street. (507)

The young doctor recognizes that he and his partner are likely to be judged from the objects that surround them (the green spectacles and the medical volume, for example). Their "innermost and peculiar sanctum" (507) portrayed in the illustration is littered with collateral evidences that these men are practitioners of the medical arts, and reckless ones at that: tonics and potions, medical volumes, and anatomical specimens (all of which are "things" that tell stories) are accompanied by empty beer bottles. Yet what is perhaps most striking about this picture is the obvious dislocation between objects and their purpose or potential significance. Sawyer and Allen, with Winkle, revel among bits of humans: Winkle's head (furthest right), is directly beneath a grislier head—a human skull. A skeletal leg reclines over the door through which Weller peers, and above the head of Allen (to the left), there is a pile of bones coffined in an enclosed shelf. We could read these vestiges, like Pickwick's mournful ivy, as *memento mori*—grim reminders of man's mortal nature. Yet the mode in which Sawyer and Allen treat the "sacred" tools of their profession indicates that this scene, like others in *The Pickwick Papers,* has a comment to make about the intrinsic value of "things"—or the lack of it. These are men who Pickwick had expected to have "*tastes* refined by reading and study" (391; italics added); he could have no idea how literally he is correct. In the illustration, Sawyer and Allen drink punch out of their scientific apparatuses, and it would not be out of place for the body parts to be used just as irreverently. This is a scene in which "things" have no intrinsic meaning, or, if they did, it has been lost among the foibles and idiosyncrasies of the scene's actors.

Uncomfortable confusions between bodies and objects also occur in an earlier scene where Sawyer and Allen discuss dissection over luncheon; the

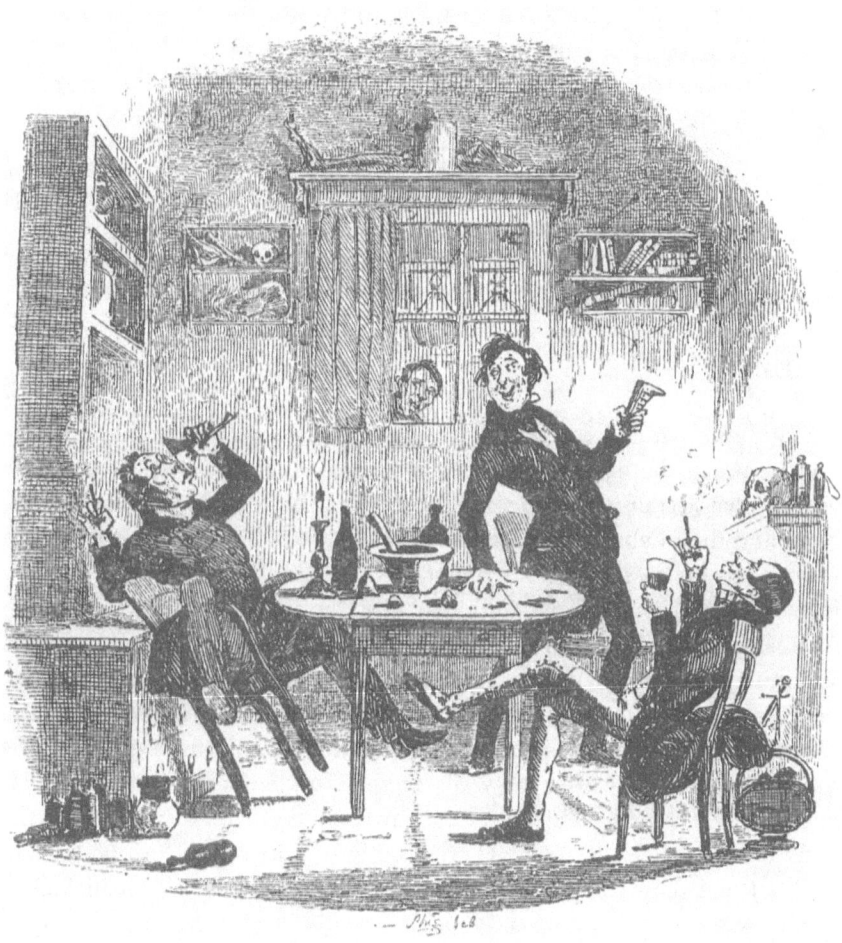

Figure 4.1. "Conviviality at Bob Sawyer's," *The Pickwick Papers* (1836–37)

reaction of Mr Pickwick offers the appropriate response which is notably absent from the students:

> "Nothing like dissecting, to give one an appetite," said Mr Bob Sawyer, looking round the table.
> Mr Pickwick slightly shuddered.
> "By the bye, Bob," said Mr Allen, "have you finished that leg yet?"
> "Nearly," replied Sawyer, helping himself to half a fowl as he spoke. "It's a very muscular one for a child's."

"Is it?" inquired Mr Allen carelessly.

"Very," said Bob Sawyer, with his mouth full.

"I've put my name down for an arm at our place," said Mr Allen. "We're clubbing for a subject, and the list is nearly full, only we can't get hold of any fellow that wants a head. I wish you'd take it."

"No," replied Bob Sawyer; "can't afford expensive luxuries."

"Nonsense!" said Allen.

"Can't, indeed," rejoined Bob Sawyer, "I wouldn't mind a brain, but I couldn't stand a whole head."

"Hush, hush, gentlemen, pray," said Mr Pickwick, "I hear the ladies."

(393–94)

Harry Stone has indicated that this scene draws uncomfortable connections between the flesh being eaten and that being discussed.[19] It recalls a well-known account of Xavier Bichat living "amidst his anatomical specimens and their debris to such an extent that it was difficult to separate the various bits on his table into lunch and experiment."[20] Bichat was famously identified by George Eliot as the man who had "left a realm large enough for many heirs" like Tertius Lydgate.[21] He was, as I noted in chapter 2, a representative of the age's emerging spirit of scientific medicine, and yet his working methods become satirized in *The Pickwick Papers* when the very men who ought to share his appreciation for the finer details show a debauched response to the tools of their trade. Combined with their misuse of their medical apparatuses, Sawyer and Allen's disrespect for the body parts they discuss indicates that "things," like bodies, are important, but they will show as little or as much as each man's whims or habits allow him to see.

"THE STROLLER'S TALE"

In the interpolated tales that break out, like a rash, on the larger narrative of *The Pickwick Papers*, the comedy of the main story is relieved by a range of parabolic narratives where morals are served up with the nourishing regularity of workhouse gruel. These stories' fantasies of moral restitution

---

19. See Stone, *The Night Side of Dickens*, 79. For additional work on Dickens's interest in cannibalism see Carey, *Violent Effigy*, 22–24.

20. Elizabeth Haigh, *Xavier Bichat and the Medical Theory of the Eighteenth Century* (London: The Wellcome Institute, 1984), 12.

21. George Eliot, *Middlemarch*, 148.

rely upon the very acts of "observation and reflection" that are absent in the characterizations of the medical students. In "The Stroller's Tale," for example, the process of interpreting objects as readable extensions of the human body functions as a means of providing narrative and moral coherence. A profligate pantomime artist, based on the son of pantomime clown Joseph Grimaldi,[22] is recompensed for his mistreatment of his wife and child whenever the former looks at him. While he languishes on his deathbed, he says to his visitor:

> I beat her, Jem; I beat her yesterday, and many times before. I have starved her, and the boy too; and now I am weak and helpless, Jem, she'll murder me for it; I know she will. If you'd seen her cry, as I have, you'd know it too. Keep her off. [. . .] There's something in her eyes wakes such a dreadful fear in my heart, that drives me mad. All last night, her large staring eyes and pale face were close to mine; whenever I turned, they turned; and whenever I started up from my sleep, she was at the bed-side looking at me. (51–52)

The story prefigures dramatic sequences both in *Oliver Twist* (1837–39), where Sikes is haunted by visions of Nancy's eyes, and in *Great Expectations* (1860–61), where Arthur Havisham's dying belief is that his undead sister haunts him:

> She's all in white [. . .] wi' white flowers in her hair, and she's awful mad, and she's got a shroud hanging over her arm, and she says she'll put it on me at five in the morning. [. . .] She's a shaking the shrowd at me! Don't you see her? Look at her eyes![23]

The concept of being haunted by one's misdemeanors, signified here by the relentlessness of the accusatory gaze, supports the traditional, "commonsense" notion that "murder will out"; in spite of their best efforts to escape their stories, Sikes and Arthur Havisham are hunted down by their guilty consciences.

In "The Stroller's Tale," however, this sort of moral reparation is underlined by the narrative's attention to detail. When Robert Seymour sent Dickens a preliminary sketch of the illustration that would accompany "The Stroller's Tale," the author had a number of suggestions on how the illustrator might improve the characters. "The furniture of the

---

22. See Charles Dickens, letter to George B. Webb, 15 May 1844, *Letters* 4, 129.
23. Charles Dickens, *Great Expectations,* ed. Robin Gilmour (1860–61; London: Dent, 1994), 309–10. Subsequent references to this edition will be given in the main body of the text.

room," however, he found "depicted, *admirably*."[24] The narrator, Jem Hutley, describes this scene as follows:

> The sick man was lying with his face turned towards the wall; and as he took no heed of my presence, I had leisure to observe the place in which I found myself.
>
> He was lying on an old bedstead, which turned up during the day. The tattered remains of a checked curtain were drawn round the bed's head, to exclude the wind, which however made its way into the comfortless room through the numerous chinks in the door, and blew it to and fro every instant. There was a low cinder fire in a rusty unfixed grate; and an old three-cornered stained table, with some medicine-bottles, a broken glass and a few other domestic articles, was drawn out before it. A little child was sleeping on a temporary bed which had been made for it on the floor, and the woman sat on a chair by its side. There were a couple of shelves, with a few plates and cups and saucers: and a pair of stage shoes and a couple of foils hung beneath them. With the exception of the little heaps of rags and bundles which had been carelessly thrown into the corners of the room, these were the only things in the apartment.
>
> I had time to note these little particulars, and to mark the heavy breathing and feverish startings of the sick man, before he was aware of my presence. (51)

Jem's encounter with the dying pantomime actor has an eerie similarity to John Mason's discovery of Seymour's body weltering in blood.[25] In both instances, descriptions of death and mortal sickness concentrate on the meaning of the "things" that surround the bodies of the men. These objects have a key role to play in the dying clown's morality drama. His surroundings, like the clothes of the boy with the baggy knees (discussed in chapter 3), tell a story that is all about sin and retribution. A bad man in life, the clown has a bad sort of end, and the fact that the objects in the room testify to this tale of poetic justice complements the views of medical writers who believed that in cases of criminal law it was justice, not the devil, that was in the detail.

---

24. Charles Dickens, letter to Robert Seymour, 14 April 1836, *Letters* 1, 145–46 (146). Italics in original.

25. At the time Dickens wrote "The Stroller's Tale" Seymour was still alive. Seymour's wife suggested some years later that Dickens's pernickety requirements tipped the fatal balance for Seymour. Peter Ackroyd is correct in expressing some doubt over this fact which has no corroborating evidence from the years when Seymour and Dickens were working together. Peter Ackroyd, *Dickens* (1990; London: Vintage, 1999), 192–93.

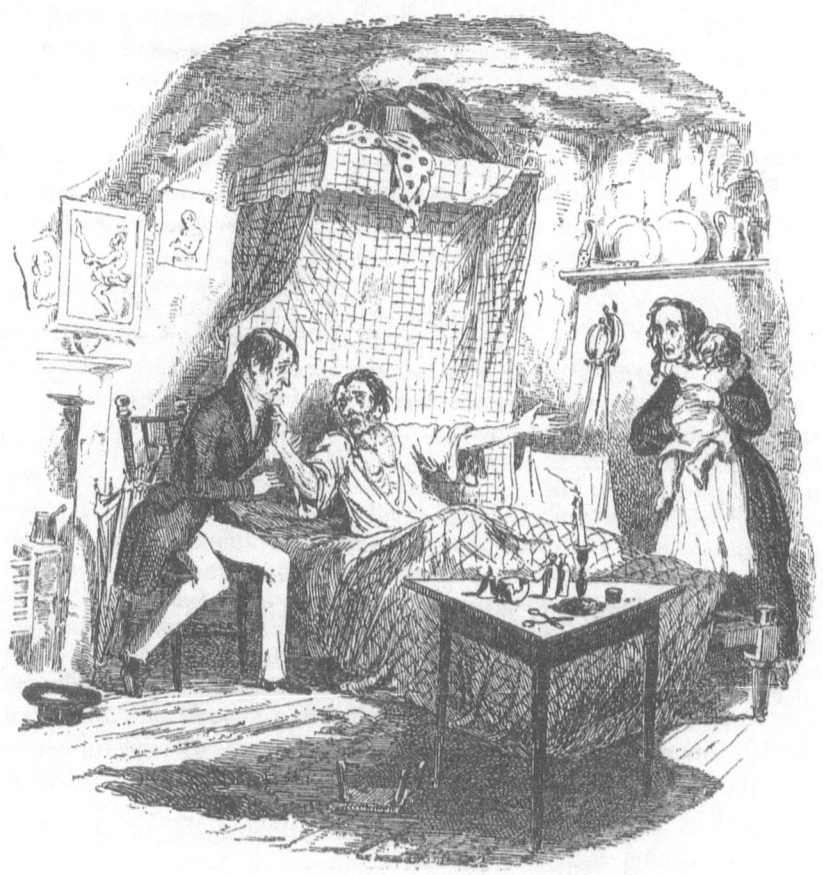

FIGURE 4.2. "The Dying Clown," *The Pickwick Papers* (1836–37). Robert Seymour's last illustration, found among his belongings after his suicide.

Yet the mode in which the above scene from "The Stroller's Tale" is narrated, through the observations of Jem, echoes the way in which the details of forensic investigations get filtered through the visions of a man who, ideally speaking, is conscious of his own will to make "things" speak. Hyppolyte Taine, "the principal theoretician of realism in France from 1855," lauded, according to Joseph T. Flibbert,

> Dickens's ability to capture the mental and emotional qualities of the environment he describes. He asserts that Dickens is not striving for precision of detail but attempting to make the environment complement the state

of mind of his characters. [. . .] According to Taine, Dickens's imagination, "déréglée, excessive, capable d'idée fixes," is selective, seizes upon the things that appeal to it, and avoids the rest.[26]

Supportive of the claim that Dickens wished his objects to have a symbolic value that would complement the larger actions of the scenes in which they appear, Taine suggests that the things "seized upon" are selected subjectively by the author. It would be difficult to imagine any other way of writing about objects in a work of fiction, yet, applied to the observant narrators and main character of *The Pickwick Papers*, Taine's idea is a useful way of interpreting the text's insistence on framing detailed descriptions through an acknowledgment of the subjectivity of observation. In "The Stroller's Tale" Jem's admissions that he "had leisure to observe" and "had time to note these little particulars" draw attention to the layer of narration through which details must pass before they reach their moral function.

LOST AND FOUND

By itself, Jem's admission of curiosity would not form much of a comment on the subjectivity of analytical observation, yet it makes up part of a text in which interpretations are never made without the influence of somebody's preformed views. In one episode based upon an event in Walter Scott's 1816 novel *The Antiquary*, Mr Pickwick stumbles upon an old stone with an inscription:

> It was at this moment that Mr Pickwick made that immortal discovery, which has been the pride and boast of his friends, and the envy of every antiquarian in this or any other country. [. . .] Mr Pickwick's eye fell upon a broken stone, partially buried in the ground, in front of a cottage-door. [. . .]
> "I can discern," continued Mr Pickwick, rubbing away with all his might, and gazing intently through his spectacles: "I can discern a cross, and a B, and then a T. This is important," continued Mr Pickwick, starting up. "This is some very old inscription, existing perhaps long before the ancient alms-houses in this place. It must not be lost." (147)

---

26. Joseph T. Flibbert, "Dickens and the French Debate over Realism: 1838–1856," *Comparative Literature* 23:1 (1971): 18–31 (29–30).

The stone is inscribed thus:

+
B I L S T
U M
P S H I
S. M.
A R K

And Mr Pickwick responds as follows:

> His eyes sparkled with delight, as he sat and gloated over the treasure he had discovered. He had attained one of the greatest objects of his ambition. In a county known to abound in the remains of the early ages; in a village in which there still existed some memorials of the olden time, he—he, the chairman of the Pickwick Club—had discovered a strange and curious inscription of unquestionable antiquity, which had wholly escaped the observation of the many learned men who had preceded him. He could hardly trust the evidence of his senses. (148)

Pickwick is right to mistrust the evidence of his senses because he is guilty of overinterpreting his find. Antiquarians have overlooked the stone because it bears modern graffiti only ("+ Bill Stumps, His Mark").

In a lead article that Dickens wrote for *Household Words* in 1850, "Three 'Detective' Anecdotes," a similar misreading occurs in the world of crime investigation. Eliza Grimwood, a woman of "handsome appearance" with "a proud way of carrying of herself," is discovered by "Inspector Wield" with her throat cut. Beneath her pillow is discovered "a pair of gentlemen's dress gloves, very dirty; and inside the lining, the letters TR, and a cross."[27] A magistrate in the story says, "There's no doubt this is a discovery that may lead to something very important," and Wield duly "look[s] at the gloves pretty narrowly."[28] In spite of this inspection, Wield discovers *by chance* that the gloves belong to a young man named Trinkle: he encounters a glove cleaner at the theater who is able to tell him whom the articles belong to. Convinced that Mr Trinkle is guilty, Wield arrests the man only to discover that he had his gloves stolen by the murdered woman.

---

27. Charles Dickens, "Three 'Detective' Anecdotes," *Household Words* 1 (1850): 577–80 (577).
28. Ibid.

This story itself foreshadows the famous case of German tailor Franz Müller in 1864, a case that Dickens commented on in his correspondence and that seems to have made some important and timely comments about the value of collateral evidence in criminal investigations. On the evening of 9 July 1864, Thomas Briggs, a senior bank clerk, was robbed and murdered in the carriage of a train heading from Central London to Chalk Farm. Briggs's murderer threw his victim out of the train, and it was the driver of the 10.20 train from Hackney Wick to Fenchurch who spotted a "dark object," which turned out to be the "body of a man," on the rails.[29] The bloodstains and the objects left in the railway carriage allowed investigators to identify the victim as Thomas Briggs; he had been robbed of his gold watch and chain and his gold-rimmed spectacles. The carriage was examined by Henry Letheby, professor of chemistry at the London Hospital, who was able to confirm from the direction of blood splatter that Briggs had been struck by a heavy object (probably his own walking stick) while dozing in the corner. Other expert witnesses testified that Briggs had been killed by a combination of blows from the stick and from head injuries he sustained in falling from the train. Yet it was a piece of circumstantial evidence that was crucial to the solving of the case: along with Briggs's bag and stick, there was left at the scene a hat that did not belong to the victim. As the prosecuting lawyer, Sergeant General R. P. Collier, said at Müller's trial:

> There was also found in that carriage a hat, and that is a circumstance of the utmost possible significance. Gentlemen [he addresses the jury], that that hat was not Mr. Briggs's is beyond all doubt. The hat was crushed, apparently as if it had been trod upon in a struggle, and Mr. Briggs's hat was not found. The conclusion appears to me inevitable that the murderer, in the hurry and excitement of the moment, took the wrong hat. [...] If you discover with certainty the person who wore the hat on that night you will have the murderer, and the case is proved almost as clearly against him as if he was seen to do it.[30]

Collier was a believer in the power of circumstantial evidence. The last sentence of this quotation highlights that strong proof of that nature was as reliable, in the lawyer's eyes, to the more "concrete" evidence of a witness. For Collier, the link between the hat and the murderer is "inevitable,"

---

29. George H. Knott (ed.), *Trial of Franz Müller* (Sidney, Wellington, Calcutta: Butterworth, 1911), xiii.

30. Unsigned, "The Murder on the North London Railway," *The Times*, 28 October 1864, 7.

and he goes some way toward justifying the reliability of circumstantial evidence:

> Undoubtedly the evidence in this case is what is called circumstantial evidence chiefly, but I may remind you that it is by circumstantial evidence that great crimes are most frequently detected. Murders are not committed in the presence of witnesses, and to reject circumstantial evidence would be to proclaim immunity to crime. [. . .] There are circumstances which give evidence which cannot be false and which cannot be mistaken.[31]

The defending lawyer, Mr Serjeant Parry, was eager to highlight the same problems of interpretation that had been hinted at, by Alexander Thomson among others, in relation to collateral evidence. Sometimes "things" tell lies, especially if we jump to conclusions based on what the most unanalytical view suggests:

> The evidence ought to be complete. There ought to be no omission, no discrepancy, no uncertainty in the evidence which is to bring home such a charge against [the defendant]. [. . .] I believe myself that circumstantial evidence, if not of the highest character, is of nearly the highest character of evidence; but only this when there is no link wanting in the chain. But if there be a doubt on the evidence laid before the jury, or anything that might cast a doubt on the evidence given, then the chain of evidence is incomplete, and the jury ought not, and cannot act upon it.[32]

Two witnesses were able to confirm that the hat found at the scene of Briggs's murder belonged to Franz Müller. Müller was also found to be in possession of the victim's hat and gold chain. The evidence led to an "inevitable" conclusion according to Collier; the jury thought so too. It took them just fifteen minutes to agree that the defendant was guilty.

Yet before the verdict and sentence were delivered, defending lawyer Parry insisted that "the facts are fairly open to interpretation."[33] Müller maintained that he had bought the hat and chain from a couple of disreputable-looking men; another witness claimed to have seen two similar-looking men in the carriage with Briggs on the night of the murder. Parry noted that only two witnesses were able to confirm that the hat found at the murder scene belonged to Müller, and both, he said, were unreliable

---

31. Ibid.
32. Unsigned, "The Murder on the North London Railway," *The Times*, 29 October 1864, 9.
33. *The Times*, 29 October 1864, 10.

because a £100 reward had been offered for evidence that would lead to the arrest of the murderer. Parry took a line that was similar to that taken by Thomson in his lectures on medical jurisprudence: all evidence, no matter how incriminating and suggestive, ought to be looked upon skeptically as a matter of course.

Unfortunately for Müller, the jury opted for the seductively black-and-white picture painted by Collier. The case became one of celebrity because it was the first murder to have been committed on the railways. As Collier said, "This is a case which has excited unusual and painful interest. It is one which, as we all know, has been canvassed and discussed in every newspaper, I might say almost every house, in the kingdom."[34] Parry added, "The crime [. . .] is almost unparalleled in this country. It is a crime which strikes at the lives of millions. It is a crime which affects the life of every man who travels upon the great iron ways of this country."[35]

When it became clear that Müller was in possession of Briggs's hat and gold chain, he was already aboard a steamer heading for New York. Police inspectors boarded a more direct ship and arrived twenty days before him. In that time, and unbeknownst to the fugitive, the story had created a stir on both sides of the Atlantic, and, echoing how New Yorkers had awaited to hear the fate of Little Nell, a large crowd gathered on the docks to see Müller arrested. Extradited to Britain, the defendant developed a love of Dickens: "He was reading 'David Copperfield.' He had been given 'Pickwick' at the commencement of the voyage, and had enjoyed the book so well, especially the account of the trial of Bardell *v.* Pickwick, that he had asked for another work by the same author."[36] The feeling of appreciation was not mutual. Dickens wrote during the trial:

> I hope that gentleman will be hanged, and have hardly a doubt of it, though croakers contrariwise are not wanting. It is difficult to conceive any other line of defence than that the circumstances proved, taken separately, are slight. But a sound Judge will immediately charge the Jury that the strength of the circumstances likes in their being put together, and will thread them together on a fatal rope.[37]

Dickens acknowledged, contrarily to Collier, that a single item of collateral evidence, like a hat left in a train carriage, did not form a substantial

---

34. *The Times*, 28 October 1864, 7.
35. *The Times*, 29 October 1864, 9.
36. Knott (ed.), *Trial of Franz Müller*, xx.
37. Charles Dickens, letter to W. W. F. De Cerjat, 25 October 1864, *Letters* 10, 443–44.

narrative by itself. Taken with other pieces of evidence, however, and strung together, circumstantial evidence could be coiled into a "fatal rope." As with his interpretation of evidence relating to spontaneous combustion, Dickens insisted on the instrumentalization of interpretation: nothing may be taken for granted by itself, he suggested implicitly; even if the case seemed cut and dried, the relevant "things" need someone to "put [them] together."

The events leading up to the German's execution formed a parallel with the author's interest in the evaluation of collateral evidence and how, written into the very act of interpretation, was a mistrust of what it means to claim truth when "things," within and without the Dickens world, are known to be untrustworthy evidence. During one of the nocturnal adventures of Mr Pickwick and Weller, for instance, a lantern gets carried past the home of "an elderly gentleman of scientific attainments" who is employed in "writing a philosophical treatise." Glancing out the window, this character

> was very much surprised by observing a most brilliant light glide through the air a short distance above the ground, and almost instantaneously vanish. After a short time the phenomenon was repeated, not once or twice, but several times: at last the scientific gentleman, laying down his pen, began to consider to what natural causes the appearances were to be assigned. (529–30)

As with Pickwick's discovery of the inscribed stone, the scientific gentleman interprets the light phenomena through a filter of anticipated greatness:

> What could they be? Some extraordinary and wonderful phenomenon of nature, which no philosopher had ever seen before; something which it had been reserved for him alone to discover, and which he should immortalise his name by chronicling for the benefit of posterity. [. . . His work] should astonish all the atmospherical wiseacres that ever drew breath in any part of the civilised globe. (530)

What this "discovery" has in common with Pickwick's stone, apart from its plain absurdity, is the fact that it is a find made out of the blue. In the field of the empirical sciences, it was common for the scientist to construct hypotheses, yet in the episodes featuring Pickwick's and the old gentleman's discoveries, scientifically minded observers create neither hypotheses nor systems of theories. Instead they are presented with unexpected "breakthroughs." The resulting lack of a trail of reasoning ought to present a unique opportunity for both men to maintain some objectivity because the "rational elements" or creative intuitions that usually infect the formulation of a hypothesis are absent.

This form of unsolicited "reasoning" defined, according to John Reese, professor of forensic and toxicological medicine, one of the key strengths of medical jurisprudence. He noted that in cases where a physician is called to investigate a crime scene, he may "perform his duty with strict impartiality, unbiassed [sic] by prejudice, and untrammeled by fear or favour."[38] In 1861 George Augustus Sala wrote an ironic article called "Notes on Circumstantial Evidence" for *Temple Bar Magazine*, saying that circumstantial evidence "in the hands of men of intellect may be so linked together by an exercise of the logical faculty as to amount to that highest moral proof, which falls only short of mathematical demonstration."[39] The practitioners of medical jurisprudence, obsessed—perhaps more than any other branch of science—with the links between evidence and interpretation, were presented, to all intents and purposes, with their objects of study independently of their own reasoning. The stone and the light phenomenon in *Pickwick* are similarly "imposed" upon their discoverers, and, based on the forensic ideals of John Reese, both men ought to be innocent of involving their feelings, as unwelcome variables, in their interpretations.

The humor of both scenes comes, however, from the fact that Pickwick and the old gentleman are guilty of overestimating their evidence. Friedrich Oesterlen suggested that "everybody has perhaps experienced the excitement produced by a new discovery or a new and striking idea," an experience, he adds, that "acts upon the feelings and imagination" as opposed to the faculty of "understanding":

> Our feelings thus wrought upon, we are no longer what we were, and what we ought to be for a calm investigation. Now, [. . .] the stimulus [may] be no more than an ardent zeal to find out, prove, or accomplish anything, slightly tinctured, perhaps, with ambition, vanity, or rivalship. [. . .] No sooner do certain feelings or tendencies preponderate, than we cease to preserve that calmness of examination which we may possess in reference to other matters, and which is so essential in our observations and researches. [. . .] We [become] satisfied with half-evidence, or with such as is false, whilst in the other case we may, perhaps, be blind to the most clear and valid reasons.[40]

---

38. John J. Reese, *Text-Book of Medical Jurisprudence and Toxicology* (Philadelphia: P. Blakiston, Son & Co., 1884), 56.
39. Sala, "Circumstantial Evidence," 91–98 (93).
40. Oesterlen, *Medicinische Logik* (*Medical Logic*), 357–58.

The farcical tableaux, where Pickwick finds an ancient engraving and the philosopher discovers extraordinary light phenomena, offer a humorous yet (especially considering the contexts that were likely to have influenced the shape of Dickens's writings) a sober indication that the interpretation of physical evidence has its pitfalls. Reese envisaged his science as a place where subjective thinking might be muted in favor of objective, out-of-the-blue discoveries, yet more thoughtful colleagues in the field of medicine, like Oesterlen, were willing to acknowledge that *human* observers will always be vulnerable to the *human* fault of dogmatic interpretation, regardless of how providentially their discoveries are made.

In his classic reading of *Bleak House*, D. A. Miller notes with reference to Jarndyce *v.* Jarndyce that "so nearly intertwined are ending and meaning that to adjourn the one seems to abjure the other."[41] Combining a farcical form, where reader sagacity clashes with character doltishness, and a decision to make a scientific "discoverer" out of his protagonist, Dickens appropriates the question of how and when we can trust the knowledge gained from an interpretation of "things," especially when those "things" are viewed as crucial points in a morally or ambition-fueled narrative with a determining *telos*. In the words of Miller, the novel "simultaneously encourages us to anticipate the end of bafflement and the acquisition of various structures of coherence."[42] At the trial of John Webster for the murder of George Parkman in 1849, the defending lawyer, E. D. Sohier, said of collateral clues that "they do not profess to present a certainty. They present a series of circumstances, from which they ask for a conclusion, that the murder was committed and by the party charged. The danger of error is multiplied on that of positive proof in proportion to the number of facts relied upon."[43] In medical jurisprudence the "end of bafflement" relies upon the interpretation of "things" as clues to a larger story. "How profound a judgment to reason upon [medical] phenomena, and to investigate these causes," wrote John Elliotson in a different context in 1830. "How cool should be the judgement to appreciate all fanciful analogies, and hypothetical suggestions!"[44] Dickens's story of the dying clown and his comments on the Müller case reveal how he saw there to be value in the analysis of objects. Reflecting on the meaning of collateral evidence may be full of

---

41. Miller, *The Novel*, 86.

42. Ibid., 89.

43. Anon., *Trial of Professor John W. Webster for the Murder of Doctor George Parkman* (New York: Stringer and Townsend, 1850), 51.

44. John Elliotson, *On Recent Improvements in the Art of Distinguishing the Various Diseases of the Heart* (London: Longman et al., 1830), 4.

pitfalls, but without space for interpretation it seems unclear, in the Dickens text, whether the gravity of "things" can be understood.

GREAT EXPECTATIONS

That Dickens continued to be fascinated by the power of detail in legal and fictional investigation is clear in the descriptions of certain trials in *Great Expectations*. The brooding advocate Mr Jaggers is unevenly successful in his forensic attention to the meaning of "things." His second appearance in the novel occurs in chapter 18, where, in a public house, he overhears Mr Wopsle reading an account of a "highly popular murder" (117) in a newspaper. Wopsle "enjoyed himself thoroughly" reenacting the inquest, "and we all enjoyed ourselves, and were delightfully comfortable. In this state of mind we came to the verdict of Wilful Murder" (118). Seeming to offer a comment about the use of murder as entertainment, the episode questions whether "Wilful Murder" is a verdict that may be reached securely by anyone, let alone a non-specialist. Jaggers's objection is based on the opposing view that an expert is required to look into the complexities of each case. "Well!" he says,

> "you have settled it all to your own satisfaction, I have no doubt? [. . .] Guilty, of course?" said he, "Out with it. Come!"
> "Sir," returned Mr Wopsle, "without having the honour of your acquaintance, I do say Guilty." Upon this we all took courage to unite in a confirmatory murmur. (118)

Jaggers then obfuscates the case:

> Do you know, or do you not know, that the law of England supposes every man to be innocent, until he is proved—proved—to be guilty? [. . .] *Do* you know that none of these witnesses have yet been cross-examined? [. . .] Tell me whether it distinctly states that the prisoner expressly said that he was instructed by his legal advisers wholly to reserve his defence? Come! Do you make that of it? [. . .] And now I ask you what you say to the conscience of that man who, with that passage before his eyes, can lay his head upon his pillow after having pronounced a fellow-creature guilty, unheard? (118–19; italics in original)

Jaggers's insistence on the case being heard from both sides is an indication of his experience in criminal trials where cross-examination could make all the difference. The weather of any particular arraignment may change in the blink of an eye, Jaggers knows, yet it is the nature of evidence and the danger of assumption that animates him the most: he insists that guilt must be proven, not assumed. Indeed, the judgment of Wopsle and his friends represents the old method of coming to a conclusion based on the myth that "truth will out" and, moreover, that matters can be taken at face value when one relies on a blind faith in the appearances of "things." Wopsle's guilty verdict, assented to by the murmurs of the rest of the group, is not unlike that of Everard Home, who took one look at Sellis's bloody corpse and assumed that the universe must have set right what the Italian's betrayal had made wrong. We are also reminded of Allen and Sawyer, whose misused or ignored tools suggest a professionalism that lies dormant. Jaggers is a different breed altogether. Experienced at law, cold and businesslike, he is part of the same analytical spirit that typifies the period's writings on medical jurisprudence. A lover of proof and evidence, he is also a master rhetorician. Pip narrates:

> We dived into the City, and came up in a crowded police-court, where a blood-relation (in the murderous sense) of the deceased with the fanciful taste in brooches, was standing at the bar, uncomfortably chewing something; while my guardian had a woman under examination or cross-examination—I don't know which—and was striking her, and the bench, and everybody present, with awe. If anybody, of whatsoever degree, said a word that he didn't approve of, he instantly required to have it "taken down." If anybody wouldn't make an admission, he said, "I'll have it out of you!" and if anybody made an admission, he said, "Now I have got you!" The magistrates shivered under a single bite of his finger. Thieves and thief-takers hung in dread rapture on his words, and shrank when a hair of his eyebrows turned in their direction. Which side he was on, I couldn't make out, for he seemed to me to be grinding the whole place in a mill; I only know that when I stole out on tiptoe, he was not on the side of the bench; for, he was making the legs of the old gentleman who presided, quite convulsive under the table, by his denunciations of his conduct as the representative of British law and justice in that chair that day. (179–80)

In *Testimony and Advocacy in Victorian Law, Literature and Theology* (2000), Jan-Melissa Schramm observes that feats of rhetorical power like Jaggers's were the antitheses of traditional assumptions that "truth will out." Jaggers's wish to have everything "taken down" and to receive testimony from the horse's mouth highlights his faith in the transforming and transformative nature of hard facts; the way in which he sends the judge's legs into convulsions is a long way from William Blackstone's faith in judges as "living oracles." Jaggers is a man who appears to have little faith in the worth of assumption, and even less trust in evidence that cannot be useful, quantifiable or forthcoming. "Take nothing on its looks," he tells Pip. "Take everything on evidence. There's no better rule" (298).

Jaggers's world is a world not of precedent, then, but of the tangible "here and now," and his representation of Molly during her criminal trial demonstrates his ability to use real clues as advocates for guilt or innocence:

> Now, Mr Jaggers shows that she had struggled through a great lot of brambles which were not as high as her face; but which she could not have got through and kept her hands out of; and bits of those brambles in question were on examination found to have been broken through, and to have little shreds of her dress and little spots of blood upon them here and there. (350–51)

Jaggers's evidence in favor of Molly is forensic in nature: the survey of the broken brambles is a fine analysis of collateral evidence. Molly's body also comes under scrutiny when she is first introduced to Pip:

> He took his hand from hers, and turned that wrist up on the table. She brought her other hand from behind her, and held the two out side by side. The last wrist was much disfigured—deeply scarred and scarred across and across. When she held her hands out, she took her eyes from Mr Jaggers, and turned them watchfully on every one of the rest of us in succession.
>
> "There's power here," said Mr Jaggers, coolly tracing out the sinews with his forefinger. "Very few men have the power of wrist that this woman has. It's remarkable what mere force of grip there is in these hands. I have had occasion to notice many hands; but I never saw stronger in that respect, man's or woman's, than these." (190)

Jaggers has a medical man's appreciation of Molly's hands, which is due, I think, to his sharing of medicine's love of reading stories from evidence. He traces his finger across the "sinews" as an anatomist might, and the strength of Molly's hands betrays a certain history and a set of character traits. In Wemmick's description of her as "a wild beast tamed" (179), the housekeeper is at once a creature of past events and present clues: once a wild beast, now tamed, her scars and submission tell stories. She is, in short, a symbol of Jaggers's forensic ability: testament to his feats of oratorical power combined with an appreciation of the complexities of anatomical and collateral evidence.

Things turn out very differently for Magwitch, which is a result of the apparent fact that he is tried using older, assumptive methods of judgment rather than the forensic feats that get Molly acquitted. In his own account of his trial in which he stands in the dock with Compeyson, he says:

> When we was put in the dock, I noticed first of all what a gentleman Compeyson looked, wi' his curly hair and his black clothes and his white pocket-handkercher, and what a common sort of a wretch I looked. When the prosecution opened and the evidence was put short, aforehand, I noticed how heavy it all bore on me, and how light on him. When the evidence was giv in the box, I noticed how it was always me that had come for'ard, and could be swore to, how it was always me that the money had been paid to, how it was always me that had seemed to work the thing and get the profit. But, when the defence come on, then I see the plan plainer; for, says the counsellor for Compeyson, "My lord and gentlemen, here you has afore you, side by side, two persons as your eyes can separate wide; one, the younger, well brought up, who will be spoke to as such; one, the elder, ill brought up, who will be spoke to as such; one, the younger, seldom if ever seen in these here transactions, and only suspected; t'other, the elder, always seen in 'em and always wi' his guilt brought home. Can you doubt, if there is but one in it, which is the one, and, if there is two in it, which is much the worst one?" And such-like. And when it come to character, warn't it Compeyson as had been to the school, and warn't it his schoolfellows as was in this position and in that, and warn't it him as had been know'd by witnesses in such clubs and societies, and nowt to his disadvantage? And warn't it me as had been tried afore, and as had been know'd up hill and down dale in Bridewells and Lock-Ups? And when it come to speech-making, warn't it Compeyson as could speak to 'em wi' his face dropping every now and then into his white pocket-handkercher—ah! and wi' verses in his speech, too—and warn't it me as could only say, "Gentlemen, this man at my side is a most precious rascal"? And when the verdict come, warn't it Compeyson as was recommended to mercy on account of good character and bad company, and giving up all the information he could agen me, and warn't it me as got never a word but Guilty? [. . .] And when we're sentenced, ain't it him as gets seven year, and me fourteen, and ain't it him as the Judge is sorry for, because he might a done so well, and ain't it me as the Judge perceives to be a old offender of wiolent passion, likely to come to worse?" (311–12)

Magwitch is unfairly treated on the basis that the law makes too many assumptions. "Can you doubt" the facts, the prosecuting lawyer asks the jury, when everything looks so clear? He almost repeats the words of Everard Home, who had had no doubt that Sellis must have cut his own throat, because, it turns out, he was an unpleasant character and—worse still—a foreigner. The power of tangible evidence in Molly's case is what saves her from a similar condemnation. In the one case Jaggers is able to marshal the powers of collateral evidence; in the other "things" are unable to quiet the voices of quack assumption and traditional views that "facts" should be judged using "common-sense." Magwitch's trial, or the story of it as recounted by the defendant himself, serves to highlight the important work that collateral evidence is expected to do in scenarios where blind prejudice and basic empiricism demand attention. In Molly's trial, evidence becomes a means through which Jaggers successfully exercises his analytical and rhetorical capabilities. Magwitch's indictment, however, is offered as a stark contrast: here, law without forensic-level interpretation is blind, impotent, and unfair.

THE PRINCE DE CONDÉ

When it came to the subject of auditing the collateral details of a death scene, writers on medical jurisprudence usually referenced the case of the Prince de Condé. The case was briefly referred to in the exchange of letters that took place between Dickens and G. H. Lewes in *The Leader* in the 1850s. Criticizing the former, as we have seen, on the nature of his evidence relating to spontaneous combustion, Lewes noted that finding a body burned did not necessarily indicate that its owner had gone the way of Mr Krook: "The persons who were in the château where the last Prince de Condé was found hanging were witnesses to the fact that he *was* found hanging, but could not testify to the point at issue—whether the Prince hanged himself or was murdered."[45] Lewes was referring to the discovery of the corpse of Condé, a seventy-four-year-old survivor of the French Revolution, hanging from a curtain pole on 27 August 1830. According to first appearances, the death was a conclusive case of suicide: "His death had been voluntary, and had been caused by strangulation." Condé must have been mentally deranged, it was added, by the "excitement occasioned by the late revolution."[46] Soon afterwards, however, there were suggestions,

---

45. Lewes, "Spontaneous Combustion," 137–38; 161–63 (137).
46. Unsigned, "Foreign Intelligence," *Hull Packet and Humber Mercury,* 7 September 1830, 2.

as Lewes indicates, that Condé had been assassinated. Unlike Robert Seymour, the prince appeared to have left no suicide note, and he had always expressed, during life, an aversion to the act of self-destruction.

Most significantly of all, medical men could reach no consensus on whether Condé had killed himself or not. The case became, according to *The Age*, "an object of great conversation";[47] medical practitioners clamoured to inspect the crime scene, to examine the body, and to give their opinions on whether or not the prince had committed suicide. According to the *London Medical Gazette*, the renowned expert Charles Marc believed that Condé *had* committed suicide; François Dubois and Auguste Gendrin, meanwhile, believed that he may have been murdered.[48]

In addition to the apparent lack of a note, and Condé's loathing of suicide, there were other indications that the prince may not have died by his own hands. To begin with, he had sustained, some years before his death, a sporting injury that precluded him from raising one hand higher than his head, suggesting that he might have had difficulty tying his own noose. What is more, when Condé's remains were discovered, they were not fully suspended from the ground. The illustration from Alfred Swaine Taylor's summary of the case in *The Principles and Practice of Medical Jurisprudence* (1865) (figure 4.3) demonstrates how the prince's feet were touching the floor when he was found. Echoing the doubts of Dubois and Gendrin, *Bell's Life in London* suggested that "nothing indicated that the weight of the body could have caused strangulation."[49] Taylor disagreed. He observed that "in order that death should take place from hanging, it is not necessary that the body should be freely and perfectly suspended. [. . .] Many cases have been since recorded in which death has taken place from hanging when the feet were in contact with the ground, or the persons were almost sitting recumbent."[50] He added that there was plenty of anatomical evidence to suggest that the prince had killed himself. The rigidity of the body, for instance, showed that he had died between the hours of 10:00 P.M. and 12:00 A.M. At this time in the evening,

> there were numerous attendants moving about near to the duke's apartments. These persons must have heard any unusual noise, which the duke

---

47. Unsigned, *The Age*, 1 January 1832, 3.
48. Unsigned, "Was the Duke of Bourbon Murdered?" *London Medical Gazette*, 31 December 1831, 485–86.
49. Unsigned, "The Prince of Condé," *Bell's Life in London and Sporting Chronicle*, 26 September 1830, 1. This article appeared five years before Dickens began writing his sketches for the same magazine.
50. Taylor, *Principles and Practice*, vol. 2, 57.

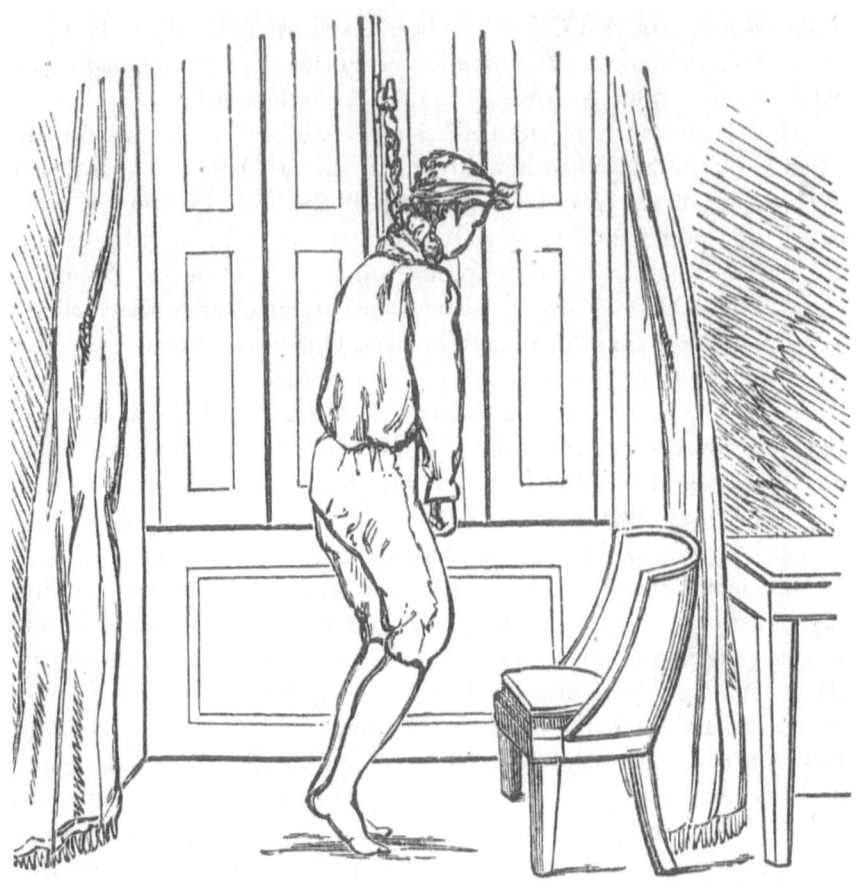

Figure 4.3. Illustration of the Prince de Condé's body as it was discovered. Alfred Swaine Taylor, *Principles and Practice of Medical Jurisprudence* (1865).

would probably have made in resisting his assailants. But no noise was heard in the apartment at that or any other time, and the presumption of this being an act of homicide was therefore strongly rebutted.[51]

There were also anatomical indications that the prince had not died from asphyxia. *John Bull* suggested:

The head had sunk upon the chest—the countenance was calm and composed—the face pale—the tongue did not protrude from the mouth, which

---

51. Ibid., vol. 1, 83.

was half open—the lips were black—the knees were pliant—the arms were hanging down—the hands were not closed, and the thumbs lay lightly upon the fingers.

To shew that these are not the appearances after hanging, we have not only the evidence of all the French surgeons who were examined, but the common experience of every man who has seen the corpse of a man hanged.

The surgeon describes the appearances which the body would have exhibited if the Prince had been hanged *alive*: the tongue would have protruded from the mouth: which would have been entirely open; the eyes would have been open, and staring from their sockets; the face would have been black, and the tongue itself swollen. Not one of these distinctive marks presented themselves.[52]

The state of the body indicated, according to this article, that the prince had been smothered, "suffocated in his bed, and then suspended to the curtain-rod" by an assassin.[53] Eager to sensationalize the story as much as possible, *John Bull* added that this was almost exactly how Burke and Hare murdered their victims in 1827 and 1828 and that it was therefore just as "terrific," "base," "damnable," and "revolting":

BURKING, callous, horrid, and detestable as the crime is when committed by ignorant, unprincipled, and wretched barbarians, receives new horrors when connected in the mind with persons moving in the station which the murderers of [Condé] may be supposed to fill. [. . .] It is, therefore, no longer a matter of doubt that the Prince was MURDERED—BURKED.[54]

The author of this piece surveys, figuratively, the scene of Condé's death with an attention to fine detail, yet many of the deductions he makes are inaccurate or doubtful. Not all of the medical witnesses agreed that the marks on Condé's body were inconsistent with hanging; Marc believed, for instance, that the prince had suspended himself from his curtain pole.[55] The link with the Edinburgh murders is also a tenuous stretch, as Burke and Hare did not hang their victims from curtain poles, nor was Condé killed in order to provide medical students with a cadaver to dissect.

---

52. Unsigned, *John Bull*, 26 December 1831, 430–32 (430, 431).
53. Ibid., 431.
54. Ibid.
55. The *London Medical Gazette* accused Marc of being "swayed by an undue political bias" because he was physician in ordinary to Louis Philippe, a relative of Condé's. See Anon., "Was the Duke of Bourbon Murdered?" 485–86.

In the 1842 edition of his *Elements of Medical Jurisprudence,* Beck stated that the corpse *did* bear the hallmarks of asphyxiation caused by suspension, and in the specialized format of a medical textbook he took the liberty of noting that when his body was found, Condé had a "semi-erection and [there had been] an emission of semen."[56] Such was thought to be typical in cases of men who had been hanged by the neck, but Beck surmised that the Frenchman's death may have been accidental: "It is a known practice with persons of this description to cause themselves to be half-hanged in order to arouse their dormant generative powers, and several have lost their lives from not being taken down in time."[57] In his *Manual of Medical Jurisprudence* (1831), Michael Ryan confirmed that "examples are recorded of both sexes, who, to excite the venereal appetite, allowed themselves to be suspended for some time; and some of them lost their lives in not having been taken down before asphyxia occurred."[58] In any case, Beck claimed that Condé had died alone, and his view was backed up by other expert commentators, including the prolific alienist Forbes Winslow who, incidentally, appeared in Dickens's Gad's Hill library with a book on insanity inscribed "with the author's compts."[59] In his 1840 book *The Anatomy of Suicide,* Winslow noted, "Conflicting as the evidence was in this case, we think no impartial mind, after maturely considering all the physical facts and moral circumstances connected with the Prince de Condé's death, can entertain any other opinion than that he sacrificed his own life."[60]

At the risk of stating the obvious, the fact that so many commentators, specialized and otherwise, disagreed on the method of Condé's death illustrates that the evidence was inconclusive. The *London Medical Gazette* observed in 1832 that "none of the explanations offered are satisfactory, and the medical jurist has hitherto been baffled in all his attempts to reconcile the circumstances to the idea either of murder or suicide."[61] It was because of disagreements over what the *body* suggested that investigators turned their attentions to the collateral evidence. When the cadaver was found, there were no suspicious footprints, no weapons, no marks of violence, but there *were* indications that the prince had had no intention to die. Most importantly, perhaps, investigators found that Condé's watch had been wound on the night he died, and he had tied a knot in his handkerchief as a reminder of something to be done the following day. The watch and the knot, the

---

56. Beck, *Elements,* 635.
57. Ibid., 637.
58. Ryan, *Manual,* 358.
59. Dickens owned Winslow's *The Incubation of Insanity* (1845). Stonehouse, *Catalogue,* 88.
60. Forbes Winslow, *The Anatomy of Suicide* (1840; Boston, Milford House, 1972), 254.
61. Unsigned, "Duke of Bourbon," *London Medical Gazette,* 21 January 1832, 608–9 (608).

Gazette claimed, demonstrated that the prince had not viewed his life to be approaching its termination: Why would a man who intended to die prepare to continue living?[62] It appears as though death had taken Condé by surprise, which is a characteristic of murders and accidents, not suicides.

The fact that the Duke's watch was still ticking indicated, most fittingly of all, that the old man's life was unfinished. In the words of Frank Kermode, the prince's life was *ticking*, but it had not yet *tocked*: "Let us take a very simple example, the ticking of a clock," Kermode writes in *The Sense of an Ending* (1967). "*Tick* is our word for a physical beginning, *tock* our word for an end."[63] *Tick* represents the beginning of a life and the continuation of it ("it keeps me ticking"), while *tock* represents closure. Taken together, *tick-tock* manifests a closed, teleological narrative—short, it is true, but with a beginning and an end. In the case of Robert Seymour, evidence (especially the suicide note) illustrates that the narrative of the illustrator's life had *tocked*. Yet there was evidence that Condé believed himself to inhabit the space between *tick* and *tock*. Like his freshly wound watch, the prince was still ticking. The idea of an uninterrupted and completed narrative structure, the "fiction" that Kermode understands through the *tick-tock* analogy was (and still is) central to the investigations of collateral evidence in cases of suspected suicide. If the circumstantial clues prove that the deceased had no plans to wind up his or her existence, then it may be surmised that the individual in question did not die voluntarily. Such, it was agreed by some, was the state of affairs with Condé.

Of course, the strongest collateral indication that an individual intends to die is a suicide note. As noted above, the fact that one of these was discovered beside Seymour's corpse enabled his inquest to reach its verdict of "mental derangement" relatively promptly and with few, if any, snags. At first it appeared that Condé had left no suicide letter, but in 1832 *The Morning Chronicle* suggested that fragments of a note were found in the grate of the prince's bedroom. It read:

> Do not take or burn anything in the chateau or the village. Do no wrong to anybody, neither to my friends nor my enemies. There is nothing for me but death. I wish happiness and prosperity to the people and to my country. Adieu for ever. I request that I may be buried in the ditch of Vincennes, near my son.[64]

---

62. Unsigned, "Was the Duke of Bourbon Murdered?" 485–86.
63. Frank Kermode, *The Sense of an Ending: Studies in the Theory of Fiction* (Oxford and New York: Oxford University Press, 1967), 44–45.
64. Unsigned, "French Papers," *Morning Chronicle*, 3 January 1832, 1.

The statement "there is nothing for me but death" indicates, seemingly definitively, that the prince was fully prepared to die, yet if there was nothing left for Condé, why did he prepare to continue living?

Whatever the cause or reason of Condé's death, the investigation was referenced repeatedly in forensic textbooks as evidence of the significance and the difficulty of the medical profession's "collateral" observations. Medical jurisprudence did not limit its focus to clues left upon anatomies, as might be expected, but it read everyday objects as though they were hieroglyphs on the secrets of human intention. Criminal behavior, it was believed, left its marks upon the scenes in which it took place, yet the wide and varied disagreements over what bodies and "things" say in conjunction with one another indicates that the act of interpretation was no simple process.

PICKWICKIAN THINGS

Dickens was a master of the art of making inanimate objects come to life for the purpose of tormenting guilty characters. We may recall, for example, the famous door-knocker in *A Christmas Carol* (1843) and the pointing Allegory in *Bleak House* (1852–53). Such hyperboles of the forensic belief in the revelatory power of "things" are often used for comic or ironic effect, such as in *The Pickwick Papers* when a chair comes to life to solve a crime and to tell stories about the dozens of posteriors it has known. Interpolated tales like this one have had a hard time of it in Dickens scholarship. K. J. Fielding called *Pickwick*'s digressions "lamentable interpolate stories,"[65] while John Butt and Kathleen Tillotson thought that the arrangement of the novel's two writing styles had "no other apparent purpose than to exhibit Boz's versatility."[66] Yet, as Robert L. Patten has noted, there do appear to be "reasons for believing that the interpolated tales are more than casually related to *Pickwick*'s main narrative. All the tales have some thematic relationship to the central plot, and [. . .] in a different dimension and mode, recapitulate the novel's principal action."[67] One thing that the stories do recapitulate in a particular and significant way is the novel's penchant for noticing small details and for putting them to work in a moral story; indeed, the tales are specifically enlightening because of their allegorical nature. The way in

---

65. Quoted in Robert L. Patten, "The Art of Pickwick's Interpolated Tales," *ELH* 34:3 (September 1967): 349–66 (349).
66. John Butt and Kathleen Tillotson, *Dickens at Work* (London: Methuen, 1957), 68.
67. Patten, "Pickwick's Interpolated Tales," 365.

which they present a character reaping what he or she has sown, compactly within the context of a short story, allows each of them to draw a clear and direct line between the interpretation of "things" and fiction's seeming insistence on moral restitution. They do not present what Gillian Piggott identifies as "simultaneous levels of meaning: the material and the immaterial, the worldly and the spiritual."[68] Rather, they present a world in which material things and immaterial morals exist in a single act of interpretation. We have already seen, for instance, how in "The Stroller's Tale" a large part of the pantomime artist's punishment consists of his being surrounded by squalid and unpleasant objects. Dickens's relentlessness of description and Jem's acts of interpretation go some way, I suggest, to recapture the forensic method of understanding guilt through a careful assessment of physical evidence. Such is also apparent in "The Story of the Goblins who Stole a Sexton," a tale in which a misanthropic gravedigger is taught the errors of his ways, like Ebenezer Scrooge, by supernatural visitants:

> [One night, Christmas eve, Gabriel Grub] was not a little indignant to hear a young urchin roaring out some jolly song about a merry Christmas, in this very sanctuary, which had been called Coffin Lane ever since the days of the old abbey, and the time of the shaven-headed monks. As Gabriel walked on, and the voice drew nearer, he found it proceeded from a small boy, who was hurrying along, to join one of the little parties in the old street, and who, partly to keep himself company, and partly to prepare himself for the occasion, was shouting out the song at the highest pitch of his lungs. So Gabriel waited till the boy came up, and then dodged him into a corner, and rapped him over the head with his lantern five or six times, just to teach him to modulate his voice. As the boy hurried away with his hand to his head, singing quite a different sort of tune, Gabriel Grub chuckled very heartily to himself, and entered the churchyard, locking the gate behind him. (381–82)

Narrated to Mr Pickwick by Mr Wardle, this tale is meticulous for its attention to setting, detail, and history. After beating the child, Grub cheerily spends the evening digging graves until he is interrupted by a spectral chuckle:

> Gabriel paused in some alarm [. . .] and looked round. The bottom of the oldest grave about him, was not more still and quiet, than the churchyard

---

68. Piggott, *Dickens and Benjamin*, 25.

in the pale moonlight. The cold hoar frost glistened on the tomb stones and sparkled like rows of gems among the stone carvings of the old church. The snow lay hard and crisp upon the ground, and spread over the thickly-strewn mounds of earth, so white and smooth a cover, that it seemed as if corpses lay there, hidden only by their winding sheets. Not the faintest rustle broke the profound tranquillity of the solemn scene. Sound itself appeared to be frozen up, all was so cold and still. (382)

Again, there is an obvious attention to detail in this scene; yet there is a key difference with the earlier scene in which the old ruins of Coffin Lane are described. Particulars in the latter are used to facilitate induction: the old abbey ruins tell a real history of shaven-headed monks. In the graveyard scene, however, details facilitate *invention*: tombstones become gems, and grave mounds are transformed into barely covered corpses. And it is at this very moment of fancy that part of the scenery comes to life to deliver Grubb's sentence:

Seated on an upright tombstone, close to him, was a strange unearthly figure, whom Gabriel felt at once, was no being of this world. [. . .] The hat was covered with the white frost, and the goblin looked as if he had sat on the same tombstone very comfortably, for two or three hundred years. He was sitting perfectly still; his tongue was put out, as if in derision; and he was grinning at Gabriel Grub with such a grin as only a goblin could call up. (384)

The goblin manifests a paradox that is inherent to all of Dickens's descriptions of the supernatural. The goblin is simultaneously not of this world yet part of its mundane furniture. Like Jacob Marley's use of the door-knocker and the spirits' use of bells in *The Chimes* (1844), Grubb's chimera uses a very common object, a tombstone, as a portal between the two worlds: this "thing," the tombstone, is a reversal of the Dickensian wish to dwell on the "romantic side of familiar things." It is a familiar side of a romantic thing that, in a way, crystallizes Dickens's appropriation of the forensic method: it is a way of getting at an interpretation through the analysis of a detail.

PIP'S FANCIES

The goblin's tombstone is a sensational rehearsal of a similar theme that is developed with greater sophistication in *Great Expectations*—a novel in which mundane objects tell stories as fantastic as Pip's embellished report on his first visit to Miss Havisham's. The idea of "things" as portals to Dickensian grotesquery is especially true of the forensic world of Jaggers where "coarse fat office-candles" are "decorated with dirty winding sheets, as if in remembrance of a host of hanged clients" (346); Mr Wemmick's costume is accessorized with trinkets he has had bequeathed by condemned criminals (178); and the lawyer's boots creak, as if conscious of their ability to tattle: "*They* laughed in a dry and suspicious way" (176; italics in original). The objects of *Great Expectations* never miss an opportunity to let slip some form of gossip, largely because the novel's world is a world of crime and punishment where interpretation is often called upon to tell tales. Take the casts of the two "famous clients" that sit on Jaggers's office wall. Pip assumes that they are regular portraits, but Wemmick tells him their history:

> "Pray," said I, as the two odious casts with the twitchy leer upon them caught my sight again, "whose likenesses are those?"
> "These?" said Wemmick, getting upon a chair, and blowing the dust off the horrible heads before bringing them down. "These are two celebrated ones, Famous clients of ours that got us in a world of credit. This chap (why you must have come down in the night and been peeping into the inkstand, to get this blot upon your eyebrow, you old rascal!) murdered his master [. . . the other] forged wills, this blade did, if he didn't also put the supposed testators to sleep too." (177–78)

These are objects that hold a lot of admonitory meaning. The way in which the clerk addresses Old Artful and suggests that he has been peeping into the inkstand takes us back into Pickwickian territory where objects come to life via the imagination of the interpreter; it also highlights how objects are never meaningless in the world of the Dickens novel—they always have a tale to tell.

Yet objects are only brought to life in the later novel through the agency of Pip's overactive fancy. The idea of Old Artful peeping into the inkwell is a good indication of how tangible things might facilitate fantasy scenarios. The tombstone belonging to Pip's parents, like that in "The Story of the Goblins who Stole a Sexton," is another conduit for imaginary elements:

> As I never saw my father or my mother, and never saw any likeness of either of them (for their days were long before the days of photographs), my first fancies regarding what they were like, were unreasonably derived

from their tombstones. The shape of the letters on my father's, gave me an odd idea that he was a square, stout, dark man, with curly black hair. From the character and turn of the inscription, "*Also Georgiana Wife of the Above,*" I drew a childish conclusion that my mother was freckled and sickly. To five little stone lozenges, each about a foot and a half long which were arranged in a neat row beside their grave, and were sacred to the memory of five little brothers of mine—who gave up trying to get a living, exceedingly early in that universal struggle—I am indebted for a belief I religiously entertained that they had all been born on their backs with their hands in their trousers-pockets, and had never taken them out in this state of existence. (1)

That Pip's deductions are fantastic is a state of affairs that does nothing to negate the novel's sense that objects tell stories when they are passed through the filter of human intellection. Pip's findings are, of course, unlikely to be true, yet they do strike the moral and affective keynotes of the novel: parenthood, benefaction, and loss. The opening of *Great Expectations* is synonymous with Pip's "first most vivid impression of the identity of *things*" (1; italics added), which is ambiguously expressed: it could be that Pip first learns to understand the nature of objects literally: "things" are a reflection of reality. In *Reading for the Plot* (1984), Peter Brooks notes that "the tracing of the [parents'] name—which [Pip] has already distorted in its application to self—involves a misguided attempted to remotivate the graphic symbol, to make it directly mimetic."[69] Secondly, and more revealingly, the words "my first most vivid impression of the *identity* of things" could mean that the boy begins to understand how "things" have identities and that these go beyond material function. The letters on the tombstones say a lot more than they are intended to say through the boy's interpretation of their materiality. The ambiguity is, I think, a telling indication that the definitions between material and moral are not that easily separated in *Great Expectations*. It is certain that this is a scene in which Pip assesses the details around him and finds in them the sad truth of his vulnerability:

> At such a time I found out for certain, that this bleak place overgrown with nettles was the churchyard; and that Philip Pirrip, late of this parish, and also Georgiana wife of the above, were dead and buried; and that

---

69. Peter Brooks, *Reading for the Plot: Design and Intention in Narrative* (Cambridge: Harvard University Press, 1984), 115–16.

Alexander, Bartholomew, Abraham, Tobias, and Roger, infant children of the aforesaid, were also dead and buried; and that the dark flat wilderness beyond the churchyard, intersected with dykes and mounds and gates, with scattered cattle feeding on it, was the marshes; and that the low leaden line beyond, was the river; and that the distant savage lair from which the wind was rushing was the sea; and that the small bundle of shivers growing afraid of it all and beginning to cry, was Pip. (1)

The style of this passage is not unlike the way the rest of the novel goes about describing Pip's perceptions: detail falls on detail in a style that gets echoed when the boy first meets Miss Havisham and he notices her whiteness, her age, and her heartbreak. In conjunction with the earlier reading of the tombstones, Pip's realization of the "identity of things" links with the awakening of a moral interpretation. "Truth" is figured in Magwitch, Pip's fairy godfather, who appears, like the sexton's goblin, among the gravestones. Magwitch serves the same function as the goblin. Though there is nothing supernatural about him, he manifests Pip's truths—as conjured from the boy's readings of the material realities of the scene. Covered in mud and water from the "dark flat wilderness" (2) which has just denoted the frightening truths that are dawning on the boy, the convict emerges, as does the goblin, from the material fabric of the scene.

When Magwitch appears later in the novel, as Pip is grown up and sharing an apartment with Herbert Pocket, the protagonist feels "a dull sense of being alone" (279), and the London weather recreates the dark wildness of the marshes:

> It was wretched weather; stormy and wet, stormy and wet; mud, mud, mud, deep in all the streets. Day after day, a vast heavy veil had been driving over London from the East, and it drove still, as if in the East there were an eternity of cloud and wind. So furious had been the gusts, that high buildings in town had had the lead stripped off their roofs; and in the country, trees had been torn up, and sails of windmills carried away; and gloomy accounts had come in from the coast of shipwreck and death. Violent blasts of rain had accompanied these rages of wind, and the day just closed as I sat down to read had been the worst of all. (279)

Like the spirits in *The Chimes* (1844), Magwitch comes in with the sound of the bells: "Saint Paul's, and all the many church-clocks in the City—some leading, some accompanying, some following—struck [eleven]. The sound was curiously flawed by the wind; and I was listening, and thinking how the wind assailed and tore it, when I heard a footstep on the stair" (280). The following scene is one in which detailed realities blend with illusions:

> The wind rushing up the river shook the house that night, like discharges of cannon, or breakings of sea. When the rain came with it and dashed against the windows, I thought, raising my eyes to them as they rocked, that I might have fancied myself in a storm-beaten light-house. Occasionally, the smoke came rolling down the chimney as though it could not bear to go out into such a night; and when I set the doors open and looked down the staircase, the staircase lamps were blown out. (278)

Notice the combination of everyday objects with imaginings: windows, doors, and staircase lamps are haunted by personified smoke and nautical chimeras. "Browned and hardened by exposure to weather" (280), Magwitch steps out of this uncanny yet real setting, and, though the night is extraordinary, the convict has the air of a being borne from the ruder elements of the everyday. As in his previous manifestation as the "reality of things," he now represents the truth of the protagonist's latest realization. "Miss Havisham's intentions towards me," Pip realizes,

> were all a mere dream; Estella not designed for me; I only suffered in Satis House as a convenience, a sting for the greedy relations, a model with a mechanical heart to practice on when no other practice was at hand; those were the first smarts I had. But, sharpest and deepest pain of all—it was for the convict, guilty of I knew not what crimes, and liable to be taken out of those rooms where I sat thinking, and hanged at the Old Bailey door, that I had deserted Joe. (288)

Like Grub's goblin, Magwitch represents the young man's conscience and his penance: he is at once Pip's reality and his moral ballast. That the convict is conjured from the details of the real world in order to acquaint the protagonist with the truth is an indication that Dickens saw the "things" of real life and "truth" to be linked. Like Gabriel Grub's goblin, however, Magwitch is a characterization that draws on an assumption created by forensic experts, though matters are expressed more imaginatively in Dickens than in any textbook on medical jurisprudence. There is a close relationship, it seems, between earthbound details and heaven-bound "truths," but it is the interpretive (and often unruly) faculties of human consciousness that get charged with the task of making sense of the connection.

THE BAGMAN'S UNCLE

Pip's fancies, which are legion and varied, belong to a Dickensian tradition of questioning the value and implication of a free imagination. The first text to deal with this issue was the "Monmouth Street" sketch, explored in chapter 3, where a boy's set of clothing leads the narrator into an imaginary pantomime. In the last of *Pickwick*'s interpolations, "The Story of the Bagman's Uncle," there is a similar interrogation of ways in which rich use of details can lead to a fictional rather than a useful or admonitory "truth." Getting incredibly drunk one evening, the eponymous uncle finds himself surrounded by ghostly mail coaches coming to life. On first entering a waste ground featuring "old worn-out mail coaches" (648), the uncle employs a forensic eye to survey the scene:

> There they stood, all huddled together in the most desolate condition imaginable. The doors had been torn from their hinges and removed, the linings had been stripped off, only a shred hanging here and there by a rusty nail; the lamps were gone, the poles had long since vanished, the iron-work was rusty, the paint worn away; the wind whistled through the chinks in the bare wood-work, and the rain, which had collected on the roofs, fell drop by drop into the insides with a hollow and melancholy sound. They were the decaying skeletons of departed mails, and in that lonely place, at that time of night, they looked chill and dismal.
>
> My uncle rested his head upon his hands, and thought of the busy bustling people who had rattled about, years before, in the old coaches and were now as silent and changed. (648)

The uncle uses forms of observation that are simultaneously sharp and sobering in their failures. Penetrating every nook of the scene, his gaze allows history to rerun in a way that is similar to how the objects surrounding the dead Condé furnished examiners with the supposed story of *his* last moments. Observe also the links between mail coaches and corpses; these are the "decaying skeletons" of the departed, "chill and dismal," compared to the "silent and changed" natures of those who once rode inside them. Thomas de Quincey later referred to the English mail-coach system as once working "in a perfection of harmony like that of heart, veins, and arteries, in a healthy animal organisation."[70] For Dickens, the same coaches, now

---

70. Thomas de Quincey, "The English Mail-Coach, or the Glory of Motion" (1849), in *Selected Essays of De Quincey* (London: Walter Scott Ltd., n.d.), 122–57 (123).

defunct, are, like Miss Havisham and the moldering remains of the dead: ghastly relicts of an old story.[71]

When the bagman's uncle falls into a slumber, he is woken by a clock striking two. Like the peals that carry Magwitch back into the life of Pip, these chimes signal the resurrection of the past:

> In one instant [. . .] the whole of this deserted and quiet spot had become a scene of most extraordinary life and animation. The mail coach doors were on their hinges, the lining was replaced, the ironwork was as good as new, the paint was restored, the lamps were alight; cushions and greatcoats were on every coach-box, porters were thrusting parcels into every boot, guards were stowing away letter-bags, hostlers were dashing pails of water against the renovated wheels; numbers of men were pushing about, fixing poles into every coach; passengers arrived, portmanteaus were handed up, horses were put to; in short, it was perfectly clear that every mail there, was to be off directly. Gentlemen, my uncle opened his eyes so wide at all this, that, to the very last moment of his life, he used to wonder how it fell out that he had ever been able to shut 'em again. (649)

Once again, the presence and function of the witness are centralized; we see an attention to detail filtered through the astonished eyes of the uncle. Even before the mail coaches resurrect, he notices every minor feature and hypothesizes about what each might tell about their past. This act of reconstructing the coaches' histories by observing their present dead state is conjured into a scene where the equipages come back to life "literally"; like the work of those investigating the death of Condé, the uncle's study of the dead allows his objects of analysis to take new life; observation becomes a form of ventriloquism.

Ventriloquists are able to make inanimate objects come to life, but never in a way that is independent of their involvement. In *The Old Curiosity Shop* (1840–41), for instance, Little Nell and her grandfather encounter two men of the "class of itinerant showmen—exhibitors of the freaks of Punch" in a graveyard. They notice

> perched cross-legged upon a tombstone behind them, [. . .] a figure of that hero himself [. . .]. His body was dangling in a most uncomfortable position, all loose and limp and shapeless, while his long peaked cap, unequally

---

71. In an article for *All the Year Round* Dickens complained that the "great stage-coaching times" had been "killed and buried" by "the ruthless railways." See Charles Dickens, "An Old Stage-Coaching House" (1863), *Journalism* 4: 269–77 (270).

balanced against his exceedingly slight legs, threatened every instant to bring him toppling down.[72]

Without the involvement of the ventriloquist, Punch is dead; limp and lifeless and lying on a tombstone, he lacks any of the vital qualities that usually have him "beaming" and "imperturbable [in] character."[73] In order to make this dead object come to life, the showman must involve himself; he must literally insert himself into it. The same might be said of the supernatural observations in *The Pickwick Papers*, with the key difference that they are given life by their observers' imaginations.

The bagman's uncle has a fantastic adventure inside one of the resurrected coaches. He manages to rescue a beautiful woman from nefarious men carrying unsubtly massive weapons, and he falls in love with his damsel. The next morning he awakes to discover that each of the coaches is, once again, "a mere shell" (659), yet he is convinced that they had come to life:

> He always said what a curious thing it was that he should have found out, by such a mere accident as clambering over the palings, that the ghosts of mail-coaches and horses, guards, coachmen, and passengers, were in the habit of making journeys regularly every night. (659)

The denouement is a good illustration of how instructive Dickens's comic technique can be. Of course, in *Pickwick*, as elsewhere, the author's humor relies upon the gap between the naivety of a character and the sagacity of his reader; we know that the uncle dreams his adventure. Yet for all its hilarity "The Story of the Bagman's Uncle" uses a hyperbolic method of recycling medical ideas as a form of questioning the relationship between the worth of objects and the role of the imagination in the interpretive process. In accordance with what medical men wrote about cases like the Prince de Condé's, the story agrees that human behavior leaves indelible traces on the objects that stage it—a collateral residue that allows the observer to reconstruct, resurrect, and restage people's behaviors. Yet the tale makes it clear how the interpretations of the observer must take part in giving life to the very spectacles they interpret. In the words of Francis Bacon, "The human understanding is like a false mirror, which, receiving rays irregularly, distorts and discolours the nature of things by mingling its

---

72. Charles Dickens, *The Old Curiosity Shop*, ed. Paul Schlicke (1840–41; London: J. M. Dent, 1995), 127.

73. Ibid.

own nature with it."[74] In the laboratory of Dickens's stories, human prehension shapes and illuminates the nature of things by mingling its own nature with it. In the more mature reflections of *Great Expectations*, the phenomenon of interpretation can also be seen to behave like a *true* mirror by giving the narrator the kinds of realizations that forensic medicine sought from a detailed attention to collateral objects.

MISS HAVISHAM

Such is apparent in the scene where Pip and Miss Havisham stare at each other for a moment through the mirror that sits on the jilted bride's dressing table. As Barbara Hardy has observed,[75] Pip is very fanciful (both as a character and a narrator), and, I add, his imaginary impulses constantly mingle with his observations. The best example of the latter occurs in his frenzied attempts to make sense of Satis House:

> It was then I began to understand that everything in the room had stopped, like the watch and the clock, a long time ago. I noticed that Miss Havisham put down the jewel exactly on the spot from which she had taken it up. [. . .] I glanced at the dressing-table again, and saw that the shoe upon it, once white, now yellow, had never been worn. I glanced down at the foot from which the shoe was absent, and saw that the silk stocking on it, once white, now yellow, had been trodden ragged. Without this arrest of everything, this standing still of all the pale decayed objects, not even the withered bridal dress on the collapsed form could have looked so like grave-clothes, or the long veil so like a shroud. (51)

> It was spacious, and I dare say had once been handsome, but every discernible thing in it was covered with dust and mould, and dropping to pieces. The most prominent object was a long table with a tablecloth spread on it, as if a feast had been in preparation when the house and the clocks all stopped together. An epergne or centre-piece of some kind was in the middle of this cloth; it was so heavily overhung with cobwebs that its form was quite undistinguishable; and, as I looked along the yellow expanse out of which I remember its seeming to grow, like a black fungus, I saw

---

74. Francis Bacon, *Novum Organum* (1620), trans. as *The New Organon* in *The Scientific Background to Modern Philosophy: Selected Readings*, ed. Michael R. Matthews (Indianapolis, IN: Hackett, 1984), 49.

75. Barbara Hardy, *Dickens and Creativity* (London: Continuum, 2008), 56–58.

speckled-legged spiders with blotchy bodies running home to it, and running out from it, as if some circumstance of the greatest public importance had just transpired in the spider community. (72–74)

As though he is performing a crime scene investigation, young Pip surveys the view ("I began to understand," "I noticed," "I glanced," "I saw," "I looked") and notes all of its decrepit particulars (the watch, the clock, the jewel, the shoe, the foot, the stocking, the veil, the "collapsed form"). Like those discovering the watch of Condé, Pip looks at the timepieces and finds them to have stopped—*tocked* as Kermode would say; and he sees that Miss Havisham's placing of certain objects in front of her, the shoe and the jewel, makes them seem like samples on a laboratory table, placed there for inspection rather than for everyday use.

All of these cues suggest that Miss Havisham and her house should undergo a forensic investigation. Everything seems dead, defunct, and decayed, yet there are signs of life, such as the spiders, that galvanize Pip's fancy. Assessing the figure of the jilted bride herself, Pip recalls:

> I saw that everything within my view which ought to be white, had been white long ago, and had lost its lustre, and was faded and yellow. I saw that the bride within the bridal dress had withered like the dress, and like the flowers, and had no brightness left but the brightness of her sunken eyes. I saw that the dress had been put upon the rounded figure of a young woman, and that the figure upon which it now hung loose, had shrunk to skin and bone. Once, I had been taken to see some ghastly waxwork at the Fair, representing I know not what impossible personage lying in state. Once, I had been taken to one of our old marsh churches to see a skeleton in the ashes of a rich dress, that had been dug out of a vault under the church pavement. Now, waxwork and skeleton seemed to have dark eyes that moved and looked at me. I should have cried out, if I could. (49)

This is the second encounter in which a collateral survey of the scene encourages the boy to cry. The first occurs in the graveyard. The later episode is sketched through the detailed observations that blend with emotional realizations. Like a forensic examiner, Pip surveys the clues of Miss Havisham's body and the scene, but their inconsistency with the vital movement of the woman's dark eyes causes him some shock as he realizes that Miss Havisham lives after her *tock*.

The description of the jilted bride's body, in particular, is a telling combination of empirical detail and panicked repetition: "I saw, I saw, I saw . . .

the *bride* within the *bridal dress* had withered like the *dress*. . . . She was dressed in rich materials—satins, and lace, and silks—all of *white*. Her shoes were *white*. And she had a long *white* veil [. . .] but her hair was *white*" (49; italics added). His eyes adjust to the scene, and Pip notices that "everything within my view which ought to be white, had been white long ago, and had lost its lustre, and was faded to yellow" (49). The conflict between the whiteness of the bridal attire and the yellowing march of time is an indicator of the marriage between what is fancied, or emoted, and what is real. Miss Havisham's wish to stop the clocks and preserve the moment of her heartbreak is an attempt to make her world composed entirely of affect, yet the perishable progress of time marks its inevitable reality upon her things.

Pip's first meeting with the jilted bride thus culminates in a "strange thing [. . .] happen[ing] to [his] fancy":

> I thought it a strange thing then, and I thought it a stranger thing long afterwards. [. . .] I saw a figure hanging there by the neck. A figure all in yellow white, with but one shoe to the feet; and it hung so, that I could see that the faded trimmings of the dress were like earthy paper, and that the face was Miss Havisham's, with a movement going over the whole countenance as if she were trying to call to me. (55)

The scene is one of some horror for the boy, though it represents the consummation of the marriage between his perception and his fancy. Although the vision is unreal, it has a weird essence of reality about it: the fact that Miss Havisham is hanging by the neck reminds us of the cadavers that were cut down from the scaffold and used for dissection; her trimmings are faded and yellow because they have been subjected to the spoiling effects of time; and the dress is like "earthy"/earth*ly* paper. The scene causes Pip some horror because, like his meeting with the jilted bride, the vision is one that cements both the emotional weight of Miss Havisham's trauma and the infectious effect it will have on him.

OBJECTIFIED GUILT

The early encounters with Miss Havisham lay the ground for an investigation that runs throughout the text: Do objects tell tales, and, if they do, how much of the imagining aspect of the mind gets in the way or is required to make sense of them? When Pip steals the pork pie from Mrs Joe's pantry, the collateral evidence is ventriloquized by Pip's guilt: "I got up and went down-stairs; every board upon the way, and every crack in every board, calling after me: "Stop thief!" and "Get up, Mrs Joe!" [. . .] I was very much alarmed by a hare hanging up by the heels, which I rather thought I caught, when my back was half turned, winking" (12). On the marshes the mist makes everything "disagreeable to [Pip's] guilty mind":

> The gates and dykes and banks came bursting at me through the mist, as if they cried as plainly as could be, "A boy with Somebody-else's pork pie! Stop him!" The cattle came upon me with like suddenness, staring out of their eyes, and steaming out of their nostrils, "Holloa, young thief!" One black ox, with a white cravat on—who even had to my awakened conscience something of a clerical air—fixed me so obstinately with his eyes, and moved his blunt head round in such an accusatory manner as I moved round, that I blubbered out to him, "I couldn't help it, sir! It wasn't for myself I took it!" Upon which he put down his head, blew a cloud of smoke out of his nose, and vanished with a kick-up of his hind-legs and a flourish of his tail. (13)

Such fancies continue into adult life. When Magwitch returns, Pip again mixes his own sense of guilt with the "reality":

> In every rage of wind and rush of rain, I heard pursuers. Twice, I could have sworn there was a knocking and whispering at the outer door. With these fears upon me, I began either to imagine or recall that I had had mysterious warnings of this man's approach. That, for weeks gone by, I had passed faces in the streets which I had thought like his. That, these likenesses had grown more numerous, as he, coming over the sea, had drawn nearer. That, his wicked spirit had somehow sent these messengers to mine, and that now on this stormy night he was as good as his word, and with me. (289)

There is a complex implication here that engages with Bacon's view that "human understanding is like a false mirror, which [. . .] distorts and discolours the nature of things by mingling its own nature with it." The accusatory floorboards, gates, wind, and whispering door, all suggest that Pip projects the nature of his own mind onto these "things." The fancies may be illusory, however, but the emotions are not. This situation is very different from the one we see in *The Pickwick Papers*, where characters discovering ancient inscriptions and new light phenomena are led astray by their own feelings. In *Great Expectations* there is something to be learned from all of

Pip's fancies. The place they take us might be emotional, but their epistemological values are real.

When Pip receives the ominous note from Wemmick, saying "DON'T GO HOME" (324), he spends the night at the Hummums, a run-down old inn in Covent Garden. Experiencing a "doleful night" (326), he turns his attention to details and "things":

> As I had asked for a night-light, the chamberlain had brought me in, before he left me, the good old constitutional rush-light of those virtuous days—an object like the ghost of a walking-cane, which instantly broke its back if it were touched, which nothing could ever be lighted at, and which was placed in solitary confinement at the bottom of a high tin tower, perforated with round holes that made a staringly wide-awake pattern on the walls. When I had got into bed, and lay there footsore, weary, and wretched, I found that I could no more close my own eyes than I could close the eyes of this foolish Argus. And thus, in the gloom and death of the night, we stared at one another. (326)

But, as at Satis House, the forensic compulsion to concentrate on details does nothing to prevent his fancies:

> When I had lain awake a little while, those extraordinary voices with which silence teems, began to make themselves audible. The closet whispered, the fireplace sighed, the little washing-stand ticked, and one guitar-string played occasionally in the chest of drawers. At about the same time, the eyes on the wall acquired a new expression, and in every one of those staring rounds I saw written, DON'T GO HOME.
>
> Whatever night-fancies and night-noises crowded on me, they never warded off this DON'T GO HOME. It plaited itself into whatever I thought of, as a bodily pain would have done. Not long before, I had read in the newspapers, how a gentleman unknown had come to the Hummums in the night, and had gone to bed, and had destroyed himself, and had been found in the morning weltering in blood. It came into my head that he must have occupied this very vault of mine, and I got out of bed to assure myself that there were no red marks about. (327)

It was common to describe corpses as "weltering in blood" in the nineteenth century, but it is still worth noting that the term is used to describe the appearance of Robert Seymour's corpse in *John Bull* (and Joseph Sellis's, discussed in chapter 1, in *The Morning Chronicle*). The image of suicide rears its mournful head because, as we saw in the cases of Seymour and the Prince de Condé, details are important in interpretations of such incidents. Pip attempts to pay close attention to the things around him at the Hummums, as he does at Satis House, but "DON'T GO HOME" plaits itself into his "reality." The note is, of course, a reality in itself, but it also takes on a disembodied form as it enters Pip's fancies. Fancies need careful control, like bodily pain, but, like the latter, they are a useful indication of something important: they focus Pip's mind on that one instruction, "DON'T GO HOME," and lead him to a correct summation that his staying away is a matter of life and death. His fancies may be absurd, then, but they are a crucial part of his understanding something concrete.

Pip's fancies are indeed a version of the forensic idea that the foibles of interpretation are unruly forces that are both a need and an anxiety for the science. As with many of Dickens's appropriations, however, the idea is exaggerated; one does not imagine many experts in medical jurisprudence fancying whispering closets, sighing fireplaces, and ticking washing-stands as part of their ordinary investigations of crime scenes. Yet the hyperboles capture the forensic tendency to introduce the factor of subjectivity as a means of putting any given investigation through a rigorous process of evaluation and discussion.

CONCLUSION

My hope is that this study has shown how an understanding of the history of forensic science—particularly its intersections with the different epistemological traditions of criminal law—allows us to better understand the games that Dickens's works play with representation. Charged with various political and humanitarian missions, these works took interpretation (emotional, scientific, religious) as both a theme and an objective. Interpretation therefore saw in the pages of Dickens's popular fictions one of its most sustained, and indeed one of its most sophisticated, anatomizations. I also hope that I have demonstrated how an ability to read Dickens—to gauge the richness of his language and his passion for description—allows for some new insights into the workings of the history of forensic medicine. Of course, Dickens will never add to the finer points of medical fact, observation, or theory; he provides no illumination, for instance, on the biology of rigor mortis; nor does he suggest better methods for processing collateral evidence. Yet his method of looking at the world by utilizing ideas and methods similar to or exactly the same as those established in medical jurisprudence has a great deal to teach us, as literary critics, as historians, and as modern readers, about the links between science, law, and perception. My book has achieved what it set out to do if the reader is able to gauge some sense of how the novel of the nineteenth century has an important place in our aim to understand what we know and how we know it. For Dickens, certainly, fiction was a place where he could engage with the complex and conflicting questions that emerged from the disagreements between varying approaches to truth. In his writings, questions of *whose* method of analysis is better suited to the investigation of a subject gets respun into considerations of absolute truth and goodness; the power of subjective interpretation; the readable quality of bodies and things; the effects of dogmatic thinking; and the power and significance of expert opinion.

The context of forensic medicine allows us to see that for Dickens, "fancy" and "imagination" were not always "against science." This has been a lazy binary that studies like mine now seek to unsettle. Indeed, medical jurisprudence, as we have seen, was a science that had a great deal of investment in the idea that the rogueries of the imagination, incited by the emotions, could be useful in encouraging a rigorous, self-policing approach to the question of interpretation. In Dickens the imagination (or "poetry," or "fancy," or whatever we like to call it) is not always set against a fact-based autocracy but often becomes useful in the quest for truth; subjective, wayward energies give a shape and a discipline to interpretation, if only by highlighting how it might go astray.

This book was written at a time when science, technology, engineering, and mathematics (the so-called STEM subjects) attracted a greater level of support than the humanities from governments, public institutions, and university management boards. Humanities research has been encouraged to make a valid account of itself and to justify what it offers, as though its extraordinary tools were a privilege enjoyed by the few rather than a necessity of the many. In this book I have sought to highlight the true importance of looking to a period when our various cultures interwove and emerged through conflict and coalition with each other. The sciences and the humanities have seemingly grown apart yet they still form codepending ends of a finely-balanced insight into the workings of justice and medical epistemologies. Privileging the sciences over the arts and humanities risks forfeiting crucial research that needs to be done on the ways we read bodies and their contexts.

On 9 November 1999 Sally Clark, a solicitor based in London, was convicted for the murder of her infant son. The weight of the case against her was comprised of the evidence of Professor Roy Meadow, a pediatrician who had risen to fame following his coinage of the term "Munchausen Syndrome by Proxy" (MSbP) and for the introduction of a number of memorable remarks on the subject of Sudden Infant Death Syndrome (SIDS). These include "There is no evidence that cot deaths run in families, but there is plenty of evidence that child abuse does" and "One cot death is a tragedy, two is suspicious, three is murder."[1] Before he took the witness stand in the trial of Clark, Meadow had a firm belief in the objective powers of statistics; Clark had lost *two* babies to SIDS, and these deaths were a clear cause for suspicion. "The chance of a cot death in a family of the social status of the Clark family is about 1 in 8,543," he said. "That means the chance of two such deaths occurring in the same family is equal to the square of that number: one chance in 73 million."[2] For ten of the twelve jury members, the statistics were seductive. Clark was given a mandatory life sentence, and two of her subsequent appeals were unsuccessful.

Three years later, however, Clark's legal team was able to access the report of the autopsy of her second child. As Leila Schneps and Coralie Colmez explain:

> No fewer than eight different colonies of the lethal bacterium *Stephylococcus aureus* had been found in Harry's body, some appearing with polymorphs, which are the cells that our bodies develop to fight off disease. [The records] showed that the baby had been suffering from a serious bacterial infection when he died, one that even could have led to meningitis. Confronted with these records, a dozen new and independent medical experts wrote reports stating that Harry most certainly could have died, and very probably *did* die naturally, from a serious infection. His death never should have been considered an unexplained crib death.[3]

The Royal Statistical Society investigated Meadow's "one in 73 million" idea, concluding that the evidence was, in the words of A. P. Dawid, vice-president of the society, "highly misleading and prejudicial."[4] Clark's conviction was eventually overturned in 2003. After suffering as she attempted to adjust to "ordinary life," she eventually died of acute alcoholic poisoning in 2007. Following another couple of cases in which Meadow gave questionable evidence, the Solicitor General of England and Wales barred him from testifying in further trials. The General Medical Council struck the professor from the medical register, though this decision was overturned in 2006.

---

1. Leila Schneps and Coralie Colmez, *Math on Trial: How Numbers Get Used and Abused in the Courtroom* (New York: Basic Books, 2013), 13.
2. Ibid., 13.
3. Ibid., 18. Italics in original.
4. A. P. Dawid, "Sally Clark Appeal," www.statslab.cam.ac.uk/~apd/SallyClark_report.doc [accessed September 2014].

Similar to the discussion that was undertaken by Dickens and G. H. Lewes on spontaneous combustion, the Clark case saw an opposition between seeming "facts" and anecdotal evidence. Before the autopsy report was uncovered by the defense team, numerous women who had similarly lost two, even three, babies to cot death wrote to Sally. The latter was vindicated by the autopsy report, and there were indications that Meadow's opinion was an unexamined premise founded, as the Royal Statistical Society suggested, on assumption rather than careful interpretation. To Meadow's strongest critics, among them his former wife, the professor was obsessed with MSbP: "He would go too far," she said in an interview with *The Evening Standard*. "He found it everywhere. He was over the top. He saw mothers with Munchausen Syndrome by Proxy wherever he looked. [. . .] Roy is a misogynist [. . .]. I don't think he likes women. [. . .] Although I can't go into details, I'm sure he has a serious problem with women."[5] Such allegations are problematic in themselves; they assume that the expert witness had to be a misogynist, an obsessive, a maniacal doctor because such personalities suit a quick assessment of his profile in the dock; they are guilty, however, of the very kind of assumption that Meadow was guilty of when it came to his "one in 73 million" statement.

What Dickens teaches us about nineteenth-century legal cases applies to the Sally Clark indictment. It is not objectivity, obsession, statistics, or science that is the enemy of truth, but the unexamined premise—the belief, in short, that an idea can be relied upon without any scrutiny of the cognitive and evidentiary journey that gets us there. We are no more objective than our Victorian forebears, and we are in as much need as they were of the careful, imaginative considerations of reality and perception that we find in the arts and humanities.

---

5. David Cohen, "He Doesn't Like Women, Says Ex-Wife," *The Evening Standard*, 23 January 2004, http://www.msbp.com/Munchausendiscredited3.htm [24 September 2014].

BIBLIOGRAPHY

JOURNALISM, LETTERS, LIBRARY

Dickens's Journalism, vol. 1: *Sketches by Boz and Other Early Papers, 1833–39*, ed. Michael Slater (London: J. M. Dent, 1996).

Dickens's Journalism, vol. 2: *"The Amusements of the People" and Other Papers: Reports, Essays and Reviews, 1834–51*, ed. Michael Slater (London: J. M. Dent, 1996).

Dickens's Journalism, vol. 3: *"Going Astray" and Other Papers from* Household Words, *1851–59*, ed. Michael Slater (London: J. M. Dent, 1998).

Dickens's Journalism, vol. 4: *"The Uncommercial Traveller" and Other Papers, 1859–70*, ed. Michael Slater and John Drew (London: J. M. Dent, 2000).

The Letters of Charles Dickens, vol. 1: 1820–39, ed. Madeline House and Graham Storey (Oxford: Clarendon Press, 1965).

The Letters of Charles Dickens, vol. 2: 1840–41, ed. Madeline House, Graham Storey, and Kathleen Tillotson (Oxford: Clarendon Press, 1969).

The Letters of Charles Dickens, vol. 3: 1842–43, ed. Madeline House, Graham Storey, and Kathleen Tillotson (Oxford: Clarendon Press, 1974).

The Letters of Charles Dickens, vol. 4: 1844–46, ed. Kathleen Tillotson and Nina Burgis (Oxford: Clarendon Press, 1977).

The Letters of Charles Dickens, vol. 5: 1847–49, ed. Graham Storey, K. J. Fielding, and Anthony Laude (Oxford: Clarendon Press, 1981).

The Letters of Charles Dickens, vol. 6: 1850–1852, ed. Graham Storey, Kathleen Tillotson, and Nina Burgis (Oxford: Clarendon Press, 1988).

The Letters of Charles Dickens, vol. 7: 1853–55, ed. Graham Storey, Kathleen Tillotson, and Angus Easson (Oxford: Clarendon Press, 1993).

The Letters of Charles Dickens, vol. 8: 1856–58, ed. Graham Storey and Kathleen Tillotson (Oxford: Clarendon Press, 1995).

The Letters of Charles Dickens, vol. 9: 1859–61, ed. Graham Storey, Margaret Brown, and Kathleen Tillotson (Oxford: Clarendon Press, 1997).

The Letters of Charles Dickens, vol. 10: 1862–64, ed. Graham Storey, Margaret Brown, and Kathleen Tillotson (Oxford: Clarendon Press, 1998).

The Letters of Charles Dickens, vol. 11: 1865–67, ed. Graham Storey, Margaret Brown, and Kathleen Tillotson (Oxford: Clarendon Press, 1999).

The Letters of Charles Dickens, vol. 12: 1868–70, ed. Graham Storey, Margaret Brown, and Kathleen Tillotson (Oxford: Clarendon Press, 2002).

J. H. Stonehouse (ed.), *Catalogue of the Library of Charles Dickens from Gadshill* (London: Piccadilly Fountain Press, 1935).

LEGAL CASES

BODLE, JOHN

The Times, 12 November 1833, 5; *The Times,* 13 November 1833, 3; *The Times,* 14 December 1833, 5; Katherine Watson, *Poisoned Lives: English Poisoners and their Victims* (London: Hambledon and London, 2004), 17–18.

CLARK, SALLY

David Cohen, "He Doesn't Like Women, Says Ex-Wife," *The Evening Standard,* 23 January 2004, http://www.msbp.com/Munchausendiscredited3.htm [24 September 2014]; A. P. Dawid, "Sally Clark Appeal," www.statslab.cam.ac.uk/~apd/SallyClark_report.doc [24 September 2014]; Leila Schneps and Coralie Colmez, *Math on Trial: How Numbers Get Used and Abused in the Courtroom* (New York: Basic Books, 2013), 2–21.

CONDÉ, PRINCE DE

Unsigned, "Foreign Intelligence," *The Hull Packet and Humber Mercury,* 7 September 1830, 2; Unsigned, "The Prince of Condé," *Bell's Life in London and Sporting Chronicle,* 26 September 1830, 1; Unsigned, *John Bull,* 26 December 1831, 430–32; Unsigned, "Was the Duke of Bourbon Murdered?" *London Medical Gazette,* 31 December 1831, 485–86; Unsigned, *The Age,* 1 January 1832, 3; Unsigned, "French Papers," *The Morning Chronicle,* 3 January 1832, 1; Forbes Winslow, *The Anatomy of Suicide* (1840; Boston: Milford House, 1972), 254; Alfred Swaine Taylor, *The Principles and Practice of Medical Jurisprudence,* 2 vols. (1865; London: J. & A. Churchill, 1894), vol. 2, 57; Unsigned, "Duke of Bourbon," *London Medical Gazette,* 21 January 1832, 608–9.

GREENACRE, JAMES

Unsigned, "The Mutilated Body," *The Morning Post,* 2 January 1837, 4; Central Criminal Court, 3 April 1837. Record: t18370403–917; Unsigned, "Phrenology," *Penny Satirist,* 29 April 1837, 4; Unsigned, "An Epitaph for Greenacre," *Penny Satirist,* 6 May 1837, 1; Unsigned, "Forensic Medicine," *The Examiner,* 7 May 1829, 9; Theodric Romeyn Beck, *Elements of Medical Jurisprudence* (1823; London: Longman et al., 1842), xv, 605–6; Albert D. Hutter, "Dismemberment and Articulation in *Our Mutual Friend,*" *Dickens Studies Annual* (1983): 135–75; David Newsome, *The Victorian World Picture: Perceptions and Introspections in an Age of Change* (1997; London: Fontana, 1998), 14.

HEYWOOD, JAMES

Unsigned, "Medical Jurisprudence: Trial for Murder.—Question of Death by Suffocation, or from Apoplexy, During Intoxication.—Contradictions in Medical Evidence," *The Lancet* 32 (1839): 896–900 (896).

MÜLLER, FRANZ

Unsigned, "The Murder on the North London Railway," *The Times*, 28 October 1864, 7; *The Times*, 28 October 1864, 7; *The Times*, 29 October 1864, 7, 9, 10; George H. Knott (ed.), *Trial of Franz Müller* (Sidney, Wellington, Calcutta: Butterworth, 1911).

REID, ROBERT

Unsigned, "High Court of Judiciary: Case of Murder," *Caledonian Mercury*, 2 July 1835. 4; John Fletcher, *Remarks on the Trial of Robert Reid for the Murder of His Wife, before the High Court of Judiciary at Edinburgh* (Edinburgh: John Carfrae and Son, 1835); Alfred Swaine Taylor, *Principles and Practice of Medical Jurisprudence*, 2 vols. (1865; London: John Churchill, 1894), vol. 1, 71.

SELLIS, JOSEPH

Unsigned, "Horrid Attempt to Assassinate H.R.H. The Duke of Cumberland," *The Morning Post*, 1 June 1810, 3; Unsigned, *The Trial of Josiah Phillips for a Libel of The Duke of Cumberland* (London: J. Hatchard, 1833), 4; [Anne Hamilton], *The Authentic Records of the Court of England, for the Last Seventy Years* (London: J. Phillips, 1832); Anne Hamilton, *Secret History of the Court of England from the Accession of George the Third to the Death of George the Fourth* (1832; London: John Dicks, 1883).

SEYMOUR, ROBERT

Anon., Untitled Article, *Bell's Life in London and Sporting Chronicle*, 24 April 1836, 1; Unsigned Report, *John Bull*, 25 April 1836, 131.

SMETHURST, THOMAS

J. Passmore Edwards, "A Plea for Dr. Smethurst," *Daily News*, 24 August 1859, 5; Unsigned, "Medical Testimony in the Smethurst and Palmer Cases," *The Morning Chronicle*, 25 August 1859, 4; Unsigned, "Our Medical Jurisprudence in Relation to Dr. Smethurst," *The Era*, 11 September 1859, 9; William Webber, "Toxicotechnia, or the Scientific Poisoning Art," *The Bury and Norwich Post and Suffolk Herald*, 1 November 1859, 4; Ian Burney, *Poison, Detection and the Victorian Imagination* (Manchester: Manchester University Press, 2006), 163–80.

MEDICAL SOURCES

Abercrombie, John, *Inquiries into the Intellectual Powers and the Investigation of Truth* (1830; Edinburgh: Waugh and Innes, 1831).

Beck, Theodric Romeyn, *Elements of Medical Jurisprudence* (1823; London: Longman et al., 1842).

Bernard, Claude, *Introduction à l'Étude de la Médecine Expérimentale*, trans. Henry Copley Greene as *An Introduction to the Study of Experimental Medicine* (1865; New York: Dover, 1957).

Bichat, Xavier, *Anatomie Générale: Appliquée à la Physiologie et à la Médecine* (1801), trans. George Hayward as *General Anatomy: Applied to Physiology and Medicine* (Boston: Richardson and Lord, 1822).

Chitty, Joseph, *A Practical Treatise on Medical Jurisprudence: with so much of Anatomy, Physiology, Pathology, and the Practice of Medicine and Surgery, as are essential to be known by Members of Parliament, Lawyers, Coroners, Magistrates, Officers in the Army and Navy* (London: Longman et al., 1834).

Christison, Robert, *A Treatise on Poisons in Relation to Medical Jurisprudence, Physiology, and the Practice of Physic* (1829; Edinburgh: Adam and Charles Black, 1845).

Cummin, William, *The Proofs of Infanticide Considered: including Dr Hunter's Tract on Child Murder, with illustrative notes; and a Summary of the Present State of Medico-Legal Knowledge on that Subject* (London: Longman et al., 1836).

Davey, J. G., "On Medical Evidence," *Association Medical Journal* (20 December 1856): 1074–77; 1089–92.

Edmunds, James, "Medical Advocates," *British Medical Journal* (2 May 1863): 465.

Elliotson, John, *Human Physiology* (London: Longman et al., 1835).

——, "On the Phrenology of Williams, and Bishop, who were Lately Executed for Murder Committed to gain Money by the Sale of Dead Bodies to Anatomical Teachers," *The Lancet* 17 (1832): 533–39.

——, *On Recent Improvements in the Art of Distinguishing the Various Diseases of the Heart* (London: Longman et al., 1830).

Fodéré, François-Emmanuel, *Traite de Medicine Legale, et d'Hygiene Publique* (1796), quoted in John Gordon Smith, *The Principles of Forensic Medicine, Systematically Arranged and Applied to British Practice* (London: Thomas and George Underwood, 1821).

Forsyth, John, *A Synopsis of Modern Medical Jurisprudence* (London: W. Benning, 1829).

Gregory, John, *Lectures on the Duties and Qualifications of a Physician* (London: Straham and Cadell, 1772).

Guy, William A., "Introductory Lecture, delivered at King's College," *Provincial Medical Journal and Retrospect of the Medical Sciences* 5 (1842): 23–32.

Harrison, James Bower, *The Medical Aspects of Death, and the Medical Aspects of the Human Mind* (London: Longman et al., 1852).

Hunter, William, "On the Uncertainty of the Signs of Murder in the Case of Bastard Children" (1784; London: J. Callow, 1818).

Inman, Thomas, "Experience in Medicine," *British Medical Journal* (6 November 1858): 923–27; 942–45.

Kinkead, R. J., "Introductory Address to the Courser of Lectures on Medical Jurisprudence," *The Lancet* (8 March 1879): 325–27.

Lair, Pierre-Aime, "On the Combustion of the Human Body, produced by the long and immoderate Use of Spiritual Liquors," *The Philosophical Magazine* 5 (1800): 133–46.

Laycock, Thomas, *Lectures on the Principles and Methods of Medical Observation and Research* (Philadelphia: Blanchard and Lea, 1857).

MacNish, Robert, *The Anatomy of Drunkenness* (1827; Philadelphia: Carey, Lea and Carey, 1828).

Male, George, *An Epitome of Juridical or Forensic Medicine; for the use of Medical Men, Coroners and Barristers* (London: Underwood, 1816).

"Mediculus," "Dissection Viewed with reference to the Resurrection," letter to the editor, *London Medical Gazette*, 25 February 1832, 789–91.

Morgagni, Giovanni Battista published *The Seats and Causes of Disease Investigated by Anatomy; containing a Great Variety of Dissections, and accompanied with Remarks* (1761; London: Longman, et al., 1822). 2 vols.

Mumford, James Gregory, *Surgical Memoirs and Other Essays* (New York: Moffat and Yard, 1908).

Mushet, William Boyd, "Pathological Contributions to Medical Jurisprudence," *British Medical Journal* (15 January 1859): 42.

Oesterlen, Friedrich, *Medicinische Logik*, trans. G. Whitley as *Medical Logic* (1852; London: Sydenham Society, 1855).

Orfila, Mathieu P., *A General System of Toxicology, or, A Treatise on Poisons* (London: E. Cox and Son, 1815).

Paris, John, and Fonblanque, Anthony, *Medical Jurisprudence*, 3 vols. (London: W. Phillips, 1823).

Percival, Thomas, *Medical Ethics; or, a Code of Institutes and Precepts, adapted to the Professional Conduct of Physicians and Surgeons* (Manchester: S. Russell, 1803).

Raynaud, Maurice, "An Address on Scepticism in Medicine," *British Medical Journal* (13 August 1881): 268–73.

Reese, John J., *Text-Book of Medical Jurisprudence and Toxicology* (Philadelphia: P. Blakiston, Son & Co., 1884).

Reynolds, J. Russell, "Lumleian Lectures, Delivered before the Royal College of Surgeons," II, *British Medical Journal* (4 May 1867): 519–20.

Ryan, Michael, *A Manual of Medical Jurisprudence and State Medicine* (1831; London: Sherwood, Gilbert and Piper, 1836).

Shenstone, William Ashwell, *Justus von Liebig, His Life and His Work* (London, Paris, New York, Melbourne: Cassell, 1901).

Smith, John Gordon, "Introductory Lecture on Medical Jurisprudence," *The Lancet* 15 (1830–31): 97–103.

———, *The Principles of Forensic Medicine, Systematically Arranged and Applied to British Practice* (London: Thomas and George Underwood, 1821).

Symonds, J. A., "On Medical Evidence in Relation to State Medicine," *British Medical Journal* (2 September 1865): 227–30.

Taylor, Alfred Swaine, *Elements of Medical Jurisprudence* (1836; London: Deacon et al., 1843).

Thomson, Alexander, "Lectures on Medical Jurisprudence" *The Lancet* (1836).

Unsigned, "Coroner's Inquest on Dr. Gordon Smith," *The Morning Post*, 17 September 1833, 3.

Unsigned review of Theodric Romeyn Beck, *Elements of Medical Jurisprudence*, *The Lancet* (12 February 1825): 172–88.

Webb, Ezekiel, *The Philosophy of Medicine* (New York: Printed for the author, 1834).

Williams, Stephen, *A Catechism of Medical Jurisprudence* (Northampton: J. H. Butler, 1835).

GENERAL NINETEENTH-CENTURY SOURCES

À Beckett, Gilbert Abbott, *The Comic Blackstone* (London: Punch, 1844).

Anon., *The Origin, Science, and End of Moral Truth; or, An Exposition of the Inward Principle of Christianity* (London: C. J. G. and F. Rivington, 1831).

———, *Trial of Professor John W. Webster for the Murder of Doctor George Parkman* (New York: Stringer and Townsend, 1850).

Austin, John, *Lectures on Jurisprudence; or The Philosophy of Positive Law*, 2 vols. (1861; London: John Murray, 1873).

Beattie, James, *An Essay on the Nature and Immutability of Truth: In Opposition to Sophistry and Scepticism* (1770; Philadelphia: Solomon Wieatt, 1809).

Blackstone, William, *Commentaries on the Laws of England*, 3 vols. (1765–69; London: Sweet et al., 1829).

Eliot, George, "The Natural History of German Life," *Westminster Review* 66 (1856): 51–79.

Forster, John, *The Life of Charles Dickens*, 2 vols. (1872–74; London: Chapman and Hall, 1876).

Hunt, Robert, *The Poetry of Science, or Studies of the Physical Phenomena of Nature* (1848; London: Reeve, Bentham and Reeve, 1849).

Knight, Charles, "The Law," *Household Words* 2 (1850): 407–8.

Lewes, George Henry, "Literature," *The Leader*, 11 December 1852, 1189.

———. *Comte's Philosophy of the Sciences: Being an Exposition of the Principles of the* Cours de Philosophie Positive *of Auguste Comte* (London: Henry G. Bohn, 1853).

———, "Spontaneous Combustion: Two Letters to Charles Dickens," *The Leader*, 5 and 12 February 1853, 137–38; 161–63.

Maine, Henry Sumner, *Ancient Law: Its Connection with the Early History of Society, and its Relation to Modern Ideas* (London: John Murray, 1861).

Marzials, Frank T., *Life of Charles Dickens* (London: Walter Scott, 1887).

Morley, Henry, "Law and Order," *Household Words* 13 (1856): 241–45.

———, "Man as a Monster," *Household Words* 9 (1854): 409–14.

Ollier, Edmund, "A Scientific Figment," *Household Words* 10 (1854): 453–56.

Poe, Edgar Allan, "Watkins Tottle and Other Sketches," in *The Fall of the House of Usher and Other Writings*, ed. David Galloway (London: Penguin, 1984), 361–63.

Poncia, F. T., "Law *v.* Medical Science," *British Medical Journal* (4 April 1863): 360.

Redford, George, letter to *The Leader*, 26 March 1853, 303–5.

Reid, Thomas, *An Inquiry into the Human Mind on the Principles of Common Sense* (1764; Edinburgh: Bell and Bradfute, 1801).

———, *Essays on the Powers of the Human Mind* (1785; London: Thomas Tegg, 1827).

R. W., letter to the editor of *Daily News*, 26 August 1859, 4.

Sala, George Augustus, "Notes on Circumstantial Evidence," *Temple Bar* 1 (1861): 91–98 (91).

Unsigned, "Boz to the *Penny Satirist*," *Penny Satirist*, 13 May 1837, 2.

———, "Life of Sir William Blackstone," *The Law Magazine* 15 (1836): 292–315.

———, "Medical Evidence," *The Legal Observer* 1 (1831): 245–47.

———, "Medical Jurisprudence," *The Law Magazine* 1 (1830): 506–27.

———, "Medical Nuts to Crack," *All the Year Round* (6 July 1861): 358–60.

———, "The Sciences, in their Relation to the Practice of the Law," *The Legal Observer* 9 (1835): 449–51.

———, "Truth," *The Portfolio* (London: William Charlton Right, 1825), 31.

Unsigned review of J. Chitty, *Practical Treatise on Medical Jurisprudence*, [. . .] *The Legal Observer* 8 (1834): 243–45.

Webb, T. E., "The Metaphysician: A Retrospect," *Fraser's Magazine* 41 (1860): 503–17.

PRIMARY SOURCES

Bacon, Francis, *Novum Organum* (1620), trans. as *The New Organon* in *The Scientific Background to Modern Philosophy: Selected Readings*, ed. Michael R. Matthews (Indianapolis, IN: Hackett, 1984).

Bunyan, John, *The Pilgrim's Progress*, ed. W. R. Owens (1678; Oxford: Oxford University Press, 2003).

Carlyle, Thomas, *Sartor Resartus: The Life and Opinions of Herr Teufelsdröckh* (1833–34; London: Routledge, n.d.).

Coleridge, Samuel Taylor, *Biographia Literaria, or Biographical Sketches of My Literary Life and Opinions* (1817; London: Dent, 1967).

De Quincey, Thomas, "The English Mail-Coach, or the Glory of Motion" (1849), in *Selected Essays of De Quincey* (London: Walter Scott Ltd., n.d.), 122–57.

Dickens, Charles, *Bleak House*, ed. Andrew Sanders (1852–53; London: J. M. Dent, 1994).

———, "Brokers' and Marine-store Shops," *The Morning Chronicle* (15 December 1834), *Journalism* 1: 176–79.

———, "Chambers," *All the Year Round* (18 August 186), *Journalism* 4: 157–69.

———, "The City of the Absent," *All the Year Round* (18 July 1863), *Journalism* 4: 260–69.

———, *David Copperfield*, ed. Malcolm Andrews (1849–50; London: J. M. Dent, 1993).

———, "A Detective Police Party (1)," *Household Words* (27 July 1850), in *Journalism* 2: 265–76.

———, "A Detective Police Party (2)," *Household Words* (10 August 1850), *Journalism* 2: 276–82.

———, "Down with the Tide," *Household Words* (5 February 1853), *Journalism* 3: 113–21.

———, "The Drunkard's Death," *Sketches by Boz* (1836), *Journalism* 1: 463–72.

———, "Full Report of the First Meeting of the Mudfog Association for the Advancement of Everything," *Bentley's Miscellany* 2 (October 1837), *Journalism* 1: 513–50.

———, "The Ghost of Art," *Household Words*, *Journalism* 2: 257–64.

———, "Gone Astray," *Household Words* (13 August 1853), *Journalism* 3: 155–65.

———, *Great Expectations*, ed. Robin Gilmour (1860–61; London: Dent, 1994).

———, "Greenwich Fair," *Evening Chronicle* (16 April 1835), *Journalism* 1: 112–19.

———, "A Little Dinner in an Hour," *All the Year Round* (2 January 1869), *Journalism* 4: 364–70.

———, "Meditations in Monmouth Street," *The Morning Chronicle* (11 October 1836), *Journalism* 1: 76–82.

———, "Night Walks," *All the Year Round* (21 July 1860), *Journalism* 4: 148–57.

———, *The Old Curiosity Shop*, ed. Paul Schlicke (1840–41; London: J. M. Dent, 1995).

———, "An Old Stage-Coaching House" (1863), *Journalism* 4: 269–77.

———, *Oliver Twist*, ed. Stephen Gill (1837–38; Oxford: Oxford University Press, 1999).

———, *Our Mutual Friend*, ed. Stephen Poole (1864–65; London: Penguin, 1997).

———, *The Pickwick Papers*, ed. Mark Wormald (1836-37; London: Penguin, 2003).

Review of Robert Hunt, *The Poetry of Science, or Studies of the Physical Phenomena of Nature*, in Slater (ed.), *Journalism* 2: 129–34.

———, "Some Recollections of Mortality," *All the Year Round* (16 May 1863), *Journalism* 4: 218–28.

———, "The Streets—Morning," *Evening Chronicle* (21 July 1835), *Journalism* 1: 49–54.

———, "Three 'Detective' Anecdotes," *Household Words* 1 (1850): 577–80.

———, "Travelling Abroad," *All the Year Round* (7 April 1860), *Journalism* 4: 83–96.

Eliot, George, *Adam Bede*, ed. Stephen Gill (1859; London: Penguin, 1985).

———, *Middlemarch*, ed. Rosemary Ashton (1871–72; London: Penguin, 1994).

Kingsley, Charles, *Alton Locke: Tailor and Poet: An Autobiography*, ed. Elizabeth A. Cripps (1850; Oxford: Oxford University Press, 1983).

Locke, John, *An Essay Concerning Human Understanding*, ed. Roger Woolhouse (1690; London: Penguin, 1997).

Smith, Albert, *The Marchioness of Brinvilliers, or The Poisoner of the Seventeenth Century*, *Bentley's Miscellany* (1845): 17–18.

Swift, Jonathan, *Gulliver's Travels*, ed. Claude Rawson and Ian Higgins (1726; Oxford: Oxford University Press, 2005).

———, "A Modest Proposal for Preventing the Children of Poor People from being a Burthen on their Parents or the Country, and for making them Beneficial to the Public" (1729), in *Major Works*, ed. Angus Ross (Oxford: Oxford University Press, 2008), 492–99.

Thackeray, William Makepeace, "Horæ Catnachianæ," *Fraser's Magazine* 19 (1839): 407–24.

Various, *The Terrific Register; or, Records of Crimes, Judgements, Providences, and Calamities*, 2 vols. (London: Sherwood, Jones and Company, 1825).

Zola, Emile, *Thérèse Raquin*, trans. Robin Buss (1867; London: Penguin, 2004).

SECONDARY SOURCES

Ackroyd, Peter, *Dickens* (1990; London: Vintage, 1999).

Alter, Robert, *Imagined Cities: Urban Experience and the Language of the Novel* (New Haven, CT: Yale University Press, 2005).

Anderson, Amanda, *The Powers of Distance: Cosmopolitanism and the Cultivation of Detachment* (Princeton, NJ: Princeton University Press, 2001).

Anger, Suzy, *Victorian Interpretation* (Ithaca, NY, and London: Cornell University Press, 2005).

Ashton, Rosemary, *G. H. Lewes: A Life* (Oxford: Oxford University Press, 1991).

Ayer, A. J., *The Problem of Knowledge: An Enquiry into the Main Philosophical Problems that enter into the Theory of Knowledge* (London: Penguin Books, 1956).

Basson, A. H., *David Hume* (London: Penguin, 1958).

Baumgarten, Murray, "Reading Dickens Writing London," *Partial Answers* 9:2 (2011): 219–31.

Ben-Yishai, Ayelet, *Common Precedents: The Presentness of the Past in Victorian Law and Fiction* (New York: Oxford University Press, 2013).

Berlin, Isiah, "The Romantic Revolution: A Crisis in the History of Modern Thought" (1960), in *The Sense of Reality: Studies in Ideas and their History*, ed. Henry Hardy (London: Chatto and Windus, 1996), 169–93.

Bevis, Matthew, "Temporizing Dickens," *The Review of English Studies* 52:206 (2001): 171–91.

Boehm, Katharina, *Charles Dickens and the Sciences of Childhood: Popular Medicine, Child Health and Victorian Culture* (Basingstoke: Palgrave Macmillan, 2013).

Bowen, John, *Other Dickens: Pickwick to Chuzzlewit* (Oxford: Oxford University Press, 2000).

Bown, Nicola, "What the Alligator Didn't Know: Natural Selection and Love in *Our Mutual Friend*," in *19: Interdisciplinary Studies in the Long Nineteenth-Century* 10 (2010), www.19.bbk.ac.uk [accessed October 2015].

Brooks, Peter, *Realist Vision* (New Haven: Yale University Press, 2005).

———, *Reading for the Plot: Design and Intention in Narrative* (Cambridge, MA: Harvard University Press, 1984).

Brown, Bill, *A Sense of Things: The Object Matter of American Literature* (Chicago: University of Chicago Press, 2003).

Buckland, Adelene, *Novel Science: Fiction and the Invention of Nineteenth-Century Geology* (Chicago: University of Chicago Press, 2013).

———, "'The Poetry of Science': Charles Dickens, Geology, and Visual and Material Culture in Victorian London," *Victorian Literature and Culture* 35 (2007): 679–94.

Burney, Ian, *Bodies of Evidence: Medicine and the Politics of the English Inquest, 1830–1926* (Baltimore, MD, and London: Johns Hopkins University Press, 2000).

———, *Poison, Detection and the Victorian Imagination* (Manchester: Manchester University Press, 2006).

Butt, John, and Tillotson, Kathleen, *Dickens at Work* (London: Methuen, 1957).

Caldwell, Janis McLarren, *Literature and Medicine in Nineteenth-Century Britain: From Mary Shelley to George Eliot* (Cambridge: Cambridge University Press, 2004).

Carey, John, *The Violent Effigy: A Study of Dickens's Imagination* (1973; London: Faber and Faber, 1991).

Carroll, David, *George Eliot and the Conflict of Interpretations: A Reading of the Novels* (Cambridge: Cambridge University Press, 1992).

Chaudhry, G. A., *The Mudfog Papers*, *The Dickensian* 70 (1974): 104–12.

Cheadle, Brian, "*Oliver Twist*," in *A Companion to Charles Dickens*, ed. David Paroissien (Oxford: Blackwell Publishing, 2008), 308–17.

Chesterton, G. K., *Charles Dickens* (1906; London: Methuen, 1943).

Chittick, Kathryn, "Dickens and Parliamentary Reporting in the 1830s," *Victorian Periodicals Review* 21 (1988): 151–60.

———, *Dickens and the 1830s* (Cambridge: Cambridge University Press, 1990).

Clark, Timothy, "Dickens through Blanchot: The Nightmare Fascination of a World without Interiority," in *Dickens Refigured: Bodies, Desires and Other Histories*, ed. John Schad (Manchester: Manchester University Press, 1996), 22–38.

Collins, Philip, *Dickens and Crime* (1962; London: Macmillan, 1965).

Connor, Steven, "All I Believed Is True: Dickens under the Influence," in *19: Interdisciplinary Studies of the Long Nineteenth Century* 10 (2010), www.19.bbk.ac.uk [accessed October 2015].

Cooter, Roger, *The Cultural Meaning of Popular Science: Phrenology and the Organization of Consent in Nineteenth-Century Britain* (Cambridge: Cambridge University Press, 2005).

Daston, Lorraine, "Objectivity and the Escape from Perspective," *Social Studies of Science* 22:4 (1992): 597–618.

Daston, Lorraine, and Galison, Peter, *Objectivity* (2007; New York: Zone Books, 2010).

Dawson, Gowan, "'By a Comparison of Incidents and Dialogue': Richard Owen, Comparative Anatomy and Victorian Serial Fiction," in *19: Interdisciplinary Studies in the Long Nineteenth Century* 11 (2010), www.19.bbk.ac.uk [accessed October 2015].

Denman, Peter, "Krook's Death and Dickens's Authorities," *The Dickensian* 82 (1986): 131–41.

Dicey, A. V., *Lectures on the Relation between Law and Public Opinion in England during the Nineteenth Century* (London: Macmillan, 1924).

Douglas-Fairhurst, Robert, *Becoming Dickens: The Invention of a Novelist* (Cambridge, MA: Belknap Press of Harvard University Press, 2011).

Drew, John, *Dickens the Journalist* (Basingstoke: Palgrave Macmillan, 2003).

Duxbury, Neil, *The Nature and Authority of Precedent* (Cambridge: Cambridge University Press, 2008).

Dyson, A. E., "Introduction," in *Dickens: Modern Judgments*, ed. A. E. Dyson (London: Macmillan, 1968).

Ellis, Harold, *A History of Surgery* (London: Greenwich Medical Media, 2001).

Eysell, Joanne, *A Medical Companion to Dickens's Fiction* (Oxford: Peter Lang, 2005).

Fielding, K. J., "Dickens and Science?" *Dickens Quarterly* 13:4 (1996): 200–216.

Fielding K. J., and Lai, Shu Fang, "Dickens's Science, Evolution and 'The Death of the Sun,'" in *Dickens, Europe and the New Worlds*, ed. Anny Sadrin (London: Macmillan, 1999), 200–211.

Flibbert, Joseph T., "Dickens and the French Debate over Realism: 1838–1856," *Comparative Literature* 23:1 (1971): 18–31.

Foucault, Michel, *Naissance de la Clinique*, trans. A. M. Sheridan as *The Birth of the Clinic* (1863; London and New York: Routledge, 2003).

Freedgood, Elaine, *The Ideas in Things: Fugitive Meaning in the Victorian Novel* (Chicago: University of Chicago Press, 2006).

Fulweiler, Howard, "'A Dismal Swamp': Darwin, Design and Evolution in *Our Mutual Friend*," *Nineteenth-Century Literature* 49 (1994): 50–74.

Gallagher, Catherine, "Marxism and the New Historicism," in *The New Historicism*, ed. Harold Veeser (New York: Routledge, 1989), 37–48.

Garcha, Amanpal, *From Sketch to Novel: The Development of Victorian Fiction* (Cambridge: Cambridge University Press, 2009).

Garrett, Peter, *Victorian Empiricism: Self, Knowledge, and Reality in Ruskin, Bain, Lewes, Spencer and George Eliot* (Canterbury, NJ: Fairleigh Dickinson University Press, 2010).

Gilbert, Pamela, K., *Cholera and Nation: Doctoring the Social Body in Victorian England* (New York: State University of New York Press, 2008).

———, *The Citizen's Body: Desire, Health, and the Social in Victorian England* (Columbus: The Ohio State University Press, 2007).

———, *Mapping the Victorian Social Body* (New York: State University of New York Press, 2004).

Gillooly, Eileen, and Deirdre David (eds.), *Contemporary Dickens* (Columbus: The Ohio State University Press, 2009).

Goodlad, Lauren, M. E., *Victorian Literature and the Victorian State: Character and Governance in a Liberal Society* (Baltimore, MD, and London: Johns Hopkins University Press, 2003).

Grant, Damian, *Realism* (London: Methuen, 1970).

Grimes, Richard L., "Masking: Towards a Phenomenology of Exteriorization" (1975), quoted in Timothy Clark, "Dickens through Blanchot: The Nightmare Fascination of a World without Interiority," *Dickens Refigured*, ed. John Schad, 22–38.

Guthrie, Douglas, *A History of Medicine* (London: Thomas Nelson and Sons, 1945).

Hack, Daniel, "'Sublimation Strange': Allegory and Authority in *Bleak House*," *ELH* 66 (1999): 129–56.

Hackenberg, Sara, "'Loitering Artfully': Reading *Flânerie* in *Our Mutual Friend*," in *Dickens: The Craft of Fiction and the Challenges of Reading*, ed. Rossana Bonadi et al. (Milan: Unicopli, 2000), 230–39.

Haigh, Elizabeth, *Xavier Bichat and the Medical Theory of the Eighteenth Century* (London: The Wellcome Institute, 1984).

Haight, Gordon S., "Dickens and Lewes," *PMLA* 71:1 (March 1956): 166–79.

———, "Dickens and Lewes on Spontaneous Combustion," *Nineteenth-Century Fiction* 10 (1955): 53–63.

Hardy, Barbara, *Dickens and Creativity* (London: Continuum, 2008).

Harris, J. W., *Legal Philosophies* (London: Butterworths, 1980).

Hollington, Michael, *Dickens and the Grotesque* (London: Croom Helm, 1984).

Hurren, Elizabeth T., *Dying for Victorian Medicine: English Anatomy and Its Trade in the Dead Poor, c.1834–1929* (Basingstoke: Palgrave Macmillan, 2012).

Hutter, Albert D., "Dismemberment and Articulation in *Our Mutual Friend*," *Dickens Studies Annual* (1983): 135–75.

Ingham, Patricia, "Dickens and Language," in *A Companion to Charles Dickens*, ed. David Paroissien (Oxford: Blackwell Publishing, 2008), 126–41.

Jaffe, Audrey, "Omniscience in *Our Mutual Friend*: On Taking the Reader by Surprise," *Journal of Narrative Technique* 17:1 (1987): 91–101.

John, Juliet, *Dickens's Villains: Melodrama, Character, Popular Culture* (Oxford: Oxford University Press, 2001).

Kaplan, Fred, *Dickens and Mesmerism: The Hidden Springs of Fiction* (Princeton, NJ: Princeton University Press, 1975).

Kawash, Samira, *Dislocating the Color Line: Identity, Hybridity, and Singularity in African-American Narrative* (Stanford, CA: Stanford University Press, 1997).

Kennedy, Meegan, *Revising the Clinic: Vision and Representation in Victorian Medical Narrative and the Novel* (Columbus: The Ohio State University Press, 2010).

Kermode, Frank, *The Sense of an Ending: Studies in the Theory of Fiction* (Oxford and New York: Oxford University Press, 1967).

Kucich, John, *Excess and Restraint: The Novels of Charles Dickens* (Athens: University of Georgia Press, 1981).

Latour, Bruno, *Science in Action* (Milton Keynes: Open University Press, 1987).

Ledger, Sally, "Dickens, Natural History, and *Our Mutual Friend*," *Partial Answers* 9:12 (2011): 363–78.

———, *Dickens and the Popular Radical Imagination* (Cambridge: Cambridge University Press, 2009).

Ledger, Sally, and Furneaux, Holly (eds.), *Charles Dickens in Context* (Cambridge: Cambridge University Press, 2011).

Lesnik-Oberstein, Karín, "*Oliver Twist:* The Narrator's Tale," *Textual Practice* 15:1 (2001): 87–100.

Levi, Albert William, *Literature, Philosophy and the Imagination* (Bloomington: Indiana University Press, 1962).

Levine, George, *Darwin and the Novelists: Patterns of Science in Victorian Fiction* (Chicago: University of Chicago Press, 1988).

———, *Dying to Know: Scientific Epistemology and Narrative in Victorian England* (Chicago and London: University of Chicago Press, 2002).

———, *Realism, Ethics and Secularism: Essays on Victorian Literature and Science* (Cambridge: Cambridge University Press, 2008).

Lucas, John, *The Melancholy Man: A Study of Dickens's Novels* (London: Methuen, 1970).

———, "Past and Present: *Bleak House* and *A Child's History of England*," in *Dickens Refigured: Bodies, Desires and Other Histories,* ed. John Schad (Manchester: Manchester University Press, 1996), 136–56.

Makras, Kostas, "Dickensian Intemperance: The Representation of the Drunkard in 'The Drunkard's Death' and *The Pickwick Papers*," in *19: Interdisciplinary Studies of the Long Nineteenth Century* 10 (2010), www.19.bbk.ac.uk [accessed October 2015].

Mangham, Andrew, *Violent Women and Sensation Fiction: Crime, Medicine and Victorian Popular Culture* (Basingstoke: Palgrave Macmillan, 2007).

Matchett, Willoughby, "The Chopped-up Murdered Man," *The Dickensian* 14 (1918): 117–19.

Midgley, Mary, *Science and Poetry* (2001; London and New York: Routledge, 2006).

Miller, Andrew H., *Novels behind Glass: Commodity Culture and Victorian Narrative* (Cambridge: Cambridge University Press, 1995).

Miller, D. A., *The Novel and the Police* (Berkeley, CA, and London: University of California Press, 1988).

Miller, J. Hillis, *Charles Dickens: The World of his Novels* (Bloomington: Indiana University Press, 1958).

———, "The Fiction of Realism: *Sketches by Boz, Oliver Twist,* and Cruikshank's Illustrations" (1971), repr. as "J. Hillis Miller on the Fiction of Realism," in *Realism,* ed. Lillian R. Furst (London and New York: Longman, 1992), 287–318.

———, "Introduction," in *Bleak House,* ed. Norman Page (London: Penguin, 1971).

Moore, Wendy, *The Knife Man: Blood, Body-Snatching and the Birth of Modern Surgery* (London: Bantam, 2005).

Morris, Christopher, "The Bad Faith of Pip's Bad Faith: Deconstructing *Great Expectations*," in *Charles Dickens,* ed. Steven Connor (Essex: Longman, 1996), 76–90.

Moye, Richard H., "Storied Realities: Language, Narrative and Historical Understanding," in *Contemporary Dickens*, ed. Eileen Gillooly and Deirdre David (Columbus: The Ohio University Press, 2009), 93–109.

Murayama, Toshikatsu, "A Professional Contest over the Body: Quackery and Respectable Medicine in *Martin Chuzzlewit*," *Victorian Literature and Culture* 30.2 (2002): 403–19.

Mussell, James, "Science," in *Charles Dickens in Context*, ed. Sally Ledger and Holly Furneaux (Cambridge: Cambridge University Press, 2011), 326–33.

Nixon, Jude V., "'Lost in the Vast Worlds of Wonder': Dickens and Science," *Dickens Studies Annual* 35 (2005): 267–333.

Nord, Deborah Epstein, *Walking the Victorian Streets: Women, Representation and the City* (Ithaca, NY: Cornell University Press, 1995).

Palmer, William J., *Dickens and New Historicism* (Basingstoke: Palgrave Macmillan, 1998).

Parham, John, "Dickens in the City: Science, Technology, Ecology in the Novels of Charles Dickens," in *19: Interdisciplinary Studies in the Long Nineteenth Century* 10 (2010), www.19.bbk.ac.uk [accessed October 2015].

Patten, Robert L., "The Art of Pickwick's Interpolated Tales," *ELH* 34:3 (September 1967): 349–66.

———, *Charles Dickens and "Boz": The Birth of the Industrial-Age Author* (Cambridge: Cambridge University Press, 2012).

Pickstone, John V., *Ways of Knowing: A New History of Science, Technology and Medicine* (Manchester: Manchester University Press, 2000).

Piggott, Gillian, *Dickens and Benjamin: Moments of Revelation, Fragments of Modernity* (Hampshire: Ashgate, 2012).

Porter, Roy, *The Greatest Benefit to Mankind: A Medical History of Humanity from Antiquity to the Present* (1997; London: HarperCollins, 1999).

Postema, Gerald J., *Bentham and the Common Law Tradition* (Oxford: Oxford University Press, 1986).

Reed, John R., *Dickens's Hyperrealism* (Columbus: The Ohio State University Press, 2010).

Richardson, Ruth, *Death, Dissection and the Destitute* (London: Penguin, 1988).

Roberts, Lissa, "Condillac, Lavoisier, and the Instrumentalization of Science," *The Eighteenth Century* 33:3 (1992): 252–71.

Rothfield, Laurence, *Vital Signs: Medical Realism in Nineteenth-Century Fiction* (Princeton, NJ: Princeton University Press, 1992).

Royle, Nicholas, "*Our Mutual Friend*," in *Dickens Refigured: Bodies, Desires and Other Histories*, ed. John Schad (Manchester: Manchester University Press, 1996), 39–54.

Rubery, Matthew, *The Novelty of Newspapers: Victorian Fiction after the Invention of the News* (Oxford: Oxford University Press, 2009).

Samuels, Ellen, *Fantasies of Identification: Disability, Gender, Race* (New York: New York University Press, 2014).

Sanders, Andrew (ed.), *Authors in Context: Charles Dickens* (Oxford: Oxford University Press, 2003).

———, *Charles Dickens: Resurrectionist* (London: Macmillan, 1982).

Schad, John, *The Reader in Dickensian Mirrors: Some New Language* (Basingstoke: Palgrave Macmillan, 1992).

Schneps, Leila, and Colmez, Coralie, *Math on Trial: How Numbers Get Used and Abused in the Courtroom* (New York: Basic Books, 2013).

Schramm, Jan-Melissa, *Testimony and Advocacy in Victorian Law, Literature and Theology* (Cambridge: Cambridge University Press, 2000).

Schwarzbach, F. S., *Dickens and the City* (London: Athlone, 1979).

Scoggin, Daniel P., "A Speculative Resurrection: Death, Money, and the Vampiric Economy of *Our Mutual Friend*," *Victorian Literature and Culture* 30:1 (2002): 99–125.

Sen, Sambudha, "Hogarth, Egan, Dickens, and the Making of an Urban Aesthetic," *Representations* 103:1 (2008): 84–106.

Shuttleworth, Sally, *Charlotte Brontë and Victorian Psychology* (Cambridge: Cambridge University Press, 1996).

Sicher, Efraim, *Rereading the City, Rereading Dickens: Representation, the Novel, and Urban Realism* (New York: AMS, 2003).

Slater, Michael, *Charles Dickens* (New Haven, CT, and London: Yale University Press, 2009).

———, *The Genius of Charles Dickens: The Ideas and Inspiration of Britain's Greatest Novelist* (London: Duckworth Overlook, 2011).

Smith, Jonathan, *Fact and Feeling: Baconian Science and the Nineteenth-Century Literary Imagination* (Madison: University of Wisconsin Press, 1994).

Smith, Karl Ashley, *Dickens and the Unreal City: Searching for Spiritual Significance in Nineteenth-Century London* (Basingstoke: Palgrave Macmillan, 2008).

Smith, Roger, *Trial by Medicine: Insanity and Responsibility in Victorian Trials* (Edinburgh: Edinburgh University Press, 1981).

Smith, Sydney, "The History and Development of Forensic Medicine," *British Medical Journal* (24 March 1951): 599–607.

Snow, C. P., *The Realists: Portraits of Eight Novelists* (London: Macmillan, 1978).

Sparks, Tabitha, *The Doctor in the Victorian Novel* (Hampshire: Ashgate, 2009).

Spilka, Mark, *Dickens and Kafka: A Mutual Interpretation* (London: Indiana University Press, 1963).

Stack, David, *Queen Victoria's Skull: George Combe and the Mid-Victorian Mind.* (London: Hambledon Continuum, 2008).

Stoehr, Taylor, *Dickens: The Dreamer's Stance* (Ithaca, NY: Cornell University Press, 1965).

Stone, Harry, *The Night Side of Dickens: Cannibalism, Passion, Necessity* (Columbus: The Ohio State University Press, 1994).

Strachan, John, "'The Mapp'd out Skulls of Scotia': *Blackwood's* and the Scottish Phrenological Society," in *Print Culture and the Blackwood Tradition, 1805–1930*, ed. David Finkelstein (Toronto: University of Toronto Press, 2006), 49–69.

Sucksmith, Peter Harvey, "The Secret of Immediacy: Dickens' Debt to the Tale of Terror in *Blackwood's*," *Nineteenth-Century Fiction* 26:2 (1971): 145–57.

Tambling, Jeremy, *Going Astray: Dickens and London* (Harlow: Pearson, 2009).

Taylor, Brooke D., "Spontaneous Combustion: When 'Fact' Confirms Feeling in *Bleak House*," *Dickens Quarterly* 27:3 (September 2010): 171–84.

Thomas, Ronald R., *Detective Fiction and the Rise of Forensic Science* (Cambridge: Cambridge University Press, 1999).

Thoms, Peter, "'The Narrow Track of Blood': Detection and Storytelling in *Bleak House*," *Nineteenth-Century Literature* 50:2 (1995): 147–67.

Tredennick, Bianca, "Some Collections of Mortality: Dickens, the Paris Morgue and the Material Corpse." *Victorian Review* 36:1 (2010).

Tromp, Marlene, *The Private Rod: Marital Violence, Sensation, and the Law in Britain* (Charlottesville, VA, and London: University of Virginia Press, 2000).

Van Whyle, John, *Phrenology and the Origins of Victorian Scientific Naturalism* (Hampshire: Ashgate, 2004).

Ventura, Hector O., "Giovanni Battista Morgagni and the Foundation of Modern Medicine," *Clinical Cardiology* 23 (2000): 792–94.

Vrettos, Athena, "Defining Habits: Dickens and the Psychology of Repetition," *Victorian Studies* 42:3 (1999): 399–426.

———, *Somatic Fictions: Imagining Illness in Victorian Culture* (Stanford, CA: Stanford University Press, 1995).

Waters, Catherine, *Commodity Culture in Dickens's Household Words: The Social Life of Objects* (Aldershot: Ashgate, 2008).

Watson, Katherine, *Forensic Medicine in Western Society: A History* (London: Routledge, 2011).

———, *Poisoned Lives: English Poisoners and Their Victims* (London: Hambledon and London, 2004).

Winyard, Ben, and Holly Furneaux, "Dickens, Science and the Victorian Literary Imagination," in *19: Interdisciplinary Studies in the Long Nineteenth Century* 10 (2010), www.19.bbk.ac.uk [accessed October 2015].

Wood, Claire, *Dickens and the Business of Death* (Cambridge: Cambridge University Press, 2015).

Wood, Jane, *Passion and Pathology in Victorian Fiction* (Oxford: Oxford University Press, 2001).

Yeo, Richard, *Defining Science: William Whewell, Natural Knowledge and Public Debate in Early Victorian Britain* (Cambridge: Cambridge University Press, 1993).

INDEX

Abercrombie, John, 72
Adam Bede (Eliot), 122
Ainsworth, William Harrison, 146
All the Year Round, 5–6, 5n11, 46, 106, 111, 116, 141, 173n148, 218n71
Alton Locke (Kingsley), 181
American Notes (Dickens), 1
Analysis of Medical Evidence (Smith), 51
anatomy, 17, 24n8, 43, 105, 134, 137, 142, 143, 145
The Anatomy of Drunkenness (MacNish), 120
Anderson, Amanda, 16, 16n37, 71, 80
Anger, Suzy, 70, 138
antihermeneutics. *See* hermeneutics
Arac, Jonathan, 161
Ariés, Philippe, 2n3
Association Medical Journal, 66
Austin, John, 31–32
autopsy. *See* post-mortem
"A Visit to Newgate" (Dickens), 1

Baumgarten, Murray, 139
Baynard, Edward, 43, 46
Beattie, James, 27
Beck, Theodric Romeyn, 48–49, 60, 174–77, 208
Beckett, Gilbert Abbott à, 32–33
Bell's Life in London, 179
Bentham, Jeremy, 32, 89

Bentley's Miscellany, 154, 170
Bernard, Claude, 71–72, 135, 159
Bianchini, Giuseppe, 121–22, 126–29
Bichat, Xavier, 107, 188
Birtwistle, John, 174–75, 177
Bishop, John, 14, 171–72
Blackstone, William, 28–29, 31–34, 36–37, 202
Blackwood's Edinburgh Magazine, 37, 171
Bleak House (Dickens) 17–18, 32–36, 32n38, 48, 94, 105, 110–11, 113n90, 117, 120–70, 199, 210; Inspector Bucket, 36, 105, 135, 162–69; Richard Carstone, 34; Court of Chancery, 32–35, 95, 157, 160; Lady Dedlock, 1, 36, 157, 159, 165–66; Sir Leicester Dedlock, 34, 164; Gridley, 34; Hortense, 36, 163–64; Jarndyce *v.* Jarndyce, 34, 199; Mr Krook, 1, 8n17, 15n35, 32, 49, 120–30; Mr Smallweed, 1; Tulkinghorn, 34–36, 156–57, 162–63, 167; Allan Woodcourt, 162, 166–70
bodies, 1–18, 2–24, 27, 36, 41–46, 50, 56, 60–61, 74–77, 83, 89–90, 95–99, 101, 107, 113–14, 128, 130, 132, 137–55, 161–62, 167–69, 174–76, 178–81, 186–90, 194, 202, 204–8, 218, 221, 228; cadaver, 6–8, 14, 24, 40, 52, 60, 98, 100, 112, 135, 137–38, 156, 207–8, 222; corpse, 2, 2n3, 5n11, 6–8, 40–44, 56, 83, 90, 98, 101, 112–14, 134, 138–41, 145, 158, 173n148, 180, 201, 204–12,

· 247 ·

217, 224; as metaphor for London, 134–37
Bodle, John, 150–51, 155, 162
Boehm, Katherina, 14n35
Bowen, John, 4, 4n7, 4n10, 89, 95
Brande, William, 155
British Association for the Advancement of Science, 170
British Medical Association, 64
British Medical Journal, 29, 52, 148
British Museum. *See* museum; British Museum
Brooks, Peter, 16n37, 130n29, 132, 214
Brown, Hannah, 174–76, 174n151
Brown, Bill, 18, 181
Buckland, Adelene, 15n35, 59, 59n107
Bunyan, John, 30–31, 90
Burdett Coutts, Angela, 169
Burke and Hare, 52, 207
Burney, Ian, 27, 58, 67, 151, 153, 155
Butler, John, 150
Butt, John, 210

cadaver. *See* bodies; cadaver
Carey, John, 1, 2n2
Carlyle, Thomas, 144–45, 149
Carroll, David, 62
Le Cat, Claude-Nicolas, 127–29
"Chambers" (Dickens), 106
Chausier, François, 47–48, 50
Cheadle, Brian, 98, 101
Cheyne, George, 43, 46
The Chimes (Dickens), 212, 215
Chitty, Joseph, 52, 63
A Christmas Carol (Dickens), 210
Christison, Robert, 51–52, 75–76, 80, 150
Cicero, 26
"The City of the Absent" (Dickens), 116–17
Clark, Sally, 227–29
Clark, Timothy, 4n7
clues, 7, 10–11, 17–18, 20, 40–41, 43, 55, 106, 112–14, 121, 134, 145–46, 168, 170, 176, 181, 199, 202, 209–10, 221
The Comic Blackstone (Beckett), 32
Commentaries on the Laws of England (Blackstone), 28–29
Comte, Auguste, 20, 73, 122
Condé, Prince de, 204–10, 217–19, 221
Condillac, Etienne Bonnot de, 82
Conrad, Joseph, 3n6
Cook, John Parsons, 26
corpse. *See* bodies; corpse

crime, 2–3, 14, 22, 25–26, 37–38, 44, 48, 50, 51, 77, 86, 93–94, 99, 101–3, 140, 145, 173, 179, 181–83, 193–98, 210, 213, 216; crime scenes, 25, 54, 73, 101–3, 179–225. *For specific crimes, see individual entries—e.g.,* murder
Cruikshank, George, 56–57, 135; "A Financial Survey of Cumberland," 57 fig 1.2
Cummin, William, 8

Daily News, 152, 154
Daston, Lorraine, 16, 16n37, 45, 47n76, 81, 82
Davey, J. G., 66
David Copperfield (Dickens), 110
death, 1–11, 2n3, 4n7, 4n10, 23–24, 35, 40–43, 46–47, 55–56, 60–61, 74–79, 83–84, 87, 89–91, 98–102, 107, 112, 128, 130, 134–35, 137–45, 140n62, 150–51, 156, 167, 170, 175, 179–80, 183–84, 190, 204–5, 207–10, 215, 218, 224, 225; of children, 6, 8–9, 40, 87, 98, 196 227–29; death masks, 182
Derrida, Jacques, 12
detective, 3, 86, 163–66, 193
"A Detective Police Party" (Dickens), 164–65
Dicey, A. V., 30
Dickens, Charles, 1–2; and bodies, 20, 98, 101, 133, 141–45, 173, 227; his death, 13, 72, 120, 122, 126, 131, 131n32; on death, 40, 92, 98, 101, 133–35, 137, 141, 144–45, 199, 218–19; and forensics, 1–20, 40, 49, 51, 54, 86, 88, 92, 96, 100, 103–6, 109, 112–13, 120, 124, 126–27, 130, 132, 137, 139–40, 143–46, 158, 160–62, 165–66, 169–70, 173, 177, 179, 181, 183, 191, 199–200, 204, 210–213, 216–217, 220, 225–227; and John Forster, 40, 107; his imagination, 1, 227; as interpreter, 19–20, 212; and journalism, 14, 132–35, 177; and law, 32–36, 125, 129, 152, 156, 158, 164, 200; and George Henry Lewes, 13, 120, 120n2, 122–23, 126–29, 172, 177, 204, 229; and London, 96, 112–13, 117–18, 130–37, 140, 139, 156–62, 169; and medicine, 3, 6–20, 49, 51, 88, 94–95, 106–7, 109, 137, 140, 142, 146, 152, 155, 158, 169, 208, 219, 226–27; and objects, 18, 108–11, 181–83, 191–92, 196–97, 199–200, 210–15, 219; and photography, 139; and science, 10–15, 16, 20, 123–25, 130, 140, 153, 165, 170, 172–73, 177, 183, 225, 227, 229; and truth, 72, 86, 88, 90, 105, 117, 125, 127, 129, 152, 156, 165, 170, 177, 227

INDEX

Dijon, Academy of, 47
Dombey and Son (Dickens), 182n12; Captain Cuttle, 1; Mr Carker, 1, 182n12
Douglas-Fairhurst, Robert, 131
"Down with the Tide" (Dickens), 111, 113, 115
Drummond, Edward, 29
"The Drunkard's Death" (Dickens), 142–45, 156, 169
Dubois, François, 205
Duke of Bourbon. *See* Prince de Condé
Duke of Cumberland, 21–25, 55–59, 61–62
Duncan, Andrew, 50–51
Duxbury, Neil, 30

Earle, Rev. J., 64
Edinburgh Medical College, 52
Edmunds, John, 77–79
Elements of Medical Jurisprudence (Beck), 48–49, 174, 208
Elements of Medical Jurisprudence (Farr), 50
Elements of Medical Jurisprudence (Taylor), 53–54, 61
Eliot, George, 14, 14n35, 122, 130n29, 131n32, 188
Elliotson, John, 51, 91, 94–95, 117, 171–72, 176–77, 199
The English Malady (Cheyne), 43
Enlightenment, 16n37, 47, 81, 91, 93, 109, 134–35, 162
epistemology, 5n10, 13, 16n37, 19–20, 34, 47, 71, 101, 103–4, 108, 112–13, 118, 156, 169, 227
Epitome of Juridical or Forensic Medicine (Male), 50, 77
Epstein Nord, Deborah, 139
The Era, 155
Essay Concerning Human Understanding (Locke), 111
Essay on the Nature and Immutability of Truth (Beattie), 27
Evans, Marian. *See* Eliot, George
The Evening Chronicle, 132–33, 135
Evening Standard, 229
evidence, 9, 13–20, 22–23, 25–29, 38, 43–47, 51, 54–62, 65–67, 73–77, 79, 81–82, 84, 100, 102, 114, 119–27, 130, 132, 137, 142, 144, 148, 150–56, 160, 169, 175–77, 180, 186, 194–98, 201–4, 207–11, 223, 226–29
Experimental Medicine (Bernard), 71

Faraday, Michael, 151
Farr, Samuel, 50

felo de se. *See* suicide
Field, Inspector, 169
Fielding, K. J., 13n32, 210
Filangieri, Gaetano, 26
Fitzjames Stephen, James, 32
Fletcher, John, 75–78, 138
Fodéré, François-Emmanuel, 48–49, 122
Fonblanque, Anthony, 40, 52, 122
forensic medicine. *See* forensics
forensics, 2–6, 8–12, 15–18, 20, 26, 33, 36, 40, 42, 45–49, 50–55, 59, 61, 68, 69, 74, 77–81, 86–87, 91–92, 94, 96, 100, 103–6, 109, 112–14, 119, 120, 127, 130, 132, 137, 139–46, 150, 155, 158, 160–71, 173–77, 179–81, 182n12, 191, 198, 200, 202–4, 210–13, 216–217, 220, 221, 224–27; medical jurisprudence, 9–10, 16–19, 45–54, 60–68, 69–85, 87–88, 92, 98, 103–5, 112, 118, 122–26, 130, 132, 137, 140, 147–50, 154–56, 174, 180–81, 183, 196, 198–99, 201, 204–10, 216, 225, 226–27; medico-legal, 3, 10, 20, 47, 53–54, 58, 62, 140
Forster, John, 7, 40, 107, 130, 152, 160
Forsyth, John, 50
Fortnightly Review, 13
Foucault, Michel, 3, 47, 47n75
Fraser's Magazine, 27, 85
Freedgood, Elaine, 18–19, 182–83
Freud, Lucien, 132
Furneaux, Holly, 13, 14n35

Galison, Peter, 16, 16n37, 47n76, 81, 82
Gendrin, Auguste, 205
General Hospital, Birmingham, 50
Géricault, Théodore, 110
Gilbert, Pamela K., 4n10, 32n38, 134
Girdwood, Gilbert, 174–77
God, 17, 28, 38, 40–41, 58, 68, 69–72, 79–80, 86, 88, 90, 92, 94–95, 103, 109, 152, 160, 166, 178
"Gone Astray" (Dickens), 158, 160
Goodlad, Lauren, 35–36, 156, 169
Gothic, 22, 37, 41, 88, 100
Grainger's Theatre, 151
Grant, Damian, 149
Great Expectations (Dickens), 1, 189, 200, 212–25; Miss Havisham, 1, 2, 213, 215–16, 218, 220–22; Jaggers, 19, 182, 200–202, 204, 213; Magwitch, 203–4, 215–16, 218, 223; Pip, 19, 201–2, 212–18, 220–25
Greenacre, James, 170–71, 173, 175–77
Gregory, John, 70, 147

Grime, Robert L., 138
Guy, William A., 45
Guy's Hospital, 53, 186

Hack, Daniel, 8n17, 126
Hamilton, Lady Anne, 25, 55–60, 62
Hard Times (Dickens), 14n35; Mr Gradgrind, 2
Hardy, Barbara, 220
Harrison, James, 11, 140
Haslam, John, 67
Helps, Sir Arthur, 131
hermeneutics, 3, 10, 19, 25, 125, 158, 160, 164–65, 193
Heywood, James, 82–85, 147
Higgins, Mary, 150
Hillis Miller, J., 3–4, 19, 91, 104–5, 139, 149, 158, 182, 184
Hints for the Examination of Medical Witness (Smith), 51
Hogarth, Mary, 40
Hogarth, William, 86, 146
Hollington, Michael, 148
Home, Sir Everard, 23–25, 54–56, 59–62, 66, 73
Household Words, 32–34, 40, 111, 125, 158, 160, 164–65, 193
Hume, David, 28
Hunter, John, 23–24, 24n8, 55, 134, 134n45, 148
Hunter, William, 8–10, 23–24, 55
Hutter, Albert D., 3n6
Huxley, Thomas Henry, 124, 124n12

The Illustrated Times, 27
Inman, Thomas, 148–49
Inquiries into the Intellectual Powers and the Investigation of Truth (Abercrombie), 72
interpretation, 3–7, 10–20, 22–23, 25–27, 29–30, 37, 42, 44–47, 50, 59, 60–82, 84–85, 98, 101, 104–5, 109–10, 112–18, 121, 126, 128–30, 132, 135, 137, 138, 144, 148–50, 153–70, 180–85, 189, 192–93, 195–200, 204, 210–16, 219–20, 225–29

Jaffe, Audrey, 3n6, 118
John Bull, 194, 206–7, 224
John, Juliet, 12n26

Kant, Immanuel, 79
Kaplan, Fred, 172
Kawash, Samira, 141
Kennedy, Meegan, 16n37, 47

Kermode, Frank, 209, 221
Ketch, John, 170, 173
King George III, 21–23, 55
King's College, London, 14
King's College Hospital, 45
Kingsley, Charles, 181
Kinkead, R. J., 68
Knight, Charles, 32
Kucich, John, 4n10

Lain, Pierre-Aime, 120n2, 121–22
The Lancet, 9, 60, 83, 171, 180
Latour, Bruno, 15n36
law, 5n10, 15, 26–37, 41–42, 46–48, 51–54, 58, 63–64, 66, 68, 72, 74, 77, 82, 85, 94, 102, 106, 109, 119, 123, 125, 127, 130, 134, 147, 153, 155, 159, 163, 165, 179, 183, 190, 200–201, 204, 226
The Law Magazine, 24
lawyer, 25, 30–31, 35, 50, 52–53, 63–67, 74, 84, 156–57, 163, 194–95, 199, 204, 213
Laycock, Thomas, 146–48
The Leader, 138–139, 145, 220
Lectures on the Duties and Qualifications of a Physician (Gregory), 70
Ledger, Sally, 3n6
legal. *See* law
The Legal Observer, 64–65
Levi, Albert William, 149
Levine, George, 14, 16, 71, 131, 145
Lewes, George Henry, 13, 15n35, 72, 96, 120, 122–29, 124n12, 131, 131n32, 153, 170, 172, 177, 204–5, 229
Liebeg, Justus von, 124–26, 125n16
Little Dorrit (Dickens); Mrs Clennam, 1; Rigaud, 1
Locke, John, 28, 111
London, 14, 24, 33, 45, 49, 51, 77, 91–100, 104–5, 11, 116–18, 131–37, 139–40, 145, 150, 156–63, 169, 173, 176, 179, 185, 194, 205, 215, 227
London Medical Gazette, 134, 205, 207n55, 208
Lucas, John, 85–86, 96

MacNish, Robert, 120–21, 120n2
Maine, Henry Summer, 30
Makras, Kostas, 142
Male, George, 48, 77
Marc, Charles, 205, 207
Marsh, James, 151, 153–55
Martineau, Harriet, 13
Mason, John, 178, 189

INDEX 251

May, James, 14
McLarren Caldwell, Janis, 169
McNaughten, Daniel, 29, 31
Meadow, Roy, 227–29
The Medical Aspects of Death (Harrison), 11
Medical Ethics (Percival), 50, 185
medical jurisprudence. *See* forensics; medical jurisprudence
Medical Jurisprudence (Paris and Fonblanque), 40, 52
medicine, 3, 6, 8, 10, 11, 13, 15, 40, 44, 45, 47, 50, 52–53, 63–64, 70–75, 78–81, 85, 94–95, 107, 109, 120, 124, 132, 134, 137, 140, 142, 146–47, 153, 176, 180, 185–86, 188–90, 202, 205, 207–8, 219
Medicinische Logik (Oesterlen), 73
medico-legal. *See* forensics; medico-legal
Middlemarch (Eliot), 109
Mill, John Stuart, 20, 72
modernism, 3, 181
Morgagni, Giovanni Battista, 134–35
Morley, Henry, 34, 40
The Morning Chronicle, 144, 152, 209, 224
The Morning Post, 21, 24, 25, 58, 59, 174n151
Moye, Richard H., 12, 12n26
The Mudfog Papers (Dickens), 170–72, 177
Murayama, Toshikatsu, 14n35
murder, 5, 8–9, 14, 15, 21–29, 38, 40–43, 52, 55, 57–58, 60–62, 73, 84, 94, 99–103, 106, 112, 119, 138–39, 150, 152, 154, 156, 162–65, 163n129, 170n138, 180, 183, 189, 193–196, 199, 200, 204–9, 213, 227–28; self murder (*see* suicide)
museum, 107; British Museum, 133
Mushet, William Boyd, 148

narrative, 10–11, 12n26, 14n35, 18, 38, 40, 59, 63, 86, 88, 89, 90, 93–94, 103–4, 108, 110, 115, 129, 132, 156, 159–60, 162–63, 178, 181, 184, 188, 189, 197, 199, 209, 210
narrator, 7–8, 11–12, 93, 101, 104, 111, 112–13, 117, 144, 146, 149, 156, 158, 162–63, 181, 190, 192, 217
Nicholas Nickleby (Dickens); Wackford Squeers, 1
"Night Walks" (Dickens), 111, 173n148

Oberstein, Karín Lesnik, 96
objectivity, 16n37, 17, 45, 71, 80, 82, 90, 98, 197, 229
objects, 18–19, 35, 37–38, 45, 50, 71, 87–89, 94, 107, 109–11, 131, 131n32, 133, 135, 137–38, 139n58, 40, 166, 170, 173, 179, 181–86, 182n12, 189–90, 192–94, 198–99, 210–14, 216–24; things, 1, 3, 4n10, 6, 11–12, 17–20, 27–28, 30, 35, 38, 45, 88, 95, 100, 106, 109–10, 112–16, 131–32, 131n32, 134, 138, 140, 145, 161, 165, 166, 179–83, 186, 188, 190–92, 195, 197, 199–201, 204, 210–16, 220, 222–25, 227
Oersterlen, Friedrich, 73, 78, 80, 118, 198–99
The Old Curiosity Shop (Dickens), 143, 218; Little Nell, 1, 8, 40, 87, 98, 196, 218; Quilp, 143
Oliver Twist (Dickens), 12n26, 17, 26, 85–103, 104, 108, 109, 117, 118, 143, 189; Bill Sikes, 42, 93, 95, 99–103, 114, 143, 189; Mr Brownlow, 85, 87, 107; Mrs Bumble, 26; Fagin, 42, 92, 93, 96, 97–100, 146, 182; Monks, 85, 96–98; Nancy, 43, 85, 95, 98, 99–103, 108, 143, 189; Oliver, 1, 87–90, 92–100, 102
Orfila, Mathieu, 48–49
The Origin, Science, and End of Moral Truth (Anon), 27
Our Mutual Friend (Dickens), 3n6, 17, 40, 103–19; John Harmon, 40, 112, 114–16; Old Harmon, 107; Bradley Headstone, 112, 118–19; Mr Inspector, 113–14, 119; Rogue Riderhood, 112, 119; Mr Venus, 1, 105–9, 111, 113, 115, 142; Silas Wegg, 1, 105–9

Paley, William, 26
Palmer, William, 26–27, 67
Parham, John, 14, 15n36
Paris, John, 40, 52, 122
Paris Morgue, 2n2, 5, 5n11, 7–8, 11, 133, 141
Parke, J., 30
Parks, John, 83
pathology, 9, 47, 47n75, 134, 144, 175
Patten, Robert L., 210
Peel, Sir Robert, 29
Penny Satirist, 173, 176
Percival, Thomas, 50, 185
perspective, 4n6, 11–12, 43, 88–89, 91, 104–5, 129
Phillips, John, 55, 57
The Philosophy of Medicine (Webb), 70
phrenology, 172–73, 177
physiology, 24, 46, 91, 107, 172
The Pickwick Papers (Dickens), 18, 178, 183–97, 187 fig. 4.1, 191 fig. 4.2, 210, 219, 223; Mr Pickwick, xiv, 183–85, 186–88, 192–93,

196–99, 211; "The Story of the Goblins who Stole a Sexton, 211–13, 215–16; "The Stroller's Tale," 188–92, 211; Sam Weller, 173, 185–86, 197; Mr Winkle, 185–86
Piggott, Gillian, 211
The Pilgrim's Progress (Bunyan), 30, 90
Poe, Edgar Allan, 37, 133
post-mortem, 11, 74, 76, 143, 150; autopsy, 7, 43, 47, 134, 134n45, 135n47, 228–29
poststructuralism, 3, 12
Practical Treatise on Medical Jurisprudence (Chitty), 52, 63
Principles of Forensic Medicine, Systematically Arranged and Applied to British Practice (Smith), 51
Principles and Practice of Medical Jurisprudence (Taylor), 206 fig 4.3, 54, 74, 140, 205
"Progress: Its Law and Cause" (Spencer), 72

Queen Charlotte, 21
De Quincey, Thomas, 165, 217

Ralph, Matthias, 173–74
Raynor, William, 84
realism, 2, 3, 10, 16n37, 17–19, 85–86, 96, 98, 99, 122–23, 130, 130n29, 132, 170, 182, 182n12, 191
"Realism in Art: Recent German Fiction" (Lewes), 122–23
Reed, John R., 14n35, 113, 182n12
Reid, Elizabeth, 114
Reid, Robert, 52, 73–77, 80, 84–85, 138, 147
Reid, Thomas, 27–28
Reinsch, Hugo, 153–55
Remarks on the Trial of Robert Reid (Fletcher), 76
Roberts, Lissa, 82
Rothfield, Lawrence, 16n37
Rothwell, Joseph, 83–84
Royal College of Physicians, 10, 52, 63
Royal College of Surgeons, 77, 152
Russell Reynolds, J., 10, 63
Ryan, Michael, 51, 79–80, 94–95, 106, 208

Sala, George Augustus, 26n13, 44, 198
Samuels, Ellen, 141
Sanders, Andrew, 2n2, 13n32
Sartor Resartus (Carlyle), 144
Schramm, Jan-Melissa, 25, 44, 63, 201
scientific realism. *See* realism

Scotland Yard, 164, 166
self-murder. *See* suicide
Sellis, Joseph, 21–25, 44, 54–62, 73, 201, 204
Seymour, Robert, 178–79, 183, 189–90, 209, 224–25
Shakespeare, William, 40
Shelley, Percy Bysshe, 55
Sketches by Boz (Dickens), 19, 135, 136 fig. 3.1, 142, 160, 182, 183
Smethurst, Thomas, 152–56, 162, 170
Smith, Albert, 154
Smith, John Gordon, 51–52, 62, 80, 137–38, 140, 143, 166
Smith, Jonathan, 73, 78
Smith, Karl Ashley, 162
Smith, Roger, 26, 63
Smith, Southwood, 169
Smith, Sydney, 52
Society of Apothecaries, 53
Socrates, 147
Spencer, Herbert, 72
spontaneous combustion, 1, 8n17, 15n35, 48, 120–30, 131n32, 153, 197, 204, 229
Stevenson, William, 57
Stoehr, Taylor, 181
Stone, Harry, 2n2, 188
"The Story of the Goblins who Stole a Sexton." *See The Pickwick Papers*
"The Streets—Morning" (Dickens), 135, 137
"The Stroller's Tale." *See The Pickwick Papers*
Sucksmith, Harvey Peter, 37
Sudden Infant Death Syndrome. *See* death; child death
suicide, 17, 24, 54–56, 61–62, 111–12, 179–81, 191, 204–5, 208–9, 224
Swift, Jonathan, 6, 31
Sydenham, Thomas, 147–48
Symonds, J. A., 64–65

Tambling, Jeremy, 135, 140
Taylor, Alfred Swaine, 53–54, 61–62, 67, 74, 140–41, 143–44, 153–56, 205–6
Taylor, Brooke D., 14n35
The Terrific Register, 36–44, 39 fig. 1.1, 46, 62, 94
testimony, 38, 44, 56, 60–61, 66, 76–77, 89, 92, 121–22, 125–28, 130, 152, 160, 174n151, 175, 177
Thackeray, William Makepeace, 85
Thérèse Raquin (Zola), 5–6, 11
things. *See* objects; things
thing theory, 18, 181

Thomas, Ronald R., 139, 162
Thoms, Peter, 163
Thomson, Alexander, 67, 142, 179–81, 185
Tillotson, Kathleen, 210
Townsend, Colonel, 43–44, 46
Traite de Medicine Legale, et d'Hygiene Publique (Fodéré), 48
"Travelling Abroad" (Dickens), 5n11, 11
Treatise on Poisons (Christison), 52, 150
Treatise on Poisons (Orfila), 48–49
Tredennick, Bianca, 2n2, 2n3, 5n11, 141
Tromp, Marlene, 93

The Uncommercial Traveller (Dickens), 5
unheimliche, 105

Ventura, Hector O., 134
Victorian, 2, 2n3, 16n37, 72, 158, 173, 229

Wakley, Thomas, 9, 180
Walker, Margaret, 82
Warren's Blacking Factory, 51
Watson, Katherine, 151
Webb, Eziekiel, 70
Webb, T. E., 27
Webber, William, 152
Westminster Hospital, 51
Westminster Review, 122, 124n12, 130n29
Westminster School of Medicine, 51
Whitehead, Alfred North, 104
Williams, Stephen, 69–70, 74–77, 90, 171
Williams, Thomas, 14
William the Conqueror, 32
Winyard, Ben, 13, 14n35
Wood, Claire, 2n3

Zola, Emile, 5–6, 11–12

www.ingramcontent.com/pod-product-compliance
Lightning Source LLC
Chambersburg PA
CBHW021139230426
43667CB00005B/177